AF695938

PATHWAY TO USMLE
A STEP 1 AND STEP 2 CK PATHOLOGY COMPANION

ALSO FROM VAYDEN ACADEMIC PRESS

⁂

PATHWAY TO USMLE — A STEP 1 AND STEP 2 CK PATHOLOGY COMPANION

Volume I · Volume III

PATHOLOGY IN PATTERNS — A RAPID-REVISION COMPANION

FRCPATH HAEMATOLOGY, FIRST PAPER

Volume 1 · Volume 2

FRCPATH HISTOPATHOLOGY, FIRST PAPER

Volume 1 · Volume 2

⁂

All titles available from Amazon worldwide
and direct from www.vaydenpress.com

PATHWAY TO USMLE

A Step 1 and Step 2 CK Pathology Companion

VOLUME 2: HAEMATOLOGY AND TRANSFUSION MEDICINE

Vishal Tayade, MD
Assistant Professor of Pathology
Grant Government Medical College and Sir J.J. Group of Hospitals, Mumbai

Published by Vayden Academic Press · vaydenpress.com

Mumbai, India

ISBN: 978-81-686730-4-5

First edition, 2026

DISCLAIMER: This book is intended as an educational supplement for medical students and physicians preparing for the USMLE Step 1 and Step 2 CK examinations. It is not a substitute for clinical judgement or current medical guidelines. Patient management decisions must be based on individual clinical assessment and current evidence-based standards of care. Neither the author nor the publisher assumes any responsibility for any adverse outcomes resulting from the use of this material.

To my parents, with gratitude.

To my teachers, who taught me to look first.

To my students, who taught me what to teach.

Preface

This book exists because I could not find one that did what I wanted. The pathology I learned, and now teach, lives in mechanism. A board question is not asking you whether you can recite a list of histological features for a disease — it is asking whether you can predict, given a molecular lesion, what the cell will do, and given a cellular phenotype, what the tissue will show. Mechanism is the only stable bridge between the two.

Each chapter begins with a Big Picture orientation, traces the dominant mechanisms, anchors every concept in a Mechanism Hook that links the molecular event to the histological finding, and ends with a block of worked clinical vignettes calibrated to the difficulty distribution of recent NBME exams. Pearls and Step 2 Pivots throughout flag the sentences that high-yield review books skip. Image Traps and Trap boxes name the recurring distractors that cost otherwise-prepared candidates points.

This is the companion I wished I had. I hope it is the one you find useful.

Vishal Tayade

Mumbai, 2026

About the Author

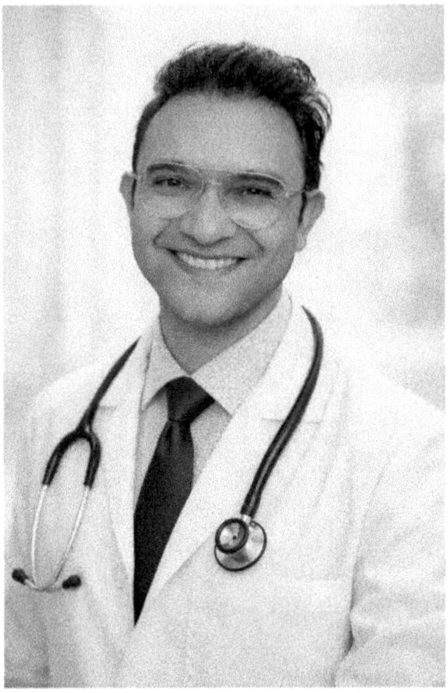

Vishal Tayade

MD Pathology · FRCPath Part 1

Vishal Tayade is Assistant Professor of Pathology at Grant Government Medical College and Sir J.J. Group of Hospitals, Mumbai, where he trains residents in surgical pathology, haematopathology, and cytopathology. He completed his MD in Pathology and training in oncopathology at Tata Memorial Centre, Mumbai. He holds Part 1 of the FRCPath, Royal College of Pathologists, London.

His academic interests sit at the intersection of pattern recognition, integrated diagnostics, and pathology education. He has published in peer-reviewed journals on haematopathology, Histopathology, cytology and laboratory diagnostics, and contributes images to the ASH Image Bank.

He is the founder of Vayden Academic Press, dedicated to writing focused, examination-grade textbooks for postgraduate pathology and laboratory medicine. The Pathway to USMLE series is his three-volume primary textbook covering general, haematological, and systemic pathology; its rapid-revision companion is Pathology in Patterns. He also publishes the FRCPath First Paper preparation volumes and the two-volume Integrated Pathology textbook.

Outside the laboratory, he writes literary fiction. His published novels include Love in Chaos, Resonance, the Dr Vishal Sarkar Mystery trilogy, and the literary novels The Chalk Line and No One Was Responsible. He lives in Mumbai.

How to Use This Book

This book is organised by organ system, in the same order in which most pathology curricula and the USMLE content outline progress.

Each chapter contains a fixed structure of teaching boxes, designed so that you can read for breadth on a first pass and for depth on later passes.

Big Picture: a single orientation paragraph that states what mechanism dominates the chapter and why.

Mechanism Hook: the molecular event tied to the histological finding. This is the highest-yield box in each chapter.

Pearl: an exam-relevant fact that appears in board questions but is often missed.

Step 2 Pivot: a fact that connects the Step 1 mechanism to a Step 2 CK clinical decision.

Image Trap: a histological pattern that looks like one disease but is actually another.

Trap: a clinical or pathophysiological scenario where the obvious answer is wrong.

Vignette: an NBME-style clinical case. Later chapters use a five-option MCQ format with worked rationale and distractor analysis; earlier chapters use a worked-stem format with diagnosis and teaching point. Ten to sixteen per chapter.

Quick Recall: a one-page-equivalent summary table of the chapter's mechanism content.

Ultra High-Yield: the fifty-to-seventy facts most likely to appear on the exam.

Table of Contents

Chapter 9 — Red Cell Disorders Part 1: Microcytic and Macrocytic Anaemias

A small red cell points to a haemoglobin synthesis defect; a large red cell points to a DNA synthesis defect or membrane lipid alteration. The MCV is the first branch point.

9.1 Big Picture and Mechanism Hooks

BIG PICTURE

Anaemia is the most common haematologic disease in the world; in clinical practice it is a manifestation, not a diagnosis. The mechanism is always one of three: decreased red cell production, increased destruction, or blood loss. The single most useful initial framework on USMLE Step 1 is the MCV-based classification — microcytic anaemias reflect defective haemoglobin synthesis (haem or globin); macrocytic anaemias reflect defective DNA synthesis or altered red cell membrane lipid; normocytic anaemias reflect acute loss or hypoproliferative states. This chapter covers the microcytic and macrocytic groups.

MECHANISM HOOK — The MCV story

The MCV is not just a number; it is a window into where erythropoiesis is failing. A small red cell tells you the cell could not put enough haemoglobin into itself — either iron is unavailable (iron deficiency, anaemia of chronic inflammation), haem synthesis is broken at the mitochondrion (sideroblastic anaemia, lead poisoning), or globin synthesis is reduced (thalassaemia). A large red cell tells you the cell divided too few times before maturing — nuclear maturation lagged behind cytoplasmic haemoglobinisation because DNA synthesis was impaired (B12 deficiency, folate deficiency, drugs that block DNA replication), or the membrane accumulated extra lipid without any DNA defect at all (alcohol, liver disease, hypothyroidism). Once the MCV places the patient on a branch, the next test is dictated by the branch: iron studies for microcytic, B12 and folate for macrocytic, with the smear refining both — pencil cells versus target cells in the microcytic group, oval macrocytes with hypersegmented neutrophils versus round macrocytes in the macrocytic group.

9.2 The MCV-Based Approach to Anaemia

The WHO defines anaemia as haemoglobin below **13 g/dL (130 g/L)** in adult men, below **12 g/dL (120 g/L)** in non-pregnant adult women, and below **11 g/dL (110 g/L)** in pregnant women. Children aged 6 months to 5 years use the same 11 g/dL threshold. Once anaemia is confirmed on a repeat sample, the MCV (mean corpuscular volume) immediately divides the differential into three workable categories. The reticulocyte count then provides a second axis — adequate marrow response (haemolysis or recent blood loss) versus inadequate response (hypoproliferation).

Classification by MCV

MCV (fL)	Category	Common Causes
< 80	Microcytic	Iron deficiency anaemia (most common); thalassaemia trait; anaemia of chronic inflammation (some cases, usually chronic and severe); sideroblastic anaemia; lead poisoning.
80–100	Normocytic	Anaemia of chronic inflammation (most common cause overall); acute blood loss; early iron deficiency; mixed deficiency (iron + B12 or folate); chronic kidney disease (reduced EPO); haemolytic anaemias; bone marrow failure (aplastic anaemia, marrow infiltration).
> 100	Macrocytic	Megaloblastic: B12 deficiency, folate deficiency, drugs that block DNA synthesis. Non-megaloblastic: chronic alcohol use, liver disease, hypothyroidism, reticulocytosis, MDS, drugs (hydroxyurea, AZT, methotrexate).

HIGH-YIELD PEARL — Mixed deficiency masks the MCV

A patient with combined iron deficiency AND B12 or folate deficiency may have a normal MCV — the microcytic tendency of iron deficiency and the macrocytic tendency of megaloblastic anaemia cancel out arithmetically. The clue is on the smear: a dimorphic population (microcytic hypochromic cells alongside macro-ovalocytes) and a markedly elevated RDW (often >18%). Common scenario on USMLE: an alcoholic with poor diet (folate low) and concurrent GI bleeding (iron low). Treat both deficiencies — and treat B12 alongside folate if there is any suspicion of B12 deficiency, never folate alone.

The reticulocyte count: the second axis

The reticulocyte percentage in an anaemic patient is misleading — a 1.5% reticulocyte count looks normal, but in the setting of haematocrit 20% it represents inadequate marrow response. Two corrections are standard. The corrected reticulocyte count multiplies the percentage by the patient's haematocrit divided by 45. The reticulocyte production index (RPI) divides the corrected count by a maturation factor (1.0 at haematocrit 45; 1.5 at 35; 2.0 at 25; 2.5 at 15) to account for the fact that prematurely released reticulocytes circulate longer than normal. An RPI above 2 indicates an adequate marrow response — haemolysis or recent blood loss. An RPI below 2 indicates a hypoproliferative process — iron, B12, or folate deficiency; chronic inflammation; renal disease; or marrow failure.

HIGH-YIELD PEARL — RDW: the early IDA flag
RDW (red cell distribution width, normal 11.5–14.5%) measures variation in red cell volume. It rises early in iron deficiency, before MCV falls, because the marrow produces a mixed population of normocytic and progressively smaller cells. A high RDW with low MCV favours iron deficiency. A normal RDW with low MCV favours thalassaemia trait — every cell is uniformly small because the genetic defect affects every cell equally. This RDW pattern is a USMLE-favoured discriminator and survives the actual differential workup as a real-world clue.

9.3 Iron Metabolism — A Mechanism Foundation

The next four entities — iron deficiency, anaemia of chronic inflammation, sideroblastic anaemia, and the thalassaemias — cannot be diagnostically distinguished without understanding iron handling. The hepcidin–ferroportin axis is testable on Step 1, central to Step 2 management decisions, and the conceptual key to interpreting iron studies in any clinical scenario.

Total body iron and turnover

A healthy adult contains about 3–4 g of iron (men) or 2–3 g (women). Of this, roughly 65% is in haemoglobin within circulating red cells, 10% in myoglobin and iron-containing enzymes (cytochromes, catalase, ribonucleotide reductase), and 20–25% in storage as ferritin and haemosiderin in macrophages and hepatocytes. The plasma transport pool — iron bound to transferrin — is tiny (about 3 mg) but the most metabolically active compartment, turning over 8–10 times per day. Daily dietary intake is 10–15 mg; only 1–2 mg is absorbed because that is the only amount the body needs to lose to replace senescent red cells. Most iron is recycled: macrophages of the spleen and liver phagocytose senescent red cells, extract haem iron, and return it to plasma.

Absorption: duodenum and proximal jejunum

Non-haem iron is in the ferric (Fe^{3+}) state in food and must be reduced to ferrous (Fe^{2+}) by duodenal cytochrome b (DcytB) at the brush border. Vitamin C and gastric acid both enhance this reduction. Once reduced, Fe^{2+} enters the enterocyte through divalent metal transporter 1 (DMT1). Haem iron is absorbed directly through a dedicated haem transporter and is far more bioavailable than non-haem iron, which is why a meat-rich diet rarely causes iron deficiency. Inside the enterocyte, iron has two fates: it is either stored as ferritin (and lost when the enterocyte sloughs into the lumen 3–5 days later) or exported across the basolateral membrane into plasma by ferroportin (FPN1) — the only known mammalian cellular iron exporter. Hephaestin then oxidises Fe^{2+} back to Fe^{3+} for loading onto transferrin.

The hepcidin–ferroportin axis

Hepcidin is a 25-amino-acid peptide hormone produced by hepatocytes — the master regulator of body iron distribution. Its single mechanism of action is to bind ferroportin and trigger its internalisation and degradation, which traps iron inside enterocytes (where it will be lost), macrophages, and hepatocytes. When hepcidin is high, body iron is trapped; when hepcidin is low, ferroportin operates freely and iron flows into plasma. Hepcidin is stimulated by high iron stores (BMP/HJV/SMAD signalling) and by inflammation (IL-6 acting through JAK/STAT3 in hepatocytes — this is the molecular basis of anaemia of chronic inflammation). It is suppressed by iron deficiency, by hypoxia, and by erythroferrone — a hormone secreted by erythroblasts during periods of high erythropoietic demand, which signals the marrow's need for iron and quiets hepcidin.

HIGH-YIELD PEARL — Hepcidin in four diseases

Iron deficiency anaemia: Hepcidin LOW → ferroportin OPEN → maximum gut absorption + maximum release of stored iron. The body responds appropriately.

Anaemia of chronic inflammation: Hepcidin HIGH (driven by IL-6) → ferroportin BLOCKED → iron trapped in macrophages despite adequate stores. This is the central pathophysiology.

HFE-hereditary haemochromatosis: Hepcidin INAPPROPRIATELY LOW (mutated HFE fails to induce hepcidin in response to iron loading) → ferroportin permanently open → unchecked absorption → parenchymal iron overload.

IRIDA (iron-refractory iron deficiency anaemia): Hepcidin CONSTITUTIVELY HIGH (loss-of-function TMPRSS6 mutation removes the brake on hepcidin) → ferroportin permanently degraded → oral iron absorption fails despite obvious iron need.

9.4 Iron Deficiency Anaemia

Iron deficiency anaemia (IDA) is the most common anaemia in the world and the most common cause of microcytic anaemia on USMLE. The diagnostic challenge is rarely confirming IDA — that is straightforward with ferritin — but identifying the source of iron loss, because in adult men and postmenopausal women, IDA is occult GI bleeding until proved otherwise. This is the reasoning step that the IMG-Trap below addresses directly.

Aetiology by demographic group

Group	Most Common Cause
Infants and toddlers	Dietary insufficiency. Cow's milk introduced before 1 year (low iron, displaces solids, may cause GI bleeding from cow-milk protein enteropathy). Preterm infants have lower stores at birth and reach the nadir earlier.
Adolescent girls	Menstrual loss + dietary insufficiency + growth-driven demand.
Premenopausal women	Menstrual loss is the dominant cause. Pregnancy doubles iron demand (20–30 mg/day late pregnancy). Multiparity and short interbirth intervals deplete stores.
Adult men	**GI blood loss until proved otherwise.** USMLE-favoured sources: colorectal cancer, gastric cancer, peptic ulcer, NSAID-induced erosions, angiodysplasia in the elderly, hookworm in endemic exposure, coeliac disease (malabsorption + occult bleeding).

Group	Most Common Cause
Postmenopausal women	**GI blood loss until proved otherwise — same workup as adult men.** Once menstrual loss has stopped, IDA in this group has the same colorectal-cancer prior as in men of the same age.
Any age	Malabsorption: coeliac disease, autoimmune atrophic gastritis (also impairs B12), Helicobacter pylori, gastric bypass or gastrectomy (loss of acid + duodenal bypass). Long-term PPI use blunts non-haem iron absorption.

Clinical features

General anaemia symptoms — fatigue, dyspnea on exertion, palpitations, headache, exercise intolerance — are non-specific. The features that point specifically to iron deficiency arise from depletion of iron-containing enzymes in epithelial tissues:

- **Pica** — compulsive consumption of non-food substances. The most specific subtype is pagophagia (ice eating); geophagia (clay/dirt) and amylophagia (starch) also occur. Pica typically resolves within days of starting iron, often before haemoglobin rises.
- **Koilonychia** — spoon-shaped nails (concave dorsal surface) in chronic severe deficiency.
- **Atrophic glossitis** — smooth, beefy red, tender tongue from loss of filiform papillae.
- **Angular cheilitis** — fissured, painful corners of the mouth.
- **Plummer–Vinson syndrome** (also called Paterson–Brown–Kelly) — IDA + dysphagia + oesophageal web + atrophic glossitis. Carries an increased risk of oesophageal squamous cell carcinoma. USMLE-favoured vignette: middle-aged woman with iron deficiency and progressive solid-food dysphagia.
- **Restless legs syndrome** — exacerbated by low iron stores (ferritin <50 ng/mL is a treatment threshold even without overt anaemia).
- **Paediatric features** — irritability, developmental delay, poor school performance, breath-holding spells. Iron deficiency in the first 2 years of life has lasting cognitive consequences even after iron repletion.

Stages and laboratory diagnosis

Iron deficiency develops in three sequential stages, each with a distinct laboratory signature. Recognising the stage matters because Stage 1 and 2 are treatable iron-deficient states without overt anaemia.

Stage	Ferritin	Serum Iron	TIBC	TSAT	Hb	MCV	Marrow Iron
1 — Iron depletion	LOW (<15 ng/mL)	Normal	Normal	Normal (>16%)	Normal	Normal	Absent (Grade 0)
2 — Iron-deficient	LOW	LOW	Raised	LOW (<16%)	Normal or	Normal	Absent

Stage	Ferritin	Serum Iron	TIBC	TSAT	Hb	MCV	Marrow Iron
erythropoiesis					borderline		
3 — Iron deficiency anaemia	LOW	LOW	RAISED (>400 µg/dL)	VERY LOW (<10%)	LOW	LOW (microcytic)	Absent

Iron studies — interpretation in detail

Test	Normal Range	In IDA	Comment
Serum ferritin	30–300 ng/mL (men); 15–200 ng/mL (women)	<15 ng/mL	**Most sensitive and specific test for IDA.** Ferritin is an acute-phase reactant — falsely normal or elevated in concurrent inflammation. In inflammatory states, a ferritin up to 100 ng/mL does NOT exclude IDA.
Serum iron	60–170 µg/dL	LOW	Highly variable; diurnal (peaks 9 AM, lowest at midnight); meaningful only in combination with TIBC.
TIBC (transferrin)	240–450 µg/dL	RAISED (>400)	**Liver upregulates transferrin synthesis in iron deficiency.** This is the key discriminator from anaemia of chronic inflammation, where TIBC is LOW or normal.
Transferrin saturation (TSAT)	20–45%	<16% (Stage 2); <10% (Stage 3)	Calculated as serum iron ÷ TIBC × 100. Most useful single iron-status index.
sTfR (soluble transferrin receptor)	0.8–1.8 mg/L	RAISED	**Reflects iron-restricted erythropoiesis.** NOT an acute-phase reactant — major advantage over ferritin in inflammation. The sTfR/log(ferritin) ratio above 2 identifies the IDA component even when ferritin is falsely normal due to inflammation.
Reticulocyte Hb	>28 pg	<28 pg	Earliest functional indicator of

Test	Normal Range	In IDA	Comment
content (Ret-He / CHr)			iron-deficient erythropoiesis; not an acute-phase reactant; particularly useful in CKD patients on ESAs.
RDW	11.5–14.5%	>15%	Anisocytosis. Rises early in IDA. Distinguishes IDA (high RDW) from thalassaemia trait (normal RDW).
Bone marrow Perls stain	Grade 2–3 storage iron	Grade 0 (absent)	Gold standard but rarely needed. Reserved for diagnostic uncertainty.

Peripheral smear

Microcytic hypochromic red cells with central pallor exceeding one-third of the cell diameter; pencil cells (elongated, cigar-shaped elliptocytes — characteristic of severe IDA on USMLE smear questions); marked anisocytosis and poikilocytosis; and in many cases reactive thrombocytosis (platelets 400–700 $\times 10^9$/L). The thrombocytosis reflects shared signalling between EPO and TPO and resolves with iron repletion. A reactive thrombocytosis without splenomegaly in a microcytic anaemia is essentially never myeloproliferative — it is iron deficiency until proved otherwise.

Treatment

Oral iron is first-line for nearly all patients. The standard preparation in the US is ferrous sulfate 325 mg tablet, which contains 65 mg of elemental iron. Other options are ferrous gluconate (36 mg elemental per 325 mg tablet) and ferrous fumarate (66 mg elemental per 200 mg tablet). Take iron on an empty stomach, with vitamin C (or orange juice) to enhance absorption; avoid concurrent calcium, antacids, tea, coffee, and PPIs, which all reduce absorption. Warn patients that stools turn black — this is iron-induced, not melena. GI side effects (nausea, constipation) limit adherence in up to 30%.

STEP 2 BRIDGE — Alternate-day iron dosing

Recent evidence shows that alternate-day single dosing (e.g., ferrous sulfate 325 mg once every other day) produces higher cumulative iron absorption than thrice-daily dosing. The mechanism is hepcidin: each oral dose raises plasma iron, induces hepcidin within 6 hours, and hepcidin then blocks absorption from the next 24-hour dose. Spacing doses 48 hours apart allows hepcidin to fall and absorption to recover. Daily dosing remains acceptable; alternate-day improves tolerance and absorption efficiency. This is now reflected in 2020 BSH and 2024 haematology guidance and is a Step 2 CK testable detail.

Reticulocyte response begins by day 5–10. Haemoglobin rises about 1 g/dL per week. Continue treatment for 3–6 months after the haemoglobin normalises to fully replete stores (ferritin >50 ng/mL).

IV iron is indicated for malabsorption (coeliac disease, post-gastric-bypass, inflammatory bowel disease), oral intolerance after a genuine trial, ongoing blood loss outpacing oral absorption, dialysis-dependent CKD on ESAs, and second-/third-trimester pregnancy with severe anaemia where oral iron cannot raise haemoglobin fast enough before delivery. Modern IV iron preparations (ferric carboxymaltose, iron sucrose, ferumoxytol, ferric derisomaltose, low-molecular-weight iron dextran) have a low rate of severe hypersensitivity (about 1 in 200,000 with modern preparations); high-molecular-weight iron dextran is no longer used. Treating the underlying cause — stopping the bleeding, treating the coeliac disease, removing the offending NSAID — is the most important step.

IMG-TRAP — Adult IDA → GI workup, not nutritional default

The trap. An adult man or postmenopausal woman presents with microcytic anaemia and confirmed iron deficiency (ferritin <15 ng/mL). The IMG candidate, drawing on training in a setting where nutritional iron deficiency, hookworm, and thalassaemia trait are pervasive, defaults to a presumed nutritional or parasitic cause and treats with oral iron alone. The wrong answer chosen on the question stem is typically "start oral iron supplementation and reassess in 3 months" or "recommend dietary counselling."

The rule. On USMLE, iron deficiency in any adult who is not menstruating is presumed to be from occult GI blood loss until disproved. The standard workup is bidirectional endoscopy — colonoscopy plus upper endoscopy (EGD) — performed in close sequence, often the same day. Colonoscopy is the priority because colorectal cancer is the most common identifiable cause and is the lesion that most demands prompt diagnosis. If both endoscopies are negative, the next steps are coeliac serology (tissue transglutaminase IgA, with total IgA), capsule endoscopy of the small bowel, and consideration of urinary blood loss in the rare case where it is sustained.

Why the trap exists. US epidemiology: occult colorectal cancer is the single most important cause of new IDA in adult men and postmenopausal women, and a missed cancer diagnosis under the assumption of nutritional iron deficiency is among the most common avoidable diagnostic errors in this group. Indian, Pakistani, Egyptian, and Sub-Saharan African residents see vastly more nutritional and parasitic IDA than they do colon cancer in their training rotations; the prior probability they bring to the bedside is calibrated to a different population than the USMLE patient.

HIGH-YIELD PEARL — The Plummer–Vinson vignette

USMLE-favoured stem: middle-aged white woman, fatigue, dysphagia for solids that worsens over months, smooth red tongue, spoon-shaped nails. Labs show iron deficiency. Best next step is barium swallow or upper endoscopy showing a postcricoid oesophageal web. Treat the iron deficiency; webs may regress with iron repletion. Important: Plummer–Vinson carries an increased risk of oesophageal and pharyngeal squamous cell carcinoma — surveillance is reasonable in patients with persistent webs.

9.5 Anaemia of Chronic Inflammation

Anaemia of chronic inflammation (ACI) — historically called anaemia of chronic disease — is the most common form of anaemia in hospitalised patients in the United States and the second most common anaemia overall after iron deficiency. It complicates chronic infection, autoimmune disease, malignancy, chronic kidney disease, and any sustained inflammatory state. The defining pathophysiologic feature is a paradox: iron stores are normal or elevated, yet iron is functionally unavailable for erythropoiesis. The hepcidin–ferroportin axis introduced in §9.3 is the single mechanism that explains this paradox.

Pathogenesis

Inflammation drives release of IL-6 and IL-1 from macrophages and endothelium. IL-6 stimulates hepcidin synthesis in hepatocytes through the JAK/STAT3 pathway. Elevated hepcidin binds ferroportin on enterocytes, macrophages, and hepatocytes; ferroportin is internalised and degraded; iron export ceases. Serum iron falls; iron is sequestered inside macrophages (visible as raised storage iron on bone marrow Perls stain); transferrin synthesis falls (cytokines downregulate the liver's transferrin output, which is why TIBC is low or normal in ACI but high in IDA); and the developing erythroblast is starved of iron despite adequate body stores. Two additional cytokine effects compound the picture: TNF-α directly inhibits BFU-E colony formation, and IFN-γ blunts erythropoietin receptor signalling on erythroid progenitors. EPO production is also slightly suppressed relative to the degree of anaemia.

Laboratory pattern

Haemoglobin is typically 9–11 g/dL (90–110 g/L); deeper anaemia in pure ACI is uncommon and warrants a search for an additional cause. MCV is usually normal — ACI is a normocytic anaemia in most cases. A microcytic ACI develops only with chronic, severe, sustained inflammation. The iron studies pattern is the diagnostic hallmark and the discriminator from IDA: serum iron LOW, TIBC LOW or normal (the cytokine-driven downregulation of transferrin), TSAT LOW, ferritin NORMAL or HIGH (acute-phase reactant). The bone marrow shows normal or increased storage iron on Perls stain, with iron trapped in macrophages and reduced incorporation into developing erythroblasts. sTfR is normal or only mildly raised — the most useful test when the picture is mixed (see Step 2 box).

STEP 2 BRIDGE — ACI in CKD — ESAs and HIF-PHIs

Anaemia of CKD has two components: reduced erythropoietin from failing kidneys AND functional iron deficiency from inflammation-driven hepcidin elevation. Treatment requires both correction of iron status (IV iron preferred over oral; ferritin target >100 ng/mL, TSAT >20%) and erythropoiesis-stimulating agents (epoetin alfa, darbepoetin alfa). Haemoglobin target is 10–11 g/dL; higher targets (>13 g/dL) increase cardiovascular events and stroke risk (TREAT, CHOIR, CREATE trials).

HIF-PH inhibitors (roxadustat, daprodustat, vadadustat) are oral agents that stabilise hypoxia-inducible factor, increasing endogenous EPO production AND suppressing hepcidin (improving iron mobilisation). Daprodustat received FDA approval in February 2023 for adult dialysis patients. They represent a paradigm shift from injectable ESAs.

HIGH-YIELD PEARL — Mixed IDA + ACI — the clinical reality

The hardest case in practice is concurrent IDA + ACI — common in inflammatory bowel disease, advanced cancer, rheumatoid arthritis, and elderly patients with multiple chronic conditions. Ferritin is the trap: in pure IDA it is <15 ng/mL, but inflammation can falsely raise it into the 30–100 ng/mL range despite genuine iron deficiency. Two solutions: (1) sTfR is NOT an acute-phase reactant; the sTfR/log(ferritin) ratio (Thomas index) above 2 identifies the IDA component even when ferritin is misleadingly normal. (2) Reticulocyte haemoglobin content (Ret-He) below 28 pg confirms iron-restricted erythropoiesis regardless of inflammation. In hospitalised patients with anaemia and an elevated CRP, do not interpret ferritin without one of these adjuncts.

9.6 Sideroblastic Anaemia

Sideroblastic anaemia is defined by the bone marrow finding of ring sideroblasts: erythroblasts with iron-laden mitochondria arranged as a perinuclear collar of blue-staining granules on Perls (Prussian blue) stain. The formal criterion is at least 5 iron granules encircling at least one-third of the nuclear circumference. Ring sideroblasts indicate a defect either in haem synthesis or in mitochondrial iron handling — iron enters the mitochondrion as it should, but cannot be incorporated into protoporphyrin IX, and accumulates in mitochondrial cristae instead. The peripheral picture is characteristically dimorphic — a mixture of hypochromic microcytic cells (the failed erythropoiesis) and normochromic normocytic cells (the surviving compensatory erythropoiesis), producing a two-population pattern on the CBC histogram and the smear. Iron studies show a distinctive pattern: serum iron HIGH or normal, TSAT HIGH, ferritin normal or HIGH — iron is in the cell but cannot reach haemoglobin.

Causes

Type	Mechanism	Distinguishing Feature
X-linked sideroblastic anaemia (XLSA)	Loss-of-function mutation in ALAS2 (5-aminolevulinic acid synthase 2; first enzyme of haem synthesis, requires pyridoxal-5-phosphate cofactor)	**Pyridoxine-responsive in ~60–70% of cases.** X-linked recessive — males severely affected; female carriers usually mild. Trial pyridoxine 50–200 mg/day for 3 months. Iron overload develops over time and may require chelation.
Lead poisoning	Lead inhibits ALAD (δ-aminolevulinic acid dehydratase) and ferrochelatase — two key enzymes of haem synthesis	**Coarse basophilic stippling on smear (characteristic).** Burton lines (gingival lead lines), abdominal colic, peripheral neuropathy (wrist drop), encephalopathy in severe paediatric exposure. Elevated blood lead level; elevated free erythrocyte protoporphyrin or zinc protoporphyrin.
Isoniazid (INH)	INH forms a hydrazone complex with pyridoxal-5-	Microcytic anaemia with ring sideroblasts after starting INH therapy.

Type	Mechanism	Distinguishing Feature
	phosphate, depleting the active B6 cofactor required by ALAS2	Routinely prevented by co-administering pyridoxine 25–50 mg/day with INH in all TB patients (also prevents peripheral neuropathy).
Chronic alcohol use	Direct mitochondrial toxin; acetaldehyde interferes with B6 metabolism	Ring sideroblasts with vacuolation of erythroid AND myeloid precursors — combination essentially specific for alcohol or copper deficiency. Reverses within 2–3 weeks of abstinence.
Copper deficiency	Copper required for cytochrome c oxidase and for the multicopper ferroxidase hephaestin	**Ring sideroblasts + neutropenia + vacuolation of myeloid precursors.** Causes: gastric bypass, excess zinc supplementation (zinc induces metallothionein in enterocytes, which sequesters copper), parenteral nutrition without copper. Treat with oral copper sulfate.
MDS with ring sideroblasts (MDS-RS)	Acquired clonal disorder of erythroid maturation. SF3B1 mutation in >80% of cases	**WHO 2022: SF3B1 mutation defines MDS with low blasts and SF3B1 mutation (no minimum ring-sideroblast threshold required).** Without SF3B1 mutation, ≥15% ring sideroblasts required for the morphologic category. ICC 2022 retains the entity name 'MDS-RS' (with the same SF3B1 and ring-sideroblast definitions), preserving the long-familiar nomenclature alongside the WHO-renamed MDS-LB-SF3B1. Older patient, persistent macrocytic anaemia, ring sideroblasts on marrow. Treat with EPO ± luspatercept (TGF-β/activin receptor ligand trap; FDA-approved for transfusion-dependent lower-risk MDS-RS).
Other drugs	Chloramphenicol, linezolid (mitochondrial protein synthesis inhibitors)	Reverse on stopping the drug. Linezolid sideroblastic anaemia is a reported toxicity at courses >2 weeks.

HIGH-YIELD PEARL — Lead poisoning — the USMLE paediatric stem

Classic vignette: child living in housing built before 1978 (US lead-paint ban), often with developmental regression, irritability, or abdominal pain. Smear shows microcytic anaemia with COARSE basophilic stippling — a characteristic that distinguishes lead from most other microcytic anaemias. Confirm with venous blood lead level. The CDC blood lead reference value was lowered in October 2021 from 5 µg/dL to 3.5 µg/dL — any value at or above this prompts case management, environmental investigation, and source removal. Chelation thresholds: succimer (DMSA, oral) for blood lead ≥45 µg/dL in children; dimercaprol (BAL) plus calcium EDTA for ≥70 µg/dL or encephalopathy. The single most important step is removing the patient from the source — chelation does not address ongoing exposure. Adults: occupational exposure (battery manufacture, smelting, ceramics, demolition) is the dominant US pattern; treat at higher thresholds.

9.7 The Thalassaemias

The thalassaemias are quantitative disorders of globin chain synthesis — the genetic code for the globin protein is intact (in contrast to the structural haemoglobinopathies like sickle cell), but the amount produced is reduced or absent. The resulting chain imbalance is the central pathology: unpaired chains precipitate within the developing erythroblast, damage the membrane, activate apoptotic pathways, and produce the dual phenotype of ineffective erythropoiesis (cells dying in the marrow) plus shortened red cell survival (cells reaching the periphery die early in the spleen). On USMLE the thalassaemias appear with two consistent demographic anchors: Mediterranean ancestry (Greek, Italian, Cypriot, Turkish, Middle Eastern) for β-thalassaemia, and Southeast Asian or Chinese ancestry for severe α-thalassaemia. Indian, Pakistani, and Bangladeshi populations have both.

Globin gene structure

Adult haemoglobin is HbA ($\alpha_2\beta_2$, ~97%); HbA_2 ($\alpha_2\delta_2$, 2–3.5%); and HbF ($\alpha_2\gamma_2$, <1%). The α-globin gene cluster is on chromosome 16 with FOUR functional copies per diploid cell (HBA1 and HBA2 on each chromosome 16). The β-globin gene is on chromosome 11 with TWO copies. The number of copies dictates the genetics of each disease — α-thalassaemia is graded by how many of four genes are deleted; β-thalassaemia by how many of two are mutated.

β-Thalassaemia

β-Thalassaemia results from point mutations or small deletions in HBB. Mutations classified as β^0 produce no β-chain at all; β^+ produce a reduced amount. The phenotype depends on the genotype:

Genotype	Clinical Phenotype	Haemoglobin	HPLC Pattern
β/β (normal)	Normal	Normal	HbA ~97%; HbA_2 2–3.5%; HbF <1%
β-thalassaemia minor (trait): β^+/β or β^0/β	Asymptomatic carrier	10–13 g/dL; mild microcytic,	**HbA_2 RAISED >3.5% (diagnostic).** HbF may be slightly

Genotype	Clinical Phenotype	Haemoglobin	HPLC Pattern
		mild/no anaemia	elevated (1–4%). Iron studies normal. RDW normal or only mildly raised. RBC count typically high (compensation).
β-thalassaemia intermedia	Moderate; transfusion-independent or rarely transfused	7–9 g/dL	HbF elevated (20–100%); HbA_2 raised; reduced HbA. Iron overload develops EVEN WITHOUT transfusions.
β-thalassaemia major (Cooley anaemia): β^0/β^0 or β^0/β^+ severe	Transfusion-dependent from infancy (~6 months — onset coincides with γ→β switch)	<7 g/dL untransfused	Predominantly HbF (>90%); HbA absent (β^0/β^0) or trace; HbA_2 raised. Massive hepatosplenomegaly, skeletal changes.

The 6-month presentation of β-thalassaemia major reflects the developmental switch from γ-globin (in HbF) to β-globin (in HbA). Before 6 months, fetal haemoglobin sustains the patient; as γ shuts down and β fails to take over, anaemia becomes profound. The marrow expands in compensation, producing the classic skeletal features: frontal bossing, maxillary hypertrophy with prominent cheekbones ("chipmunk facies"), and the "hair-on-end" appearance on skull X-ray (radial striations from diploic-space expansion). Massive ineffective erythropoiesis suppresses hepcidin via erythroferrone, driving iron overload from gut absorption alone — even before any transfusion. Once transfusions begin, iron deposition accelerates, with cardiac, hepatic, and endocrine consequences as the leading causes of death by the third decade if unchelated.

α-Thalassaemia

α-Thalassaemia results predominantly from gene deletions rather than point mutations. Severity tracks with the number of deleted α-genes:

Genotype	Common Name	Clinical Picture	HPLC
αα/αα	Normal	—	Normal
-α/αα (1 gene deleted)	Silent carrier	No clinical features	Normal adult HPLC; trace Hb Bart's at birth only
--/αα (cis) or -α/-α (trans)	α-thalassaemia trait	Mild microcytosis; mild or no anaemia	**HbA_2 NORMAL — critical distinction from β-trait.**

Genotype	Common Name	Clinical Picture	HPLC
			Adult HPLC normal. Diagnosis requires GAP-PCR or MLPA for common α-deletions. Cis genotype (--/αα), common in Southeast Asians, carries reproductive risk for HbH or hydrops; trans (-α/-α), common in Africans, does not.
--/-α (3 genes deleted)	HbH disease	Moderate haemolytic anaemia (Hb 7–10 g/dL); splenomegaly; chronic course with episodic exacerbations	HbH (β_4 tetramers) 10–40% on HPLC. "Golf-ball" inclusions on supravital staining (precipitated β-tetramers).
--/-- (4 genes deleted)	Hb Bart's hydrops fetalis	Stillbirth or neonatal death; incompatible with postnatal life unless intrauterine transfusion	Hb Bart's (γ_4 tetramers) 80–95%. No functional α-chains; γ-tetramers have very high oxygen affinity and cannot release oxygen to tissues.

HIGH-YIELD PEARL — β-trait vs α-trait — same MCV, different HbA_2

β-thalassaemia trait: HbA_2 >3.5% on HPLC is diagnostic. Mediterranean, Middle Eastern, South Asian ancestry common.

α-thalassaemia trait: HbA_2 NORMAL (and may be slightly low). Adult HPLC entirely normal. Diagnosis is by exclusion (microcytic anaemia + normal iron studies + normal HPLC + appropriate ancestry) or by molecular testing (GAP-PCR/MLPA for common α-deletions).

USMLE clue: When the question gives a microcytic patient with normal RDW, normal iron studies, and normal HPLC — α-thalassaemia trait is the answer. The trap is offering "iron deficiency" as an option for a patient whose ferritin is normal.

Critical caveat: Iron deficiency suppresses HbA_2 synthesis. A patient with concurrent IDA and β-thal trait may have a falsely normal HbA_2. Always exclude iron deficiency before interpreting HPLC for thalassaemia screening.

Smear features and skeletal findings

All thalassaemia syndromes share a microcytic hypochromic picture with target cells (codocytes), basophilic stippling, and anisopoikilocytosis. β-Thalassaemia major adds nucleated red blood cells, marked target cells, marked anisopoikilocytosis, and (after splenectomy) Howell–Jolly bodies and Pappenheimer bodies. The MCV is disproportionately low for the degree of anaemia — a patient with thalassaemia trait may have an MCV of 65 fL with haemoglobin 11.5 g/dL, far more microcytic than expected for that haemoglobin in IDA. The Mentzer index (MCV ÷ RBC count) below 13 favours thalassaemia; above 13 favours IDA — useful as a screening discriminator but not diagnostic. The high RBC count in thalassaemia trait reflects compensation: many small cells maintain haemoglobin near normal.

Management of transfusion-dependent thalassaemia

STEP 2 BRIDGE — Modern thalassaemia therapy

Hypertransfusion: Maintain pretransfusion Hb >9–10 g/dL to suppress ineffective erythropoiesis, prevent skeletal expansion, and allow normal growth. Begin around age 6 months in β-major.

Iron chelation: Mandatory once ferritin >1000 ng/mL or after 10–20 transfusions. Options: deferoxamine (subcutaneous infusion, classical agent), deferasirox (oral, first-line in many centres), deferiprone (oral, cardiac iron preferential).

Luspatercept: Activin receptor ligand trap — binds GDF11 and other TGF-β superfamily ligands that block late erythroid maturation. FDA-approved 2019 for adult β-thalassaemia and 2020 for lower-risk MDS-RS. Reduces transfusion burden in transfusion-dependent β-thalassaemia.

Allogeneic HSCT: Curative; matched-sibling outcomes best in children before iron-overload organ damage.

Gene therapy: Betibeglogene autotemcel (Zynteglo, lentiviral β-globin) FDA-approved August 2022 for transfusion-dependent β-thalassaemia. Exagamglogene autotemcel (Casgevy, CRISPR-Cas9 edit of BCL11A enhancer to reactivate HbF) FDA-approved January 2024 for β-thalassaemia.

9.8 Microcytic Anaemia — Distinguishing Features

The four microcytic anaemias — IDA, ACI, sideroblastic, and thalassaemia trait — can be separated using a small panel of laboratory tests. The discriminator table below is the single most testable summary in the chapter; commit it to memory.

Feature	IDA	β-Thalassaemia Trait	ACI (microcytic)	Sideroblastic
MCV	Very low (often <70 fL)	Mildly low (65–75 fL); disproportionately low for the degree of anaemia	Mildly low (rare; usually normocytic)	Variable; often dimorphic

Feature	IDA	β-Thalassaemia Trait	ACI (microcytic)	Sideroblastic
RDW	RAISED (>15%)	Normal	Normal or mildly raised	RAISED (dimorphic)
RBC count	Low	Often HIGH (compensation)	Low or normal	Variable
Serum iron	LOW	Normal	LOW	Normal or HIGH
TIBC	RAISED (>400)	Normal	LOW or normal	Normal
TSAT	<10%	Normal (~30%)	Low (<16%)	HIGH
Ferritin	<15 ng/mL	Normal or raised	Normal or HIGH	Normal or HIGH
HbA_2 (HPLC)	Normal (or falsely low)	RAISED >3.5% (diagnostic)	Normal	Normal
BM Perls iron	Absent (Grade 0)	Normal/increased	Increased; iron in macrophages	Ring sideroblasts
Smear clue	Pencil cells; severe hypochromia	Target cells; basophilic stippling	Mildly hypochromic; target cells	Dimorphic; basophilic stippling (lead)

HIGH-YIELD PEARL — The 30-second microcytic algorithm

Step 1 — Ferritin. Below 15 ng/mL: IDA (find the source — see IMG-Trap §9.4). Above 100 ng/mL with low TSAT: ACI. In between: ferritin alone is not enough — use sTfR/log(ferritin) ratio or Ret-He.

Step 2 — If ferritin is normal/raised and TSAT is high: Sideroblastic anaemia. Look for the cause (lead, INH, alcohol, copper deficiency, MDS-RS in the elderly). Marrow Perls confirms ring sideroblasts.

Step 3 — If ferritin is normal and iron studies are unremarkable: HPLC for thalassaemia. HbA_2 >3.5% confirms β-trait. HbA_2 normal with appropriate ancestry and microcytosis suggests α-trait — confirm with α-deletion molecular testing.

Step 4 — Smear. Coarse basophilic stippling: lead. Pencil cells: IDA. Target cells: thalassaemia or liver disease. Dimorphic population: sideroblastic or mixed deficiency.

9.9 B12 and Folate — Why Megaloblastic, Why Neurologic

The macrocytic anaemias break cleanly into two groups by the same morphologic question that defined the chapter: did the cell divide enough times before maturing? Megaloblastic anaemias answer no — DNA synthesis was impaired, the nucleus could not keep up with cytoplasmic haemoglobinisation, and the resulting cell is large because it skipped one or more divisions. Non-megaloblastic macrocytosis answers a different question — the cell divided normally but accumulated excess membrane lipid, or it simply is a bigger young cell (reticulocyte) released early in compensation. The macroovalocyte and the hypersegmented neutrophil belong to the megaloblastic group; the round macrocyte belongs to the non-megaloblastic group. Before the lab tests, the smear has already separated them.

MECHANISM HOOK — The methyl trap and why neurologic signs come only with B12

DNA synthesis requires the conversion of dUMP to dTMP by thymidylate synthase, using 5,10-methylene-tetrahydrofolate (5,10-methylene-THF) as the methyl donor. When this reaction fails, dTMP falls, uracil is misincorporated into DNA in place of thymidine, and the resulting repair attempts further fragment replication — producing the open, lacy chromatin and nuclear–cytoplasmic asynchrony of the megaloblast. The folate cycle requires that 5-methyl-THF (the form in which folate circulates in plasma) be converted back to THF by methionine synthase, a B12-dependent enzyme. When B12 is deficient, methionine synthase stalls, all circulating folate becomes trapped as 5-methyl-THF, and the cell experiences functional folate deficiency despite adequate folate stores — the methyl trap. This is why B12 deficiency causes a megaloblastic anaemia identical to folate deficiency. But B12 has a second job that folate does not: as adenosylcobalamin, B12 is the cofactor for methylmalonyl-CoA mutase, which converts methylmalonyl-CoA to succinyl-CoA. When B12 is deficient, methylmalonyl-CoA accumulates, methylmalonic acid (MMA) rises in serum, and abnormal odd-chain fatty acids are incorporated into myelin — producing subacute combined degeneration of the dorsal columns and lateral corticospinal tracts. Folate deficiency does not affect this pathway. MMA is therefore the most specific test for B12 deficiency, and neurologic signs are unique to B12 deficiency. The cardinal warning follows directly: never treat suspected B12 deficiency with folate alone — folate may correct the anaemia by partially bypassing the methyl trap, but neurologic damage progresses unchecked and may become irreversible.

B12 absorption — a five-step pathway

Vitamin B12 (cobalamin) is found exclusively in animal-derived foods (meat, fish, dairy, eggs); it is not synthesised by plants, which is why strict vegans require supplementation. Total body stores are 2–5 mg, predominantly hepatic, with daily requirements of 2 µg — stores last 3–4 years after intake stops, which is why B12 deficiency from any cause develops slowly. Absorption is uniquely complex:

- **Step 1 — Stomach:** Gastric acid and pepsin release dietary B12 from food protein. (PPIs, gastrectomy, and atrophic gastritis impair this step.)
- **Step 2 — Stomach:** Released B12 binds salivary haptocorrin (formerly called R-binder), which protects B12 through the acidic stomach environment.
- **Step 3 — Duodenum:** Pancreatic proteases degrade haptocorrin, releasing B12, which then binds intrinsic factor (IF) — a glycoprotein secreted by gastric parietal cells. (Pernicious anaemia destroys parietal cells; total gastrectomy removes them physically; both abolish IF.)
- **Step 4 — Terminal ileum:** The B12–IF complex is recognised by the cubilin–amnionless (cubam) receptor on enterocytes and absorbed. (Crohn's disease, ileal resection, and Diphyllobothrium latum infestation block this step.)

- **Step 5 — Plasma:** Inside the enterocyte, B12 is released and bound to transcobalamin II (TC-II), which delivers it to tissues. About 1% of any oral B12 dose is absorbed by passive diffusion alone — the basis for high-dose oral B12 therapy in some pernicious anaemia patients.

Folate absorption — short and simple

Folate is absorbed in the proximal jejunum without requiring intrinsic factor. Body stores are only 5–20 mg; daily requirement is 400 µg; deficiency develops in 3–4 months when intake stops. Sources are green leafy vegetables, legumes, fruits, and (in the US) fortified grain products — folic acid fortification of cereal grain products has been mandatory in the US since January 1998 and has virtually eliminated dietary folate deficiency in the general population. Folate is heat-labile; prolonged cooking destroys 50–90%.

9.10 Megaloblastic Anaemia — Diagnostic Approach

Peripheral smear and bone marrow

The hallmark on smear is the macroovalocyte (oval macrocyte) — a large oval red cell, larger than the nucleus of a small lymphocyte, distinct from the round macrocytes of liver disease. Hypersegmented neutrophils are the most specific peripheral finding: 5% or more of neutrophils with five or more lobes, OR any single neutrophil with six or more lobes, is virtually diagnostic of megaloblastic anaemia. WBC and platelet counts are often mildly reduced in moderate-to-severe deficiency — pancytopenia from a single nutritional deficiency is possible. The bone marrow is hypercellular with marked erythroid hyperplasia. Megaloblasts show nuclear–cytoplasmic dissociation: the nucleus retains open, lacy, stippled chromatin (immature) while the cytoplasm is already fully haemoglobinised (mature). Giant metamyelocytes and giant band forms are characteristic in the granulocytic series. Because DNA synthesis is impaired across all dividing cells, ineffective haematopoiesis is massive — many cells die in the marrow (intramedullary haemolysis), causing very high LDH and elevated indirect bilirubin that biochemically mimic haemolytic anaemia, but with a NEGATIVE direct antiglobulin test.

Discriminating B12 from folate deficiency

Test	B12 Deficiency	Folate Deficiency	Comment
Serum B12	LOW (<200 pg/mL definite; 200–300 borderline)	Normal	Borderline B12 (200–300) requires reflex MMA testing.
Serum folate	Normal or HIGH (folate trapped as 5-methyl-THF)	LOW (<2 ng/mL deficient)	Serum folate is volatile — a single hospital meal can normalise it. RBC folate is the tissue-store index.
RBC folate	Normal	LOW (<150	More reliable index of tissue

Test	B12 Deficiency	Folate Deficiency	Comment
		ng/mL)	folate than serum.
Methylmalonic acid (MMA)	ELEVATED (most specific test)	Normal	**MMA elevation is unique to B12 deficiency.** Folate does not participate in the methylmalonyl-CoA mutase pathway. Use MMA when B12 is borderline.
Homocysteine	ELEVATED	ELEVATED	Elevated in BOTH; not discriminating. Also elevated in renal disease and MTHFR polymorphism.
Neurologic features	PRESENT (subacute combined degeneration; peripheral neuropathy; cognitive change)	ABSENT	Most reliable clinical discriminator. Can occur WITHOUT anaemia.
LDH	Markedly elevated (intramedullary haemolysis)	Markedly elevated	Both — non-discriminating. May mislead toward haemolytic anaemia.
Indirect bilirubin	Mildly elevated	Mildly elevated	Both — same mechanism (intramedullary cell death).

HIGH-YIELD PEARL — Subacute combined degeneration (SACD)

Sites of damage: Posterior columns of the spinal cord (loss of vibration sense and proprioception; positive Romberg sign; sensory ataxia) and lateral corticospinal tracts (upper motor neuron signs — hyperreflexia, spasticity, extensor plantar responses). Peripheral neuropathy and dementia may also occur.

Critical principle: Neurologic disease can occur WITHOUT anaemia, and vice versa. The dissociation is particularly seen when concurrent high folate intake corrects the haematologic defect (folate partially bypasses the methyl trap and feeds DNA synthesis) without addressing B12 deficiency. The marrow recovers; the nervous system does not. Patients with adequate folate but undetected B12 deficiency present with isolated neurologic disease.

Treatment caveat: Replace B12 first, or simultaneously with folate. Never folate alone in an unspecified macrocytic anaemia.

HIGH-YIELD PEARL — Schilling test — historical context only

The Schilling test (radiolabeled oral B12 ± oral IF, with measurement of urinary excretion to localise the absorption defect) was used historically to distinguish pernicious anaemia (corrected by adding IF) from terminal ileum disease (not corrected by IF). It is no longer performed in the US — radiolabeled cobalt is unavailable, and the test has been superseded by anti-intrinsic-factor antibody testing for pernicious anaemia and clinical/imaging assessment for ileal disease. Older USMLE questions may reference the Schilling test for historical context; current practice uses serum B12, MMA, and antibody testing.

9.11 Pernicious Anaemia and Other Causes of B12 Deficiency

Pernicious anaemia (PA) is the most common cause of B12 deficiency in adults in the United States. It is an autoimmune destruction of gastric parietal cells (Type A atrophic gastritis), resulting in loss of intrinsic factor secretion and gastric acid secretion. Highest prevalence is in older adults of Northern European descent (typical onset >60 years), with associations to other autoimmune diseases — Hashimoto thyroiditis, type 1 diabetes, vitiligo, Addison disease, and primary biliary cholangitis. Family history is positive in 20–30%.

Pathogenesis

Antiparietal-cell antibodies and anti-intrinsic-factor antibodies are the serologic markers. Parietal cells reside in the gastric body and fundus; their progressive destruction produces atrophic gastritis confined to those regions (Type A — distinct from H. pylori–associated antral atrophic gastritis, Type B). Loss of acid produces achlorhydria and reactive hypergastrinaemia (G-cells in the antrum, freed from acid-mediated negative feedback, secrete excess gastrin). Loss of IF abolishes terminal-ileum absorption of dietary B12. Two consequences extend beyond the anaemia: (1) a 3-fold elevated risk of gastric adenocarcinoma, mandating consideration of upper endoscopy at diagnosis and surveillance thereafter; (2) an elevated risk of gastric Type 1 carcinoid tumours (driven by sustained hypergastrinaemia stimulating ECL cells in the gastric body).

Diagnostic antibodies

Antibody	Sensitivity	Specificity	Comment
Anti-intrinsic-factor (IF)	~50–70%	~99%	**Highly specific — a positive result confirms PA.** Two types: Type 1 (blocking) prevents B12–IF binding; Type 2 (binding) reacts with formed B12–IF complex. Negative result does not exclude PA (50% miss rate).
Antiparietal-cell (APC)	~85–90%	~50% (low)	More sensitive than anti-IF, but found in 15% of healthy older adults and in many with non-PA atrophic gastritis. Not diagnostic on its own.

Antibody	Sensitivity	Specificity	Comment
Serum gastrin	—	—	Markedly elevated (>200 pg/mL) — supportive but not diagnostic. Reflects ECL-cell stimulation; predicts carcinoid risk.
Pepsinogen I	—	—	Low — reflects loss of chief cells in gastric body. Useful adjunct in equivocal cases.

Treatment of PA

STEP 2 BRIDGE — B12 replacement — IM and oral

Standard regimen: Cyanocobalamin or hydroxocobalamin 1000 μg IM once daily for 1 week (loading), then weekly for 4 weeks, then monthly for life (or 1000 μg every 3 months in some protocols).

High-dose oral alternative: Cyanocobalamin 1000–2000 μg orally once daily can be used in patients without neurologic features and with good adherence — about 1% is absorbed by passive diffusion independent of IF, sufficient at this dose to maintain repletion. Studies show non-inferiority in stable PA without neurologic involvement.

Haematologic recovery: Reticulocyte response peaks day 5–10. Haemoglobin rises ~1 g/dL per week. Monitor potassium during recovery — the rapid expansion of red cell mass demands K^+, and severe hypokalaemia can develop.

Neurologic recovery: Months, often incomplete if treatment is delayed. Damage from sustained subacute combined degeneration may be permanent.

Other causes of B12 deficiency

Cause	Mechanism	Clinical Clue
Strict vegan diet	B12 is animal-source only; not synthesised by plants	Years of strict veganism; mild to moderate deficiency; readily corrected with oral supplement.
Gastrectomy or gastric bypass	Loss of acid (food-bound B12 not released) and loss of IF	May present years after surgery. Routine B12 monitoring is standard postoperative care; supplementation often required for life.
Crohn's disease or ileal resection	Terminal ileum is the absorption site for the B12–IF complex	History of Crohn's, surgical resection of distal ileum, or radiation. Concurrent fat malabsorption.
Diphyllobothrium latum (fish	Tapeworm absorbs free B12 from the gut lumen	Raw or undercooked freshwater fish (Great Lakes, Scandinavia, Eastern

Cause	Mechanism	Clinical Clue
tapeworm)		Europe). Now uncommon in the US; classic exam association.
Long-term metformin	Inhibits calcium-dependent uptake of the B12–IF complex by ileal enterocytes	Mild deficiency in 10–30% of long-term users; check B12 annually in patients on metformin >4 years, especially with concurrent peripheral neuropathy that might be misattributed to diabetes.
Long-term PPIs	Reduced gastric acid impairs release of food-bound B12	Years of PPI use; mild deficiency; clinical consequences debated but real in the elderly.
Nitrous oxide (N_2O)	Irreversibly oxidises the cobalt of B12, inactivating methionine synthase. Does NOT lower serum B12.	**Serum B12 normal but MMA elevated.** Recreational "whippits" use is the dominant US scenario; chronic dental and anaesthetic exposure also reported. May precipitate acute megaloblastic crisis or subacute combined degeneration in patients with marginal pre-existing B12 status. USMLE-favoured vignette: young adult with paresthesias and macrocytosis admitting to nitrous oxide canisters.

IMG-TRAP — Macrocytic anaemia in older US patient — pernicious anaemia, not folate

The trap. An older adult, often of Northern European descent, presents with macrocytic anaemia, fatigue, and possibly mild peripheral neuropathy or cognitive change. The IMG candidate, drawing on training in a setting where dietary folate deficiency in elderly populations is common (cooking practices that destroy folate, cereal-heavy diets, tea-with-meals patterns reducing folate absorption, no national food fortification), defaults to nutritional folate deficiency and chooses "start oral folic acid 5 mg daily."

The rule. On USMLE, macrocytic anaemia in an older US adult is presumed to be pernicious anaemia / B12 deficiency until proven otherwise. The first-line workup is serum B12 (with reflex MMA and homocysteine if 200–300 pg/mL). Low B12 with elevated MMA points to true B12 deficiency; anti-intrinsic-factor antibody is highly specific (~99%) for pernicious anaemia. Treat with parenteral cobalamin — never folate alone, which masks the anaemia while neurologic damage from undetected B12 deficiency continues to progress.

Why the trap exists. Three factors converge in US epidemiology: mandatory grain folic-acid fortification since 1998 has virtually eliminated dietary folate deficiency in the general population; pernicious anaemia has its highest prevalence in older Northern European-descent patients (the demographic the USMLE patient is drawn from); and the autoimmune background (Hashimoto thyroiditis, type 1 diabetes, vitiligo) is more prevalent in this population. The opposite epidemiology — folate deficiency dominant, PA uncommon — characterises the South Asian elderly populations many IMG candidates trained on. The USMLE answer is calibrated to US epidemiology, not to either training population's prior.

9.12 Folate Deficiency

Folate deficiency produces a megaloblastic anaemia indistinguishable on smear and marrow from B12 deficiency, but without neurologic features and without elevation of MMA. In the United States, mandatory folic acid fortification of grain products since January 1998 has virtually eliminated dietary folate deficiency in the general adult population; the entities below are the residual scenarios where folate deficiency still occurs.

Cause	Mechanism	USMLE Vignette
Chronic alcohol use	Poor dietary intake; impaired absorption; impaired utilisation (ethanol interferes with folate enterohepatic recirculation)	**Most common cause of folate deficiency in the US.** Alcoholic with macrocytic anaemia, peripheral neuropathy, and AST:ALT >2:1.
Pregnancy	Doubled folate demand for fetal neural-tube development and expanding red cell mass	Routine 400 µg preventive supplementation periconceptionally; 4 mg therapeutic dose if prior pregnancy with neural tube defect. Inadequate folate increases risk of NTDs (anencephaly, spina bifida).
Haemolytic anaemia	Increased erythropoietic demand depletes stores	Sickle cell disease, hereditary spherocytosis, thalassaemia. Daily folate supplement is standard care.
Malabsorption	Tropical sprue (jejunal folate absorption); coeliac disease; short bowel syndrome	Chronic diarrhoea + macrocytic anaemia + responsive to folate.
Methotrexate (MTX)	Inhibits dihydrofolate reductase → blocks regeneration of THF from DHF	**Functional folate deficiency; rescue with FOLINIC ACID (leucovorin), not folic acid.** Folinic acid bypasses the DHFR block; folic acid alone cannot rescue MTX toxicity.
Trimethoprim	Inhibits bacterial DHFR with weaker effect on human	Long-term TMP-SMX (HIV prophylaxis, recurrent UTI).

Cause	Mechanism	USMLE Vignette
	DHFR	Megaloblastic features can develop.
Phenytoin (and phenobarbital)	Impaired folate absorption; possible hepatic enzyme induction effect	Long-term anticonvulsant use; routine folate supplementation often coadministered.
Sulfasalazine	Competitively inhibits folate absorption	IBD or rheumatoid arthritis on sulfasalazine — supplemental folic acid is given routinely.

HIGH-YIELD PEARL — MTX rescue — folinic acid (leucovorin), NOT folic acid
This is a high-yield distinction. Methotrexate inhibits dihydrofolate reductase (DHFR), blocking conversion of DHF back to THF. Folic acid (the dietary form) requires DHFR for activation — it cannot be rescued through a blocked enzyme. Folinic acid (5-formyl-THF, leucovorin) is already past the block and directly enters the active folate pool. Use leucovorin for high-dose MTX rescue, MTX overdose, and severe MTX toxicity. The same logic applies to TMP-SMX haematologic toxicity. Folic acid (1 mg daily) is appropriate as routine prophylaxis for low-dose weekly MTX in rheumatoid arthritis and psoriasis — it competes with MTX for cellular uptake and reduces mucositis and haematologic toxicity without abolishing therapeutic efficacy.

9.13 Non-megaloblastic Macrocytosis

Not all macrocytosis is megaloblastic. Non-megaloblastic macrocytosis shows round (not oval) macrocytes, no hypersegmented neutrophils, and no megaloblastic change in the marrow. The mechanism is altered red cell membrane composition or accelerated reticulocyte release, not impaired DNA synthesis. The smear is the cheapest discriminator: round macrocytes with no hypersegmented neutrophils essentially excludes B12 or folate deficiency.

Cause	Mechanism	USMLE Clue
Chronic alcohol use	Direct toxic effect on red cell membrane (altered lipid composition); often coexists with folate deficiency	**Most common cause of macrocytosis in US adults.** MCV usually 100–108 fL; mild or no anaemia; may have macrocytosis without anaemia. Vacuolated myeloid precursors on marrow.
Liver disease	Altered membrane lipid (excess cholesterol and phospholipid loaded onto red cell membrane)	Round macrocytes; target cells; in advanced cirrhosis, spur cells (acanthocytes from cholesterol asymmetry); abnormal LFTs; no megaloblastic marrow.
Hypothyroidism	Mechanism uncertain; possibly reduced	Mild macrocytosis; elevated TSH. Always check for concurrent B12

Cause	Mechanism	USMLE Clue
	erythropoietic drive; may coexist with autoimmune PA	deficiency — both can be present in the autoimmune polyendocrinopathy spectrum.
Reticulocytosis	Reticulocytes are physiologically larger than mature red cells; brisk reticulocytosis (post-bleed, post-haemolysis, response to therapy) raises MCV	Polychromasia on smear; elevated reticulocyte count; LDH and indirect bilirubin elevated if haemolysis.
MDS	Dysplastic erythropoiesis; abnormal nuclear maturation in clonal stem cell disease	Older patient; macrocytic anaemia with cytopenias in other lineages; dysplasia on marrow; clonal cytogenetics or somatic mutations (SF3B1, TET2, ASXL1, splicesome).
Drugs (hydroxyurea, AZT/zidovudine, 5-FU, cytarabine)	Inhibit DNA synthesis pathways distinct from B12/folate (ribonucleotide reductase, reverse transcriptase, thymidylate synthase)	Drug history. Hydroxyurea in sickle cell, MPN, or CML; AZT in HIV; 5-FU in colorectal/breast cancer. Macrocytosis without overt megaloblastic features.
Pregnancy (mild)	Mild physiologic macrocytosis from increased erythropoietic drive in 3rd trimester	Mild; resolves postpartum. Pathologic macrocytosis in pregnancy points to true folate deficiency.

HIGH-YIELD PEARL — MCV >115 fL — narrow the differential

Mild macrocytosis (MCV 100–110 fL) has a long differential including alcohol, liver disease, hypothyroidism, reticulocytosis, and drugs. MCV above 115 fL substantially narrows the differential to: B12 deficiency, folate deficiency, MDS (especially MDS-RS with SF3B1), and rare drugs at high cumulative dose (hydroxyurea, AZT). Below 110 fL, the smear and reticulocyte count are essential to direct workup; above 115 fL, B12 + folate + MMA + reticulocyte count is the immediate next step.

9.14 Buzzwords and Visual Cues

The cues below are USMLE-favoured single-phrase stems and visual signs. Each maps to one or two diagnoses. Memorise the mapping; in the question stem, recognising the cue often arrives at the answer faster than working through the laboratory differential.

Buzzword / Visual Cue	Most Likely Diagnosis
Pencil cells (elongated cigar-	Iron deficiency anaemia

Buzzword / Visual Cue	Most Likely Diagnosis
shaped elliptocytes)	
Pagophagia (compulsive ice eating)	Iron deficiency
Koilonychia (spoon-shaped nails)	Iron deficiency
Plummer–Vinson: dysphagia + atrophic glossitis + iron deficiency	Iron deficiency with oesophageal web
Coarse basophilic stippling	Lead poisoning (also seen in thalassaemia, sideroblastic anaemia, MDS)
Burton lines (gingival lead lines)	Lead poisoning
Wrist drop / foot drop in adult with abdominal colic	Lead poisoning (peripheral neuropathy)
Hair-on-end skull X-ray	β-thalassaemia major (or severe sickle cell)
Frontal bossing + chipmunk facies in child	β-thalassaemia major
Target cells	Thalassaemia, liver disease, post-splenectomy, HbC disease, IDA
HbA_2 > 3.5% on HPLC	β-thalassaemia trait (diagnostic)
High RBC count with microcytic anaemia	Thalassaemia trait (compensation)
Mentzer index < 13 (MCV ÷ RBC count)	Thalassaemia trait
Hb Bart's (γ_4 tetramers) on neonatal HPLC	α-thalassaemia hydrops fetalis (4-gene deletion)
HbH inclusion bodies / "golf-ball" cells on supravital stain	α-thalassaemia, HbH disease (β_4 tetramers, 3-gene deletion)
Ring sideroblasts on Perls stain	Sideroblastic anaemia (any cause)
Ring sideroblasts + neutropenia + myeloid vacuolation	Copper deficiency (or chronic alcohol use)
Macroovalocytes + hypersegmented neutrophils (≥5 lobes)	Megaloblastic anaemia (B12 or folate deficiency)
Subacute combined degeneration of cord (posterior columns + lateral CST)	B12 deficiency

Buzzword / Visual Cue	Most Likely Diagnosis
Beefy red tongue (atrophic glossitis)	B12 deficiency or iron deficiency
Glove-and-stocking sensory loss in macrocytic anaemia	B12 deficiency peripheral neuropathy
Anti-intrinsic-factor antibody positive	Pernicious anaemia (highly specific)
Methylmalonic acid (MMA) elevated	B12 deficiency (NOT folate)
Whippits / recreational nitrous oxide	Functional B12 deficiency (serum B12 may be normal; MMA elevated)
Diphyllobothrium latum (fish tapeworm)	B12 deficiency (parasitic — raw freshwater fish)
Folinic acid (leucovorin) for rescue	Methotrexate toxicity (NOT folic acid alone)
Round macrocytes without hypersegmented neutrophils	Non-megaloblastic macrocytosis (alcohol, liver, hypothyroid, retic)
Spur cells (acanthocytes) in cirrhotic patient	Spur cell anaemia of advanced liver disease
Reactive thrombocytosis (400–700 $\times 10^9$/L) with microcytic anaemia	Iron deficiency anaemia

9.15 USMLE Vignettes

Ten USMLE-style vignettes covering the chapter. Read each stem before reading the answer, then verify the teaching point. The full set covers all four microcytic entities, both major macrocytic entities, and the high-yield discriminations.

VIGNETTE 1

Stem. A 32-year-old woman presents with 4 months of progressive fatigue and dyspnea on climbing stairs. She reports heavy menstrual periods lasting 7–8 days with passage of clots. Examination: pallor, smooth tongue, brittle nails. Haemoglobin 8.6 g/dL, MCV 68 fL, RDW 18.5%, RBC count 3.2 million/µL. Ferritin 8 ng/mL, TIBC 485 µg/dL, TSAT 5%, serum iron 22 µg/dL.

Diagnosis / Best next step. Iron deficiency anaemia from menorrhagia.

VIGNETTE 2

Stem. A 57-year-old man presents for routine evaluation. He reports no symptoms. He is on no medications, eats a balanced diet, and consumes minimal alcohol. Labs: Hb 10.4 g/dL, MCV 72 fL, RDW 17.2%, ferritin 9 ng/mL, TIBC 470 µg/dL, TSAT 5%. Stool guaiac is negative on a single sample.

Diagnosis / Best next step. Best next step: COLONOSCOPY plus upper endoscopy (bidirectional endoscopy). Iron supplementation alone is the wrong

Start oral ferrous sulfate (alternate-day single dose preferred). Refer for gynaecologic evaluation of menorrhagia (consider endometrial biopsy if >45 or risk factors; consider hormonal management or LNG-IUD).

Teaching point. Premenopausal women with IDA: identify and treat the source of bleeding (menstrual is most common). The high RDW + low MCV pattern is the classic IDA fingerprint. Reactive thrombocytosis is common.

answer.

Teaching point. Adult IDA in a man (or postmenopausal woman) is presumed to be from occult GI blood loss until proved otherwise. Negative stool guaiac on a single sample does not exclude colorectal cancer — bleeding is intermittent. Colonoscopy is the priority because colorectal cancer is the most common identifiable cause and the lesion that most demands prompt diagnosis. This is IMG-Trap #8 from §9.4.

VIGNETTE 3

Stem. A 48-year-old woman presents with 6 months of progressive difficulty swallowing solids — initially bread, now most solids. She has noticed fatigue and a sore tongue. Examination: pallor, smooth red tongue without papillae, fissuring at the corners of the mouth, and koilonychia. Haemoglobin 9.2 g/dL, MCV 70 fL, ferritin 6 ng/mL. Barium swallow shows a thin postcricoid web.

Diagnosis / Best next step. Plummer-Vinson syndrome (Paterson-Brown-Kelly) — triad of iron deficiency anaemia, dysphagia, and oesophageal web with atrophic glossitis. Treat the iron deficiency; the web may regress with iron repletion. Endoscopic dilation if persistent dysphagia.

Teaching point. Plummer-Vinson carries an increased risk of oesophageal and pharyngeal squamous cell carcinoma. Surveillance endoscopy is reasonable in patients with persistent webs. The iron deficiency is the central pathology — treat it.

VIGNETTE 4

Stem. A 68-year-old woman with longstanding rheumatoid arthritis on methotrexate and prednisone presents with fatigue. Examination: synovitis of the hands and wrists; no jaundice or splenomegaly. Haemoglobin 9.8 g/dL, MCV 86 fL, RDW 13.4%, ferritin 280 ng/mL, TIBC 220 µg/dL, TSAT 12%, CRP 6.0 mg/dL. Reticulocyte count 1.2%.

Diagnosis / Best next step. Anaemia of chronic inflammation from active RA. Optimise disease control (consider escalating DMARD therapy with rheumatology). Avoid empiric iron supplementation. Reassess once inflammation is controlled.

Teaching point. ACI: low iron, LOW or normal TIBC (the cytokine-driven discriminator from IDA), normal-to-elevated ferritin, normal MCV in most cases. The pathology is iron sequestration by hepcidin, not iron deficiency. Treating with iron alone fails; treating the underlying inflammation succeeds.

VIGNETTE 5

Stem. A 4-year-old boy living in a home built in 1962 is brought in for behavioural regression and recurrent abdominal pain. His mother notes he sometimes eats paint

VIGNETTE 6

Stem. A 28-year-old man of Greek descent presents for preconception counselling with his fiancée. He is asymptomatic. Routine labs: Hb 12.4 g/dL, MCV 65 fL, chips peeling from the windowsill. Examination: irritable, mildly pale, no organomegaly. Hb 9.2 g/dL, MCV 70 fL. Smear: microcytic anaemia with COARSE basophilic stippling. Blood lead level 56 µg/dL.

Diagnosis / Best next step. Lead poisoning. Begin oral succimer (DMSA) and immediate environmental investigation with source removal. Notify public health authorities.

Teaching point. Coarse basophilic stippling on smear in a child living in pre-1978 housing is lead poisoning until proved otherwise. Chelation thresholds in children: succimer for blood lead ≥45 µg/dL; dimercaprol (BAL) plus calcium EDTA for ≥70 µg/dL or encephalopathy. The most important step is removing the patient from the source — chelation does not fix ongoing exposure. The CDC blood lead reference value was lowered in October 2021 to 3.5 µg/dL (any value at or above this triggers case management).

RBC count 6.8 million/µL, RDW 13.5%, ferritin 130 ng/mL, TSAT 32%. HPLC: HbA 92%, HbA_2 5.4%, HbF 1.2%.

Diagnosis / Best next step. β-thalassaemia trait. Genetic counselling and partner screening are critical: if both partners carry β-thal trait, each pregnancy carries 25% risk of β-thalassaemia major.

Teaching point. The combination is diagnostic: microcytic anaemia with HIGH RBC count, normal RDW, normal iron studies, and HbA_2 > 3.5% on HPLC. The high RBC count reflects compensatory erythropoiesis (many small cells). This pattern in a Mediterranean-ancestry patient is β-trait until proved otherwise. Iron supplementation is contraindicated (no deficiency; risks iron overload).

VIGNETTE 7

Stem. A 30-year-old Filipino-American woman is found on routine labs to have Hb 11.5 g/dL, MCV 72 fL, RDW 13.0%, RBC count 5.2 million/µL. Ferritin 95 ng/mL, TSAT 28%. HPLC: HbA 96%, HbA_2 2.4%, HbF 0.5% — entirely normal.

Diagnosis / Best next step. α-thalassaemia trait. Confirm with GAP-PCR for common α-deletions (—SEA, —α3.7, —α4.2). Genetic counselling because the —SEA cis deletion (common in Southeast Asians) carries reproductive risk for HbH disease or hydrops fetalis if both partners carry it.

Teaching point. α-thalassaemia trait gives a normal adult HPLC — the diagnosis is by exclusion (microcytic anaemia + normal iron studies + normal HPLC + appropriate ancestry) or by molecular testing. The cis (--/αα) versus trans (-α/-α) genotype matters for

VIGNETTE 8

Stem. A 72-year-old woman of Northern European descent presents with 6 months of progressive fatigue and recent onset of paresthesias in both feet. Her daughter notes mild forgetfulness and unsteady gait. Examination: pallor, smooth beefy red tongue, reduced vibration sense at the ankles, positive Romberg sign. Hb 9.0 g/dL, MCV 118 fL, RDW 17%. Smear: macroovalocytes and hypersegmented neutrophils. B12 145 pg/mL, folate 8 ng/mL (normal), MMA elevated, anti-intrinsic-factor antibody positive.

Diagnosis / Best next step. Pernicious anaemia with subacute combined degeneration. Begin parenteral cyanocobalamin (1000 µg IM daily for 1 week, then weekly for 4 weeks, then monthly for life). Do NOT give folate alone.

Teaching point. This is IMG-Trap #2

genetic counselling: cis carries severe-offspring risk, trans does not. The Southeast Asian cis pattern is the high-risk one.

from §9.11. The older Northern European-descent patient with macrocytic anaemia and neurologic findings is pernicious anaemia until proved otherwise. Anti-IF antibody is highly specific (~99%). Folate alone would mask the anaemia while the neurologic damage progressed — never folate alone in unspecified macrocytic anaemia.

VIGNETTE 9

Stem. A 22-year-old man presents with 3 weeks of progressive paresthesias, gait unsteadiness, and difficulty buttoning his shirt. He admits to recreational use of nitrous oxide canisters ("whippits") for the past 2 months — multiple canisters daily. Examination: reduced vibration and proprioception, hyperreflexia, positive Romberg sign. Hb 11.8 g/dL, MCV 105 fL. Serum B12 320 pg/mL (normal range), but methylmalonic acid markedly elevated, homocysteine elevated.

Diagnosis / Best next step. Functional B12 deficiency from chronic nitrous oxide exposure with subacute combined degeneration. Stop nitrous oxide. Begin parenteral cobalamin replacement.

Teaching point. Nitrous oxide irreversibly oxidises the cobalt of B12, inactivating methionine synthase. Serum B12 may be entirely normal because the molecule is present but functionally inactive. MMA elevation is the diagnostic clue. The recreational use scenario is increasingly common in the US and well-represented on USMLE.

VIGNETTE 10

Stem. A 65-year-old woman with longstanding Crohn's disease (s/p ileal resection 10 years ago) presents with worsening fatigue. Hb 9.0 g/dL, MCV 92 fL (normocytic), RDW 19.2%. Smear: dimorphic population — small hypochromic cells alongside large oval macrocytes. Ferritin 22 ng/mL, TSAT 14%, B12 180 pg/mL, folate 6 ng/mL, MMA elevated.

Diagnosis / Best next step. Mixed iron + B12 deficiency on a background of inflammatory bowel disease and ileal resection. Treat both deficiencies. Parenteral cobalamin (ileal absorption is lost) plus IV iron (preferred over oral in IBD).

Teaching point. Mixed deficiency masks the MCV — the microcytic effect of iron deficiency and the macrocytic effect of B12 deficiency cancel out, producing a deceptively normocytic MCV. The clue is the dimorphic smear and the markedly elevated RDW (>18%). In any patient with normocytic anaemia and very high RDW, suspect mixed deficiency. Ferritin in low-normal range with concurrent inflammation may understate iron deficiency — sTfR/log(ferritin) ratio confirms it.

9.16 Closing Discriminators

Five closing distinctions worth carrying into the exam. Each compresses a recurring USMLE comparison.

HIGH-YIELD PEARL — Discriminator 1 — IDA vs β-thalassaemia trait

RDW: RAISED in IDA (>15%); normal in thal trait.

RBC count: Low in IDA; HIGH in thal trait (compensation).

MCV per gram of Hb: Disproportionately low in thal trait (MCV 65 with Hb 11.5); proportionate in IDA.

Iron studies: Low ferritin, high TIBC, low TSAT in IDA; all normal in thal trait.

HPLC: HbA_2 >3.5% in β-trait (diagnostic). Normal in IDA — but rule out coexistent IDA before interpreting (iron deficiency suppresses HbA_2).

HIGH-YIELD PEARL — Discriminator 2 — IDA vs ACI

TIBC: HIGH (>400) in IDA; LOW or normal in ACI. Single best discriminator.

Ferritin: <15 ng/mL in IDA; normal or HIGH (acute-phase reactant) in ACI.

BM Perls iron: Absent (Grade 0) in IDA; increased macrophage iron in ACI.

When mixed (IDA + ACI): Use sTfR/log(ferritin) ratio (Thomas index) > 2 OR Ret-He < 28 pg to identify the IDA component despite inflammation.

HIGH-YIELD PEARL — Discriminator 3 — B12 vs folate deficiency

MMA: Elevated in B12 deficiency; normal in folate deficiency. Most specific test.

Homocysteine: Elevated in BOTH; not discriminating.

Neurologic features: Present only in B12 deficiency. SACD, peripheral neuropathy, cognitive change.

Treatment principle: Never folate alone in unspecified macrocytic anaemia — folate may correct anaemia while B12 neurologic damage progresses.

HIGH-YIELD PEARL — Discriminator 4 — Megaloblastic vs non-megaloblastic macrocytosis

Macroovalocytes: Megaloblastic (B12, folate). Round macrocytes: non-megaloblastic (alcohol, liver, hypothyroid).

Hypersegmented neutrophils (≥5 lobes in ≥5%, or any ≥6 lobes): Megaloblastic only.

MCV magnitude: MCV >115 fL strongly favours megaloblastic (or MDS). MCV 100–110 is non-discriminating.

LDH and indirect bilirubin: Markedly elevated in megaloblastic (intramedullary haemolysis); negative DAT distinguishes from immune haemolytic anaemia.

IMG-TRAP — IMG-Trap recap — both traps in one place

IMG-Trap #8 (Adult IDA): Adult man or postmenopausal woman with iron deficiency = occult GI blood loss until proved otherwise. First step: bidirectional endoscopy (colonoscopy + EGD), not iron supplementation alone. Colorectal cancer is the leading concern.

IMG-Trap #2 (Older adult macrocytic anaemia): Older US adult with macrocytic anaemia ± neurologic features = pernicious anaemia / B12 deficiency until proved otherwise. First step: serum B12 (with reflex MMA if borderline), then anti-IF antibody. Folate alone is wrong — masks anaemia while neurologic damage progresses.

Common thread. US epidemiology differs from training-country epidemiology. The default presumption in both stems is dictated by US prevalence (colorectal cancer for the first; pernicious anaemia for the second), not by training-country prior probability (parasitic/nutritional iron deficiency; nutritional folate deficiency).

9.17 Quick Recall — One-Page Compression

QUICK RECALL — ONE-PAGE COMPRESSION

1. Framework. MCV first (microcytic <80 / normocytic 80–100 / macrocytic >100). Reticulocyte count second (RPI >2 = adequate response; <2 = hypoproliferative).

2. Hepcidin axis. Hepcidin HIGH → ferroportin blocked → iron trapped (ACI, haemochromatosis with appropriate hepcidin response, IRIDA). Hepcidin LOW → ferroportin open → iron flowing (IDA, hypoxia-driven, HFE-haemochromatosis with inappropriately low hepcidin).

3. IDA diagnosis. Ferritin <15 ng/mL highly specific. TIBC HIGH, TSAT <10% in established IDA. RDW raised (>15%). Pencil cells on smear. Reactive thrombocytosis common.

4. IDA workup in adults. Adult man or postmenopausal woman = bidirectional endoscopy. Premenopausal woman = gynaecologic + GI evaluation as indicated. (IMG-Trap #8.)

5. ACI key. Iron LOW, TIBC LOW or normal (cytokine-driven), ferritin normal or HIGH. Treat the inflammation; iron alone fails.

6. Sideroblastic. Ring sideroblasts on Perls. Iron HIGH, TSAT HIGH (iron in cell, not in haem). Causes: XLSA (ALAS2; pyridoxine-responsive), lead, INH, alcohol, copper deficiency, MDS-RS (SF3B1).

7. Lead poisoning. Coarse basophilic stippling. Burton lines, abdominal colic, peripheral neuropathy. CDC reference value 3.5 µg/dL (lowered Oct 2021). Succimer at ≥45 µg/dL; BAL + EDTA at ≥70 or encephalopathy.

8. β-thal trait. HbA_2 >3.5% on HPLC. Normal RDW, high RBC count. Iron studies normal. (Exclude IDA first — iron deficiency suppresses HbA_2.)

9. α-thal trait. HbA_2 NORMAL. Adult HPLC normal. Diagnosis by GAP-PCR for α-deletions. Cis (--/αα) carries reproductive risk; trans (-α/-α) does not.

10. The methyl trap. B12 deficiency traps folate as 5-methyl-THF → functional folate deficiency → megaloblastic anaemia. Serum folate may be elevated despite functional deficiency.

11. MMA = B12 only. Methylmalonic acid is elevated in B12 deficiency, not folate deficiency. Most specific test when B12 borderline (200–300 pg/mL).

12. SACD. B12 deficiency damages posterior columns (loss of vibration/proprioception; positive Romberg) and lateral corticospinal tracts (UMN signs). Can occur WITHOUT anaemia.

13. PA antibodies. Anti-IF: ~50–70% sensitive, ~99% specific (use to confirm). Anti-parietal-cell: more sensitive, low specificity (not diagnostic alone).

14. Older US adult macrocytic anaemia. Pernicious anaemia until proved otherwise. Never folate alone. (IMG-Trap #2.)

15. Folate antagonists. Methotrexate, trimethoprim, phenytoin, sulfasalazine. MTX rescue is FOLINIC ACID (leucovorin), not folic acid.

16. Non-megaloblastic macrocytosis. Round macrocytes, no hypersegmented neutrophils. Causes: alcohol, liver disease, hypothyroidism, reticulocytosis, drugs (hydroxyurea, AZT, 5-FU).

End of Chapter 9. Haemolytic anaemias and the membrane/enzyme/haemoglobin defects continue in Chapter 10.

Chapter 10 — Red Cell Disorders Part 2: Haemolytic Anaemias and Haemoglobinopathies

Haemolysis is destruction outpacing production. The DAT divides every case into two halves: immune above the line; membrane, enzyme, haemoglobin, mechanical, or PNH below it.

10.1 Big Picture and Mechanism Hooks

BIG PICTURE

Haemolytic anaemia is anaemia from accelerated red cell destruction at a rate exceeding the marrow's capacity for compensatory production. The marrow can ramp output 6–8 times normal; clinical anaemia develops only when red cell lifespan falls below approximately 15–20 days (normal 120 days). The diagnostic workflow asks three questions in order: (1) Is haemolysis really occurring? — confirmed by the haemolytic screen. (2) Is destruction intravascular or extravascular? — different lab signature, different cause list. (3) Is the mechanism immune or non-immune? — the DAT (Coombs test) is the single most important branch point. This chapter walks each branch.

MECHANISM HOOK — The haemolysis triad — three lab signatures of one event

Every haemolytic anaemia leaves three biochemical fingerprints that together confirm haemolysis before any cause-specific test is run. First, increased red cell destruction: serum LDH rises (released from lysed cells), indirect bilirubin rises (haem catabolism), and in intravascular haemolysis plasma free haemoglobin appears in serum and urine. Second, reduced red cell lifespan: serum haptoglobin falls — the liver synthesises haptoglobin to scavenge free haemoglobin, and once consumed it is not replaced quickly, making haptoglobin the most sensitive single marker of haemolysis. Third, compensatory production: the reticulocyte count rises (RPI >2), polychromasia appears on the smear, and in severe cases nucleated red cells are released into the periphery. The triad is not specific to any single aetiology — sickle cell disease, autoimmune haemolysis, hereditary spherocytosis, and DIC all produce it — but it confirms that haemolysis is happening, which is the prerequisite for asking the next two questions. Two pitfalls are worth noting up front: a low haptoglobin without other evidence of haemolysis can occur in advanced liver disease (synthetic failure) or hereditary low haptoglobin (about 2% of individuals of African descent), and not every reticulocytosis is haemolysis — recent blood loss and the recovery phase of nutritional anaemia therapy both raise reticulocytes without ongoing destruction.

10.2 The Haemolytic Screen — Confirming Haemolysis

The haemolytic screen is the minimum laboratory panel for any suspected haemolytic anaemia. The six tests below — LDH, indirect bilirubin, haptoglobin, reticulocyte count, plasma free haemoglobin, and urine haemosiderin — together establish whether haemolysis is occurring and provide initial classification (intravascular vs extravascular). The peripheral smear is examined in parallel: morphology often points to the diagnosis (spherocytes, schistocytes, sickle cells, bite cells, target cells, agglutination) before the chemistry returns.

Test	Direction in Haemolysis	Comment
LDH	RAISED (often markedly so in intravascular)	Sensitive but non-specific — also rises in muscle injury, hepatocyte damage, malignancy, intramedullary haemolysis (megaloblastic anaemia).
Indirect (unconjugated) bilirubin	RAISED	Reflects haem catabolism. Conjugated fraction normal unless concurrent liver disease.
Haptoglobin	LOW or absent	**Most sensitive marker of haemolysis.** Falsely low in liver disease (synthetic failure) and hereditary low haptoglobin (~2% of African-descent individuals). Acute-phase reactant — falsely raised in inflammation, may mask haemolysis.
Reticulocyte count (with RPI)	RAISED (RPI >2 = adequate response)	Compensatory marrow response. Polychromasia on smear is the morphologic correlate. Falsely low in concurrent iron/B12/folate deficiency, parvovirus B19, or marrow failure.
Plasma free haemoglobin	RAISED in intravascular haemolysis	Pink-tinged plasma on visual inspection. Normal in extravascular haemolysis (Hb stays inside macrophages).
Urine haemosiderin (Rous test)	POSITIVE in chronic intravascular haemolysis	Free Hb passes the glomerulus, is reabsorbed by renal tubular cells as haemosiderin; tubular cells slough into urine 5–7 days later. Useful when intravascular haemolysis is suspected but episodic.
Peripheral smear (always)	Diagnostic morphology	Spherocytes (HS, warm AIHA), schistocytes (MAHA), sickle cells (SCD), bite cells/Heinz bodies (G6PD), target cells (thalassaemia, HbC, liver), agglutination (cold AIHA), nucleated RBCs (severe haemolysis or marrow stress).

HIGH-YIELD PEARL — LDH plus low haptoglobin — the practical screen

In a busy hospital workflow, LDH and haptoglobin together provide >95% diagnostic yield for haemolysis. LDH rises early; haptoglobin falls early. If both are abnormal in the right direction with reticulocytosis and indirect hyperbilirubinaemia, haemolysis is essentially confirmed; the next test (DAT) starts the cause-finding workflow. If LDH and haptoglobin are both normal in a stable anaemic patient, haemolysis is unlikely — pursue another mechanism (production failure, blood loss, dilution).

Schumm test (methemalbumin) is rarely ordered today but is a high-yield exam fact: positive in chronic intravascular haemolysis once haptoglobin has been exhausted and free Hb is oxidised to methaemoglobin and bound to albumin. Modern equivalents are urine haemosiderin (Rous) and direct measurement of plasma free Hb.

10.3 Intravascular vs Extravascular Haemolysis

Once haemolysis is confirmed, the next branch is anatomic: where is destruction occurring? Intravascular haemolysis is rupture inside the bloodstream, releasing free haemoglobin into plasma. Extravascular haemolysis is phagocytosis of damaged red cells by macrophages of the spleen, liver, and bone marrow — Hb stays inside the macrophage and is processed normally to bilirubin. The lab pattern is distinct enough that intravascular haemolysis can be recognised from chemistry and urinalysis alone.

Feature	Intravascular	Extravascular
Site of destruction	Within blood vessels (complement lysis, mechanical fragmentation, oxidative)	Macrophages of spleen, liver, bone marrow (erythrophagocytosis)
Plasma free haemoglobin	RAISED (pink plasma)	Normal or minimally raised
Haptoglobin	Absent (consumed rapidly)	Low (consumed slowly)
Haemoglobinuria	Present (dark/red urine)	Absent
Urine haemosiderin (Rous)	POSITIVE (chronic intravascular)	Negative
Methemalbumin (Schumm)	Positive in chronic intravascular	Negative
LDH	Very high	Mildly elevated
Indirect bilirubin	Elevated	Elevated
Reticulocytes	Raised	Raised
Splenomegaly	Usually absent	Often present (RBCs trapped in cords of Billroth)

Feature	Intravascular	Extravascular
Key causes	PNH; ABO-mismatched transfusion; severe G6PD crisis; cold agglutinin disease (severe); MAHA (TTP, HUS, DIC); mechanical valve haemolysis; severe malaria (blackwater fever); march haemoglobinuria; PCH	Warm AIHA; hereditary spherocytosis; sickle cell disease; thalassaemia; hereditary elliptocytosis; cold agglutinin disease (mild); pyruvate kinase deficiency

HIGH-YIELD PEARL — All haemolysis raises LDH, indirect bilirubin, and reticulocytes; intravascular adds three

Universal markers of haemolysis (any type): LDH up, indirect bilirubin up, reticulocytes up, haptoglobin down.

Add for intravascular only: haemoglobinaemia (pink plasma), haemoglobinuria (dark/red urine), positive urine haemosiderin (Rous test) in chronic cases. Methemalbumin via Schumm test is positive in chronic intravascular haemolysis once free Hb has been oxidised.

Splenomegaly: Suggests extravascular pattern (RBCs trapped in splenic cords). Notably absent in PNH (intravascular) and most acute intravascular causes.

10.4 The DAT-Based Approach — First Branch Point

The direct antiglobulin test (DAT, also called the direct Coombs test) is the single most important branch point in any haemolytic anaemia workup. The DAT detects antibody (IgG) or complement fragments (C3d) bound to the patient's red cells in vivo. A positive result establishes immune haemolysis; a negative result redirects the workup to non-immune mechanisms (membrane, enzyme, haemoglobinopathy, mechanical, or PNH). Both branches share the universal haemolytic screen above; only the cause-finding tests differ.

DAT methodology

The patient's red cells are washed and then incubated with antihuman globulin reagent. Polyspecific reagent contains anti-IgG plus anti-C3d and is the standard initial test. If positive, monospecific reagents (anti-IgG only and anti-C3d only) localise the bound species. Modern column-agglutination (gel card) methodology has largely replaced tube technique in clinical labs — the principle is the same, but read-out is more reproducible and can detect weak coating that tube methods miss.

DAT pattern → most likely diagnosis

DAT (polyspecific)	Monospecific Reagents	Most Likely Diagnosis
Positive	IgG only	Warm AIHA (idiopathic or secondary); methyldopa-type drug-induced AIHA

DAT (polyspecific)	Monospecific Reagents	Most Likely Diagnosis
Positive	IgG + C3d	Warm AIHA with complement activation; SLE-associated AIHA; immune-complex DIIHA
Positive	C3d only	**Cold agglutinin disease.** IgM dissociates from RBCs at 37 °C during the wash step, leaving only the bound C3d. Also seen after PCH episodes once complement has been deposited.
Negative	—	Non-immune haemolysis (HS, HE, G6PD, PK, haemoglobinopathies, MAHA, PNH); rare DAT-negative AIHA (~5% of clinical AIHA — low-affinity IgG, IgA, or IgM warm AIHA)

DAT-positive workup (immune)

A positive DAT triggers the immune-haemolysis workflow: warm vs cold AIHA distinction (clinical and serologic), drug history (methyldopa, fludarabine, penicillin high-dose IV, quinidine), search for an underlying cause (CLL, SLE, lymphoma, infection, post-transfusion). Treatment is mechanism-specific: corticosteroids ± rituximab for warm AIHA; cold avoidance + rituximab + sutimlimab for cold agglutinin disease; transfusion (least-incompatible units) for life-threatening anaemia. These entities are detailed in §10.10–10.12.

DAT-negative workup (non-immune)

A negative DAT in confirmed haemolysis directs the workup to the non-immune mechanisms — each with its own diagnostic test:

- **Membrane disorders** (spherocytes on smear; MCHC >36 g/dL flag; EMA binding test — §10.5)
- **Enzyme disorders** (bite cells / Heinz bodies on smear during crisis suggest G6PD; PK enzyme assay for chronic non-spherocytic haemolytic anaemia — §10.6)
- **Haemoglobinopathies** (sickle cells, target cells, basophilic stippling; HPLC — §10.7–10.9)
- **Mechanical / microangiopathic** (schistocytes on smear; ADAMTS13 activity — §10.14)
- **PNH** (unique combination of intravascular haemolysis + venous thrombosis at unusual sites + cytopenias; FLAER flow cytometry — §10.13)

HIGH-YIELD PEARL — DAT-negative is not "no antibody"

About 5–10% of clinically classical AIHA is DAT-negative. Three mechanisms account for false-negative DAT: (1) low-affinity IgG that dissociates during the antiglobulin wash — diagnosed by enzyme-treated red cell DAT or column DAT; (2) IgA-mediated AIHA — standard polyspecific reagent (anti-IgG + anti-C3d) does NOT include anti-IgA; request specifically; (3) IgM warm AIHA (rare) — IgM dissociates at 37 °C during the wash step. In any patient with confirmed haemolysis (raised LDH, low haptoglobin, raised reticulocytes), no alternative cause, and a DAT-negative result, a steroid trial is justified — about 5–10% of warm AIHA presents this way.

Inverse trap: A positive DAT does not always mean clinical AIHA. Up to 1% of healthy blood donors and 8% of hospitalised patients have a positive DAT without haemolysis ("DAT-positive without AIHA"). Always interpret DAT alongside the haemolytic screen — antibody coating without compensatory reticulocytosis or rising bilirubin is a serologic finding, not a disease.

10.5 Hereditary Membrane Disorders

Hereditary spherocytosis (HS) is the most common inherited haemolytic anaemia in populations of Northern European ancestry. It results from mutations in genes encoding the proteins that anchor the lipid bilayer to the underlying spectrin–actin cytoskeleton — ankyrin (ANK1, ~50% of cases), band 3 (SLC4A1, ~25%), α-spectrin (SPTA1), β-spectrin (SPTB), and protein 4.2 (EPB42). When the anchoring is defective, the bilayer vesiculates progressively, the cell loses surface area relative to volume, and the resulting sphere lacks deformability. Spherocytes cannot squeeze through the narrow fenestrations of the splenic cords of Billroth and are removed by macrophages — pure extravascular haemolysis. Most cases are autosomal dominant (~75%) or de novo mutations (~25%); autosomal recessive forms are typically more severe.

Clinical features

The classic triad is anaemia, jaundice, and splenomegaly. Severity ranges from incidentally detected mild haemolysis to transfusion-dependent disease in the rare recessive forms. Common presentations include neonatal jaundice (often the presenting feature, sometimes requiring exchange transfusion), pigment gallstones from chronic bilirubin overload (cholecystectomy combined with splenectomy if both are indicated), and aplastic crisis with parvovirus B19 infection — a sudden Hb fall with reticulocytopenia (zero or near-zero retics, distinguishing aplastic crisis from sequestration or accelerated haemolysis).

Diagnosis

Test	Principle	Interpretation	Comment
MCHC on CBC	Cellular dehydration as membrane is lost	**MCHC > 36 g/dL is the characteristic analyzer flag.** Combined with low MCV and spherocytes on smear, this is diagnostic in the right clinical context. HS is the only common condition that reliably elevates MCHC.	First clue — often present on routine CBC.
Peripheral smear	Direct visualisation	Spherocytes (small, dense, no central	Cannot distinguish HS from warm AIHA on

Test	Principle	Interpretation	Comment
		pallor); polychromasia from reticulocytosis	smear alone — DAT separates them (negative in HS, positive in warm AIHA).
EMA binding test	Eosin-5-maleimide binds band 3 and RhAG; fluorescence by flow cytometry	Reduced fluorescence (>21% below mean) confirms HS	**PREFERRED modern test.** Sensitivity ~93%; not affected by recent transfusion; rapid (hours); requires only ~100 µL blood.
Osmotic fragility test (OFT)	Spherocytes lyse at higher salt concentrations than normal cells	Increased fragility confirms spherocytes	Older test; sensitivity ~68%; AFFECTED by recent transfusion (donor cells dilute the result); pre-incubation at 37 °C for 24 h improves sensitivity in mild cases. Largely replaced by EMA.
SDS-PAGE of membrane proteins	Identifies specific protein deficiency	Ankyrin, band 3, spectrin, or protein 4.2 reduced	Research / specialist centres. Rarely needed for clinical diagnosis.

Treatment

STEP 2 BRIDGE — Splenectomy in HS — when and how

Indications: Moderate-to-severe HS with symptomatic anaemia (Hb persistently <10 g/dL), poor growth in children, or recurrent need for transfusion. Mild HS (compensated, asymptomatic) does not require splenectomy.

Pre-splenectomy preparation: Pneumococcal conjugate (PCV15 or PCV20) followed by polysaccharide (PPSV23) ≥8 weeks later; H. influenzae type b (Hib) vaccine; meningococcal ACWY conjugate plus serogroup B vaccine. All vaccines given ≥2 weeks before elective splenectomy when possible. Booster pneumococcal at 5-year intervals.

Post-splenectomy: Penicillin V prophylaxis (250 mg twice daily) is recommended for at least 2 years post-op and through childhood; lifelong in some protocols. Patients counselled about overwhelming post-splenectomy infection (OPSI) — fever in an asplenic patient is a medical emergency requiring empiric IV antibiotics.

Outcome: Splenectomy dramatically reduces or abolishes haemolysis. Spherocytes persist on smear (the membrane defect is unchanged) but their lifespan now approaches normal. Concurrent cholecystectomy if symptomatic gallstones — combined laparoscopic procedure is standard.

Folate supplementation: Daily folate 1 mg in chronic haemolysis to prevent megaloblastic crisis from folate depletion.

Other membrane disorders

Hereditary elliptocytosis (HE) results from mutations in α-spectrin (SPTA1) or protein 4.1 (EPB41) that destabilise spectrin tetramer formation, weakening lateral membrane stability. Most cases are mild — compensated haemolysis with ≥25% elliptocytes on smear (normal <5%). Hereditary pyropoikilocytosis (HPP) is a severe recessive variant with neonatal haemolytic anaemia and red cells that lyse at 45 °C (vs 49 °C for normal cells). Hereditary stomatocytosis encompasses cation leak disorders producing slit-shaped central pallor; the dehydrated form (xerocytosis) has DECREASED osmotic fragility (cells resist osmotic stress because they are already volume-depleted). Southeast Asian ovalocytosis (SAO, SLC4A1 mutation) produces rigid oval cells that resist invasion by Plasmodium falciparum — a population-level malaria-protective polymorphism.

HIGH-YIELD PEARL — Spherocytes and the DAT — the indispensable second test
Spherocytes on a peripheral smear can result from either hereditary spherocytosis OR warm autoimmune haemolytic anaemia (warm AIHA) — the two morphologies are essentially identical. The DAT separates them: NEGATIVE in HS (membrane defect, no antibody), POSITIVE in warm AIHA. This is one of the most testable second-test discriminations on USMLE: "young patient with spherocytes and family history of jaundice" + DAT-negative = HS; "middle-aged patient with new spherocytes" + DAT-positive = warm AIHA. The MCHC pattern is also informative: HS is the only common cause that consistently raises MCHC > 36 g/dL.

10.6 Enzyme Disorders — G6PD and PK

Two RBC enzyme deficiencies dominate the USMLE differential: G6PD (oxidative, episodic, X-linked) and PK (chronic, autosomal recessive). They are mechanistically distinct and tested with very different vignette patterns.

G6PD deficiency — pathway and clinical scenarios

Glucose-6-phosphate dehydrogenase is the rate-limiting first enzyme of the hexose monophosphate (pentose phosphate) shunt. Its product, NADPH, regenerates reduced glutathione (GSH), which is the red cell's primary defence against oxidative stress. Without G6PD, oxidant exposure (drugs, infections, fava beans) overwhelms GSH, haemoglobin is oxidised to methaemoglobin and then denatured into Heinz bodies that attach to the inner membrane. Splenic macrophages "bite" out the Heinz bodies as red cells transit, producing the characteristic bite cells (degmacytes) and blister cells on the smear. Severe oxidant exposure causes intravascular haemolysis; milder exposures cause extravascular destruction. The disease is X-linked — males hemizygous and severely affected; female carriers usually mild via lyonisation (X-inactivation), but some heterozygotes have clinically significant deficiency depending on the X-inactivation skew.

Variant	Activity	Population	Severity
Class I	Severely deficient	Sporadic	Chronic non-spherocytic haemolytic anaemia (CNSHA) — haemolyses WITHOUT triggers. Most severe class.
Class II — Mediterranean	<5%	Mediterranean, Middle East, South Asia, India	Severe acute haemolysis with strong oxidant triggers. Favism (acute haemolysis after fava beans) is classic.
Class III — A-	10–60%	African American, sub-Saharan African	Self-limited acute haemolysis with strong triggers; older RBCs preferentially lysed; younger RBCs (with higher G6PD) survive. Haemolysis stops despite continued exposure.
Class IV–V	Normal or raised	—	Clinically silent.

Triggers

Drugs: antimalarials (primaquine, tafenoquine), dapsone, sulfa antibiotics (TMP-SMX, sulfasalazine), nitrofurantoin, nalidixic acid, phenazopyridine, rasburicase, methylene blue (high dose). **Foods:** fava beans (Class II Mediterranean — favism — within 24–48 hours of ingestion). **Infections:** the most common precipitant of all, independent of any drug. Hepatitis A and B, pneumonia, salmonellosis, and typhoid are classic precipitants on USMLE.

Diagnosis

Test	Principle	Interpretation	Pitfall
Quantitative G6PD enzyme assay	Spectrophotometric NADPH generation rate	<10% activity = severe; 10–60% = moderate; >60% normal	**FALSELY NORMAL during acute haemolytic crisis.** Most G6PD-deficient cells are already lysed; circulating cells are reticulocyte-enriched (younger RBCs have HIGHER G6PD). Test ≥3 months after the episode.
Beutler fluorescent spot test	G6PD-dependent NADPH	Non-fluorescent spot = deficient	Qualitative; same pitfall during crisis (false-

Test	Principle	Interpretation	Pitfall
	fluoresces under UV		normal).
Smear during crisis	Direct visualisation	Bite cells, blister cells, Heinz bodies (only on supravital stain)	Heinz bodies NOT visible on routine Wright/Romanowsky stain — require crystal violet or new methylene blue.

HIGH-YIELD PEARL — Never test G6PD during acute haemolysis

This is one of the most testable conceptual errors on USMLE. During an acute haemolytic crisis: (1) the most G6PD-deficient red cells have already been lysed and removed from circulation; (2) the remaining cells are predominantly young reticulocytes, which physiologically have HIGHER G6PD activity than mature red cells (younger cells make more enzyme). Both the quantitative assay and the Beutler spot test can therefore appear FALSELY NORMAL when the patient is acutely haemolysing. The correct approach: confirm the diagnosis clinically (smear with bite cells, history of trigger), treat the acute event, and retest enzyme activity ≥3 months later when the reticulocyte count has normalised. In females with intermediate results, testing male family members can confirm the diagnosis when lyonisation makes the proband's value ambiguous.

Methaemoglobinaemia in G6PD deficiency: If a G6PD-deficient patient develops drug-induced methaemoglobinaemia, methylene blue is INEFFECTIVE (its conversion to leucomethylene blue requires NADPH, which is the deficiency) and can paradoxically worsen oxidative haemolysis. Use ascorbic acid orally for mild cases; exchange transfusion for severe.

Pyruvate kinase (PK) deficiency

PK deficiency is the second most common red cell enzyme defect after G6PD. It is autosomal recessive (PKLR gene) and produces a CHRONIC (not episodic) haemolytic anaemia — no oxidant trigger required. PK catalyzes the final ATP-generating step of glycolysis; its deficiency leaves the red cell ATP-depleted, with loss of membrane deformability and sodium-pump failure. ATP-depleted cells ("echinocytes," or burr cells) become rigid and are removed extravascularly by the spleen. Splenectomy is partially effective and produces a paradoxical RISE in reticulocyte count post-operatively — the spleen had been actively removing the youngest, most ATP-depleted cells, and removing the spleen extends their survival. Mitapivat, an oral activator of red cell pyruvate kinase, was approved by the FDA in February 2022 for transfusion-dependent and not-transfusion-dependent PK deficiency in adults; it directly augments residual enzyme activity and reduces transfusion requirement.

10.7 Sickle Cell Disease — Molecular Mechanism

Sickle cell disease (SCD) is the most common serious haemoglobinopathy in the United States. Approximately 100,000 Americans live with SCD, with prevalence concentrated in the Black/African American population: about 1 in 365 Black births, with carrier frequency of approximately 1 in 13. Universal newborn screening identifies SCD before 1 year of age in all 50 US states. The disease is the prototypical example of a single point mutation producing a multisystem clinical syndrome through one mechanism — haemoglobin polymerisation on deoxygenation.

The HbS mutation

HbS results from a single point mutation in codon 6 of the β-globin gene (HBB): GAG → GTG, substituting valine for glutamic acid at position 6 of the β-chain. Glutamic acid is hydrophilic and negatively charged; valine is hydrophobic. The substitution changes the surface chemistry of the molecule without altering its overall structure. Each red cell still synthesises haemoglobin tetramers normally; oxygen binding is normal at high pO_2; and HPLC shows a single major HbS peak with HbA absent (in HbSS). The clinical disease arises entirely from what happens when HbS is deoxygenated.

MECHANISM HOOK — Why deoxygenation triggers polymerisation

In oxygenated HbS (R-state), the valine substitution at β6 sits inside the tetramer's surface and is functionally hidden. When HbS gives up oxygen (T-state), the conformational change exposes the hydrophobic valine and creates a complementary hydrophobic acceptor pocket on an adjacent β-chain. The valine of one HbS molecule fits into the pocket of the next — the nucleation step. Once nucleation occurs, additional HbS molecules add rapidly, building long, stiff polymer fibres that distort the red cell from biconcave disc into elongated crescent. In oxygenated blood, the polymer dissociates and the cell may resume near-normal shape. With repeated cycles, membrane damage becomes cumulative and irreversibly sickled cells (ISCs) appear — these stay deformed regardless of oxygenation. ISCs are rigid, non-deformable, and abnormally adherent to vascular endothelium; they cannot squeeze through small vessels and they slow flow upstream, deoxygenating more HbS, recruiting more polymerisation, and generating the vaso-occlusive crisis. Polymerisation happens ONLY in the deoxygenated state, which explains every clinical feature: vaso-occlusion targets tissues with the highest oxygen extraction (bone marrow, spleen, kidney medulla, retina, lung in the setting of any pulmonary process); dehydration accelerates sickling by raising intracellular HbS concentration (concentration-squared dependence of polymerisation); acidosis right-shifts the dissociation curve and increases deoxygenated HbS; high altitude and anaesthesia produce hypoxia that initiates crisis. The same logic explains every modifier that prevents polymerisation: HbF (γ-chain has no β6 valine) physically dilutes HbS at the molecular level and cannot enter the polymer — this is why hydroxyurea, which induces γ-globin expression and raises HbF, is the most effective disease-modifying drug in SCD; HbA in trait (HbAS) dilutes HbS the same way at physiologic oxygen tensions; co-inheritance of α-thalassaemia lowers MCHC and reduces the probability of HbS–HbS contact. Voxelotor was a polymerisation inhibitor that bound HbS in the oxygenated state — but Pfizer voluntarily withdrew it worldwide in September 2024 after post-marketing data showed an imbalance of vaso-occlusive crises and fatal events; the FDA confirmed the withdrawal, the EMA suspended marketing authorisation, and patients have transitioned to alternative therapy. New patients are no longer started on voxelotor.

Sickle cell genotypes

Genotype	HbS (%)	HbA (%)	HbF / Other	Clinical
HbAA (normal)	0	97	HbA_2 2–3.5%; HbF <1%	Normal.
HbAS (trait)	35–45	55–60	Normal HbA_2 and HbF	Asymptomatic at normal oxygen. Risk: renal medullary carcinoma (rare), exercise-related sudden death in extreme conditions, haematuria from papillary infarct, splenic infarction at high altitude. NO chronic anaemia, NO crises at sea level.
HbSS (sickle cell disease)	85–95	0	HbF variable (high if hydroxyurea-treated)	Chronic haemolytic anaemia (Hb 6–8 g/dL); recurrent vaso-occlusive crises; functional asplenia by age 5; baseline reticulocytosis.
HbSC	45–50	0	HbC ~45–50%	Milder than HbSS. Notable for proliferative retinopathy and avascular necrosis of femoral head.
HbS/β^0-thal	70–85	0	HbF 5–30%; HbA_2 raised (>3.5%)	Clinically similar to HbSS. Raised HbA_2 on HPLC is the discriminator.
HbS/β^+-thal	50–80	5–30	HbF 5–20%; HbA_2 raised	Milder than HbSS — some HbA present.
HbS/HPFH	70–80	0	HbF 20–30% (pancellular)	Mild. High HbF protects against polymerisation.

IMG-TRAP — Sickle cell demographics in the US patient

The trap. An IMG candidate sees a Black or African American patient with severe pain in bones, chest, back, or abdomen — and treats sickle cell disease as just one item on a broad differential alongside community-acquired pneumonia, peptic ulcer disease, urinary tract infection, or musculoskeletal pain. In the candidate's training environment, SCD is concentrated in specific tribal populations of central and eastern India and is uncommon in routine clinical practice; the prior probability the candidate brings to the bedside is calibrated to that population.

The rule. On USMLE, the demographic anchors for SCD are explicit and consistent: African American or Black patient with acute severe pain — vaso-occlusive crisis until proved otherwise; Black paediatric patient with sudden splenic enlargement, hypotension, and Hb drop — splenic sequestration; Black patient with fever, chest pain, hypoxia, and a new pulmonary infiltrate — acute chest syndrome (not just CAP); Black child with fever and absent vaccinations — encapsulated organism sepsis in functional asplenia. Newborn screening identifies SCD universally before age 1, so by adulthood the diagnosis is established — vignettes assume baseline disease and ask about acute management or chronic prophylaxis.

Why the trap exists. US SCD prevalence in the Black population is approximately 1 in 365 births with a carrier frequency of about 1 in 13 — high enough that any unexplained pain syndrome, anaemia, or stroke in a Black US patient must include SCD at the top of the differential. Indian SCD epidemiology is concentrated in tribal populations (Chhattisgarh, Odisha, Madhya Pradesh, Maharashtra, Gujarat) with sickle gene prevalence of 10–33% in those communities, but is uncommon in non-tribal regions. IMG candidates trained outside the tribal belt see SCD infrequently and may underweight the demographic signal. The USMLE provides demographic information deliberately — when the patient is identified as Black or African American with otherwise unexplained pain, anaemia, or stroke, sickle cell is statistically likely AND test-favourable.

HIGH-YIELD PEARL — Modifiers of sickling — three that reduce, none that prevent

1. HbF (most potent). γ-chains lack the β6 valine and cannot enter the polymer. HbF dilutes HbS at the molecular level. Hereditary persistence of fetal haemoglobin (HPFH) co-inherited with HbSS dramatically reduces severity. Hydroxyurea induces HbF — first-line disease-modifying therapy.

2. HbA (in trait). HbA dilutes HbS in HbAS (sickle trait). Polymerisation does not occur at physiologic oxygen tensions. HbAS is generally clinically silent.

3. α-thalassaemia co-inheritance. Reduces MCHC. Polymerisation rate has a concentration-squared dependence on HbS — even modest reductions in MCHC substantially reduce sickling.

Voxelotor — formerly a fourth modifier, now withdrawn. Voxelotor stabilised the oxygenated R-state of HbS to prevent polymerisation. Pfizer voluntarily withdrew it worldwide in September 2024 after post-marketing data showed excess vaso-occlusive crises and fatal events. The FDA confirmed the withdrawal; the EMA suspended marketing authorisation. Voxelotor is no longer used and should not be selected on current USMLE.

10.8 Sickle Cell Disease — Crises and Management

Acute crises are the dominant clinical presentation of HbSS. Five acute syndromes account for most emergency presentations and are testable by stem pattern on USMLE.

Crisis	Mechanism	Clinical Pattern	Key Lab / Workup
Vaso-occlusive (painful) crisis	Microvascular occlusion by sickled cells → tissue ischaemia	Severe pain in bones, joints, back, chest, abdomen. Most common crisis. Hb unchanged from baseline.	Leukocytosis common (inflammatory, not infectious); inflammatory markers elevated. Hb stable. Treat: IV fluids, IV opioids, oxygen if hypoxic, address triggers.
Acute chest syndrome (ACS)	Multifactorial: vaso-occlusion in pulmonary vasculature, infection, fat embolism from infarcted bone marrow	**New pulmonary infiltrate + fever and/or respiratory symptoms.** Most common cause of death in SCD adults. Rapid progression possible.	Hypoxia (SpO_2 <90%); new infiltrate on CXR; elevated WBC. Treat: simple or exchange transfusion; antibiotics (atypical coverage with macrolide); analgesia; oxygen; bronchodilators.
Aplastic crisis	Parvovirus B19 infects erythroid progenitors via P antigen receptor → halts erythropoiesis	Sudden Hb fall WITHOUT reticulocytosis. Pallor, congestive cardiac failure if severe.	**Reticulocytes near ZERO — distinguishes from sequestration.** Parvovirus B19 IgM/PCR. Self-limited 7–10 days. Transfusion support. Isolate from pregnant healthcare workers.
Splenic sequestration	Acute trapping of sickled cells + large blood volume in spleen	Sudden painful splenomegaly + rapid Hb drop + hypovolaemic shock. Most common in children <5 years (HbSC patients into adulthood).	**Reticulocytes RISING — distinguishes from aplastic crisis.** Acute Hb drop ≥2 g/dL. Emergency volume resuscitation + transfusion. Splenectomy considered for recurrent episodes.
Stroke	Large-vessel occlusion (typically MCA territory). Most common ages 2–5 and 30s–40s.	Acute neurologic deficit; seizures; loss of consciousness. Medical emergency.	**Emergency exchange transfusion to reduce HbS to <30%.** MRI/CT brain. Chronic transfusion or HSCT prevents recurrence. Transcranial Doppler screening for stroke risk in children (TCD ≥200 cm/s = high risk → primary prophylaxis with chronic transfusion).

HIGH-YIELD PEARL — Aplastic vs sequestration crisis — the reticulocyte count is the discriminator

Aplastic crisis: Parvovirus B19 → erythroid progenitor infection → reticulocytes near ZERO → Hb falls because production stopped. Self-limited 7–10 days. Transfusion support.

Sequestration crisis: Blood physically trapped in spleen → reticulocytes RAISED (marrow responds normally) → Hb falls because cells are pooled, not destroyed. Volume resuscitation + transfusion. Recurrent → splenectomy.

Both show rapid Hb fall with potential for cardiac failure. The reticulocyte count separates them on USMLE — and a parvovirus-positive serology in any patient with chronic haemolytic anaemia (SCD, HS, thalassaemia) is essentially diagnostic of aplastic crisis.

Disease-modifying and chronic management

STEP 2 BRIDGE — SCD chronic management — vaccinations, prophylaxis, hydroxyurea, gene therapy

Penicillin prophylaxis: Penicillin V 125 mg twice daily from 2 months to 3 years; 250 mg twice daily ages 3–5; continued past 5 years in patients with prior pneumococcal sepsis or splenectomy. Reduces pneumococcal sepsis dramatically; functional asplenia is established by ~age 5 in HbSS.

Vaccinations (universal): Pneumococcal conjugate (PCV15 or PCV20) full series + PPSV23 at 2 years with booster at 5 years; Hib full series; meningococcal conjugate ACWY (start at 2 months) + meningococcal serogroup B (≥10 years); annual influenza; COVID per current schedule. Standard paediatric vaccines as scheduled.

Hydroxyurea: First-line disease-modifying drug. Recommended for all HbSS and HbS/β^0-thal patients from 9 months of age (NHLBI guideline; WHO recommendation). Starting dose 15–20 mg/kg/day; titrate to 30–35 mg/kg/day or maximum tolerated dose. Mechanism: induces fetal haemoglobin (HbF) — γ-chains cannot enter HbS polymer. Reduces vaso-occlusive crises, ACS, transfusion need, hospitalisation, and mortality.

L-glutamine (Endari): FDA-approved 2017 for SCD. Reduces vaso-occlusive crisis frequency. Mechanism: improves NAD redox status, reduces oxidative stress in sickled cells.

Crizanlizumab (Adakveo): Anti-P-selectin monoclonal antibody. Reduces vaso-occlusive crisis frequency by blocking sickled cell adhesion to endothelium. IV monthly.

Voxelotor — WITHDRAWN. Pfizer voluntarily withdrew voxelotor worldwide in September 2024 after post-marketing data showed an imbalance of vaso-occlusive crises and fatal events. The FDA confirmed the withdrawal; the EMA suspended marketing authorisation. Voxelotor should not be selected on current USMLE.

Curative therapy — HSCT: Allogeneic HSCT from matched sibling donor; best outcomes in children before organ damage; matched unrelated donor and haploidentical protocols expanding access.

Curative therapy — gene therapy: Two FDA approvals in December 2023. Lovotibeglogene autotemcel (Lyfgenia) is a lentiviral vector adding a modified anti-sickling β-globin. Exagamglogene autotemcel (Casgevy) is a CRISPR-Cas9 edit of the BCL11A enhancer that reactivates fetal haemoglobin. Both require autologous HSC collection, ex vivo modification, and myeloablative conditioning. Sustained transfusion independence and crisis reduction in clinical trials.

10.9 Other Haemoglobinopathies

HbC, HbE, and unstable haemoglobins

Variant	Mutation	Phenotype	USMLE Anchor
HbC	β-globin codon 6: GAG → AAG (Glu → Lys)	HbCC: mild haemolytic anaemia, target cells (40–90%), splenomegaly. Haemoglobin C crystals visible in RBCs (rod-shaped or hexagonal). HbAC: silent.	African ancestry. Mild compared to HbSS.
HbE	β-globin codon 26: GAG → AAG (Glu → Lys); also activates cryptic splice site → behaves like mild β^+-thalassaemia	HbEE: mild microcytic anaemia, no severe haemolysis. HbE/β^0-thal: most severe — clinically equivalent to β-thal major.	Southeast Asian ancestry (Thailand, Cambodia, Northeast India, Bangladesh). HbE/β-thal is the most common severe thalassaemia worldwide.
Unstable haemoglobins (HbKöln, HbZürich)	Mutations in hydrophobic core or haem pocket destabilise tetramer	Chronic congenital non-spherocytic haemolytic anaemia. Heinz bodies on supravital stain. Episodic exacerbations with oxidant stress.	Heat instability test (lyse at 50 °C, normal lyse at 49 °C). Isopropanol precipitation test (unstable Hb precipitates in 25% isopropanol).

Acquired haemoglobin disorders

Disorder	Mechanism	Clinical Clue	Treatment
Methaemoglobinaemia	Iron oxidised from Fe^{2+} to Fe^{3+} → cannot bind O_2. Acquired: dapsone, nitrites, benzocaine (topical anaesthetic —	**Cyanosis with NORMAL pO_2.** Chocolate-brown blood. Pulse oximetry reads ~85% regardless of true	Methylene blue 1–2 mg/kg IV (mechanism: provides electrons via NADPH-

Disorder	Mechanism	Clinical Clue	Treatment
	neonates and dental procedures), aniline dyes, well-water nitrates (infants <6 mo). Congenital: cyt b5 reductase deficiency.	saturation — UNRELIABLE. Co-oximetry required.	dependent reduction). NOT IN G6PD DEFICIENCY (NADPH-dependent step is the deficiency; methylene blue may worsen oxidative haemolysis). Alternative: ascorbic acid orally; severe → exchange transfusion or hyperbaric O_2.
Carbon monoxide poisoning	CO binds Hb 200× more avidly than O_2 → reduces O_2-carrying capacity AND left-shifts O_2 dissociation curve (impaired tissue release)	**Pulse oximetry FALSELY NORMAL — CO-Hb absorbs light similarly to O_2-Hb.** Headache, dizziness, confusion, syncope, coma. Cherry-red lips/skin (rare and late finding). Sources: smoke inhalation, faulty heating, indoor combustion in poorly ventilated spaces.	100% oxygen via non-rebreather (reduces CO half-life from ~5 hours to ~60–90 minutes). Hyperbaric oxygen for severe (loss of consciousness, focal neurologic deficits, pregnancy, age <1 year, persistent symptoms after 100% O_2).

10.10 Warm Autoimmune Haemolytic Anaemia

Warm AIHA is the most common form of autoimmune haemolytic anaemia. IgG autoantibodies bind red cell surface antigens at 37 °C — typically directed against broad Rh-related determinants rather than a single antigen. IgG-coated cells are recognised by Fcγ receptors on splenic macrophages, which remove the antibody along with a portion of membrane in each pass — progressive loss of surface area produces spherocytes that are eventually phagocytosed entirely. The picture is therefore predominantly EXTRAVASCULAR haemolysis. IgG subclasses that fix complement (IgG1, IgG3) add an intravascular component.

Causes

Category	Examples	Comment
Idiopathic (primary)	—	~50% of warm AIHA cases.

Category	Examples	Comment
Lymphoproliferative	Chronic lymphocytic leukaemia (CLL), non-Hodgkin lymphoma (DLBCL, follicular)	**CLL is the most common haematologic association.** Always evaluate for underlying B-cell malignancy in adult-onset warm AIHA. Lymph node exam, peripheral smear for lymphocytosis, flow cytometry if suspicion.
Autoimmune	SLE, rheumatoid arthritis, autoimmune hepatitis	SLE is a classic association — DAT may be positive even without overt haemolysis.
Drug-induced (autoantibody type)	Methyldopa, levodopa, fludarabine, cladribine, penicillin (high-dose IV — hapten type)	Methyldopa causes true autoantibody — clinically and serologically identical to idiopathic warm AIHA. Continues for weeks after drug stopped.
Infection	Mycoplasma (cold-type more common), EBV, viral hepatitis	Less common than cold-type post-infectious AIHA.
Common variable immunodeficiency (CVID)	Recurrent infections, low immunoglobulins, AIHA, ITP	Evans syndrome (combined AIHA + ITP) often seen in CVID.

Treatment

STEP 2 BRIDGE — Warm AIHA — first-, second-, third-line

First-line: Prednisone 1 mg/kg/day (or equivalent IV methylprednisolone) for severe presentation. Response in 70–80%; taper over weeks–months once Hb stabilises.

Second-line: Rituximab (anti-CD20, depletes antibody-producing B cells) — increasingly used early in management. Splenectomy — historically second-line; less commonly used now given rituximab availability.

Refractory: Cyclosporine, mycophenolate mofetil, azathioprine, IVIG (modest benefit). Fostamatinib (oral SYK inhibitor) is FDA-approved for chronic ITP and has been studied off-label in refractory warm AIHA, though the Phase 3 FORWARD trial (2022) did not meet its primary endpoint of durable haemoglobin response in the overall study population.

Transfusion: Do NOT withhold transfusion in life-threatening anaemia. Crossmatch will show pan-reactivity (the autoantibody reacts with all donor cells). Use "least incompatible" units. Communicate clearly with the blood bank.

Folate: 1 mg daily (chronic haemolysis depletes folate). Monitor for thrombosis — AIHA carries elevated VTE risk.

10.11 Cold AIHA and Paroxysmal Cold Haemoglobinuria

Cold-reactive immune haemolysis comprises two distinct entities with different antibodies, mechanisms, and treatments. Both share a positive DAT for C3d only — the antibody dissociates from red cells during the 37 °C wash step of the antiglobulin test, leaving only complement on the surface.

Feature	Cold Agglutinin Disease (CAD)	Paroxysmal Cold Haemoglobinuria (PCH)
Antibody class	IgM (monoclonal in primary CAD; polyclonal in post-infectious)	IgG biphasic — Donath–Landsteiner antibody
Thermal optimum	0–4 °C; agglutinates up to 30 °C in significant disease	Binds at 0–15 °C; activates complement at 37 °C
DAT	C3d ONLY (IgM washes off at 37 °C)	C3d (after complement activation by biphasic IgG)
Antigen specificity	Anti-I (adult I antigen) — primary CAD, Mycoplasma pneumoniae. Anti-i (fetal i antigen) — EBV / infectious mononucleosis.	Anti-P (P antigen / globoside; GLOB blood group system)
Haemolysis site	Mostly extravascular (C3b-coated cells removed by hepatic Kupffer cells); some intravascular at high titers	**INTRAVASCULAR — brisk, with haemoglobinuria.** Donath-Landsteiner antibody completes complement to MAC at body temperature.
Clinical	Acrocyanosis on cold exposure (cold-induced agglutination in peripheral circulation); chronic mild anaemia; cold-induced exacerbations	Acute haemoglobinuria after cold exposure in children post-viral illness (adenovirus, measles, varicella, mumps, IM). Historical: late congenital syphilis (now rare).
Diagnostic test	Cold agglutinin titer (>1:1000 at 4 °C; thermal amplitude — highest temperature at which agglutination still occurs — predicts severity better than titer)	Donath–Landsteiner test: patient serum + O-group RBCs incubated at 4 °C for 30 min then 37 °C for 60 min; haemolysis confirms biphasic IgG anti-P.
Treatment	Cold avoidance (mainstay). Rituximab (depletes monoclonal B cells in primary CAD). Sutimlimab (anti-C1s; FDA-approved 2022 for primary CAD). Steroids and splenectomy generally NOT effective.	Self-limited typically (post-viral). Cold avoidance during episode. Supportive transfusion. Rare complication of viral illness.

HIGH-YIELD PEARL — Cold AIHA exam pitfall — "DAT IgG-negative, C3d-positive" is positive for cold AIHA

A common exam trap: the monospecific DAT in cold agglutinin disease reads "IgG negative, C3d positive." Students sometimes conclude that no antibody is present. This is wrong — the IgM autoantibody IS present in vivo, but it dissociates from the red cell during the 37 °C wash step of the test (IgM binding is temperature-dependent and reversible). The complement fragment C3d, by contrast, remains covalently bound. The DAT result is therefore an artifact of the assay's wash conditions; the disease is real. The correct interpretation: positive DAT for C3d only with a clinical picture of cold-induced agglutination, haemolysis, and a Mycoplasma- or EBV-positive history (or a monoclonal IgM gammopathy in primary CAD) confirms cold agglutinin disease.

Mycoplasma association: M. pneumoniae infection produces polyclonal anti-I cold agglutinins in up to 60% of patients. Clinically significant haemolysis is uncommon but classic on USMLE — the stem describes a patient with atypical pneumonia developing dark urine and haemoglobinuria after cold exposure.

10.12 Drug-Induced Immune Haemolytic Anaemia

Drug-induced immune haemolytic anaemia (DIIHA) operates by three distinct mechanisms. Recognising the mechanism from the drug name is testable on USMLE.

Mechanism	Prototype Drug(s)	Process	DAT Pattern	Resolution
Hapten / drug adsorption	High-dose IV penicillin (rare with current dosing); cefotetan	Drug binds covalently to RBC membrane; antibodies form against drug–membrane complex; IgG-coated cells cleared by spleen.	IgG positive; C3d variable	Resolves rapidly after drug stopped (drug clears).
Immune complex ("innocent bystander")	Quinidine, quinine; ceftriaxone (especially in children)	Drug–antibody immune complexes deposit on RBCs and activate complement; cells lysed as bystanders.	**C3d predominantly.** Same mechanism causes thrombocytopenia ("quinidine thrombocytopenia" — heparin-induced thrombocytopenia is a separate entity).	Resolves rapidly after drug stopped.

Mechanism	Prototype Drug(s)	Process	DAT Pattern	Resolution
Autoantibody	Methyldopa, levodopa, fludarabine, cladribine, β-lactams (penicillin G high-dose IV)	**Drug induces formation of true RBC autoantibodies — clinically and serologically identical to idiopathic warm AIHA.** DAT remains positive for weeks–months after drug stopped because antibodies persist.	IgG positive (warm AIHA pattern)	Continues after drug stopped (weeks). Steroids may be needed for clinically significant haemolysis. Fludarabine -induced AIHA can be severe and persistent — often a CLL patient who develops AIHA in the setting of fludarabine therapy.

10.13 Paroxysmal Nocturnal Haemoglobinuria

PNH is a rare clonal haematopoietic stem cell disorder in which the affected cells lack GPI-anchored proteins on their surface. The acquired somatic mutation in the X-linked PIGA gene disrupts the first enzyme of glycosylphosphatidylinositol (GPI) anchor biosynthesis, producing cells that cannot attach more than 20 GPI-linked proteins to their plasma membrane. Two of those missing proteins — CD55 and CD59 — are the red cell's primary defences against autologous complement. CD55 (decay accelerating factor) accelerates decay of C3 and C5 convertases on the RBC surface; CD59 (membrane inhibitor of reactive lysis, also called protectin) blocks insertion of the membrane attack complex (C5b-9). In their absence, complement spontaneously assembles on PNH red cells, producing CHRONIC INTRAVASCULAR haemolysis — the defining feature of the disease. The DAT is NEGATIVE (no antibody is involved; the mechanism is uncontrolled autologous complement).

Clinical triad and unusual features

The classic triad is (1) Coombs-negative intravascular haemolytic anaemia, (2) venous thrombosis at unusual sites, and (3) cytopenias from underlying marrow failure or aplastic anaemia. The thromboses are characteristic and high-yield: hepatic veins (Budd–Chiari syndrome), portal and mesenteric veins, cerebral venous sinuses, and dermal veins (Mondor disease). Up to 50% of patients with aplastic anaemia harbour a PNH clone (small or large) — the clones expand because GPI-deficient HSCs are relatively resistant to immune-mediated destruction in aplastic anaemia, an immune-escape phenomenon. Smooth muscle dystonia from nitric oxide scavenging by free plasma haemoglobin produces oesophageal spasm, abdominal pain, erectile dysfunction, and pulmonary hypertension — all relieved by complement inhibition. Morning haemoglobinuria (the historical name of the disease) occurs in only a minority of patients and is not required for diagnosis.

Diagnosis

Test	Principle	Interpretation	Comment
FLAER flow cytometry	Fluorescent aerolysin binds GPI anchors directly on granulocytes and monocytes	FLAER-negative cells = GPI-deficient (PNH clone)	**GOLD STANDARD.** Reports clone size as % of granulocytes. Highly sensitive (clones ≥0.01% detectable). Granulocytes/monocytes preferred over RBCs because they are not selectively lysed.
CD55 + CD59 flow on RBCs	Direct measurement of GPI-anchored proteins	Type III cells (no CD55/CD59), Type II (partial), Type I (normal)	Supplementary. RBC clone size underestimates true clone because complement has selectively lysed the most-deficient cells.
CD24 (granulocytes) + CD14 (monocytes)	Alternative GPI markers on white cells	Used in international consensus PNH testing protocol	Combined with FLAER; assesses both white cell populations per 2009 international guidelines.
Ham acid serum test (historical)	Complement-mediated lysis of PNH cells in acidified normal serum	Positive in PNH; negative in normal	Replaced by FLAER. Historical answer choice on older USMLE materials; current answer is FLAER.

Treatment — complement inhibition revolution

STEP 2 BRIDGE — PNH treatment — anti-C5, anti-C3, anti-Factor B

Eculizumab (anti-C5): First in class. Blocks C5 cleavage → prevents both C5a (proinflammatory) and C5b-9 (MAC). Dramatically reduces intravascular haemolysis and thrombosis; transformed PNH from a fatal disease to a manageable chronic illness. IV every 2 weeks.

Ravulizumab: Long-acting anti-C5; same efficacy as eculizumab; IV every 8 weeks. Quality-of-life advantage.

Pegcetacoplan (anti-C3): FDA-approved 2021. Inhibits proximal complement at C3 — addresses C3-mediated extravascular haemolysis that develops in ~10–30% of patients on terminal C5 inhibitors (residual haemolysis after C5 blockade). Subcutaneous twice weekly.

Iptacopan (anti-Factor B, oral): FDA-approved December 2023. First oral monotherapy for PNH. Inhibits the alternative pathway at Factor B. Alternative to anti-C5/C3 in adults; may reduce treatment burden.

MANDATORY meningococcal vaccination: All terminal complement inhibitors (eculizumab, ravulizumab) block MAC formation, eliminating the host's primary defence against Neisseria meningitidis. Meningococcal sepsis carries dramatically elevated risk on these agents — vaccination (ACWY conjugate + serogroup B) is required ≥2 weeks before starting therapy. Penicillin prophylaxis is added in some protocols. Pegcetacoplan and iptacopan require pneumococcal vaccination as well (proximal pathway inhibition affects pneumococcal defence).

HSCT: Only curative treatment. Reserved for severe marrow failure or refractory disease; not first-line because complement inhibition has dramatically improved survival.

HIGH-YIELD PEARL — PNH clone in aplastic anaemia — what it means

Up to 50% of aplastic anaemia patients have a detectable PNH clone (any size) on FLAER flow cytometry. The presence of a clone in aplastic anaemia (1) supports an autoimmune pathogenesis — GPI-deficient stem cells are relatively resistant to the T-cell-mediated immune attack that destroys normal HSCs, and the resistant clone expands; (2) predicts response to immunosuppressive therapy (ATG + cyclosporine) — clone-positive aplastic anaemia patients respond better than clone-negative; (3) requires monitoring for clinical PNH evolution as the clone enlarges. A clone of ≥1% of granulocytes with clinical features (intravascular haemolysis, thrombosis, marrow failure) defines classical PNH; smaller clones without symptoms are subclinical and managed expectantly with serial FLAER monitoring.

10.14 Microangiopathic Haemolytic Anaemia — TTP, HUS, DIC, HELLP

Microangiopathic haemolytic anaemia (MAHA) is defined by mechanical fragmentation of red cells as they are sheared through damaged or partially occluded microvasculature. The hallmark on smear is the schistocyte — helmet-shaped, triangular, or comma-shaped fragment cells. The MAHA triad is schistocytes plus thrombocytopenia plus DAT-negative haemolysis; once recognised, the clinical question is which thrombotic microangiopathy (TMA) underlies it. ADAMTS13 activity is the discriminator: less than 10% defines TTP; normal activity redirects to HUS, DIC, HELLP, malignant hypertension, mechanical valve haemolysis, or transplant-associated TMA.

Schistocyte counting

Per ICSH 2012 guidelines, a schistocyte must show one of: (1) two pointed ends (helmet, triangular), (2) dense and irregular staining with at least one pointed end, or (3) a straight or concave "cut" border. The clinical threshold is ≥1% schistocytes on manual count of 1000 red cells. Up to 0.5% may be seen in normal blood, burns, cardiac surgery, or severe infection. Automated analyzer schistocyte flags require manual confirmation.

Comparing the four major TMAs

Feature	TTP	STEC-HUS	Atypical HUS (aHUS)	DIC	HELLP
Pathogenesis	Severe ADAMTS13 deficiency (acquired IgG inhibitor in >95%; rare hereditary Upshaw–Schulman). Ultra-large vWF multimers persist → platelet-rich microthrombi.	Shiga toxin from E. coli O157:H7 → endothelial Gb3 receptor → renal endothelial apoptosis	Alternative complement pathway dysregulation (Factor H, I, MCP, B, C3 mutations)	Systemic activation of coagulation by an underlying trigger (sepsis, malignancy, obstetric)	Pre-eclampsia spectrum; placental endothelial injury
ADAMTS13	<10% (severely deficient)	Normal	Normal (>10%)	Normal	Normal
Renal	Mild-moderate (Cr <3× normal)	SEVERE (oliguria, dialysis common)	SEVERE; chronic risk	Variable	Variable
Neurologic	COMMON (50–80%): confusion, seizures, focal deficits	Uncommon	Variable	Variable	Headache
Prodrome	None typical	Bloody diarrhoea 5–10 d prior	None	Underlying illness (sepsis, cancer)	Pregnancy / postpartum
Coagulation	Normal PT/APTT/fibrinogen	Normal	Normal	Prolonged PT/APTT, low fibrinogen, very high D-dimer	Mildly abnormal
Platelet	Often <20	Often <30	$<30 \times 10^9$/L	Variable	Often <100

Feature	TTP	STEC-HUS	Atypical HUS (aHUS)	DIC	HELLP
count	×10^9/L	×10^9/L			×10^9/L, falling rapidly
Treatment	**TPE IMMEDIATELY on suspicion.** Rituximab for refractory; caplacizumab (anti-vWF) reduces time to platelet recovery. NO platelet transfusions.	Supportive; dialysis if needed. NO antibiotics (increase toxin release). Eculizumab in severe/atypical cases.	Eculizumab (anti-C5) — dramatically effective. Meningococcal vaccination required.	Address trigger; supportive (FFP, cryoprecipitate, platelets, packed RBCs).	Delivery is definitive (or delivery of placenta if postpartum).

HIGH-YIELD PEARL — TTP — start TPE before the ADAMTS13 result returns

Rule: Therapeutic plasma exchange (TPE) is started IMMEDIATELY on clinical suspicion of TTP — do NOT wait for the ADAMTS13 result, which may take 24–72 hours to return. Untreated TTP carries 90% mortality; promptly treated TTP, 10–20%.

Mechanism: TPE removes the ADAMTS13 inhibitor (autoantibody) AND replaces functional ADAMTS13 from donor plasma. If TPE is not immediately available, FFP infusion is a temporising measure (provides ADAMTS13 but does not remove inhibitor).

Adjuncts: Rituximab for refractory or relapsing acquired TTP. Caplacizumab (anti-vWF nanobody) blocks ULvWF binding to platelets and significantly reduces time to platelet normalisation and organ damage; FDA-approved 2019.

DO NOT transfuse platelets in TTP unless life-threatening haemorrhage. Platelet transfusion in TTP can worsen microvascular thrombosis ("fuel to the fire") and accelerate organ injury.

PLASMIC score: A clinical scoring system (platelets, haemolysis markers, MCV, INR, creatinine, cancer history, transplant history) that predicts likelihood of severe ADAMTS13 deficiency. Score ≥6 → high probability of TTP → start TPE without waiting for ADAMTS13.

HIGH-YIELD PEARL — STEC-HUS — no antibiotics
Shiga toxin-producing E. coli (STEC, most commonly O157:H7) causes typical HUS in children 1–5 years old, classically following bloody diarrhoea after exposure to undercooked ground beef, unpasteurised dairy, contaminated water, or petting zoo. Antibiotic treatment of STEC infection INCREASES Shiga toxin release (bacterial lysis releases stored toxin) and worsens HUS — a classic USMLE point. Supportive care: hydration, transfusion if severe, dialysis as needed. Eculizumab is reserved for severe atypical cases or when complement-mediated mechanisms are suspected.

10.15 Buzzwords and Visual Cues

Single-phrase USMLE cues for haemolytic anaemias and haemoglobinopathies. Each maps to one or two diagnoses. The cue often arrives at the answer faster than working through the differential.

Buzzword / Visual Cue	Most Likely Diagnosis
Spherocytes + DAT NEGATIVE + family history	Hereditary spherocytosis
Spherocytes + DAT POSITIVE	Warm AIHA
MCHC > 36 g/dL	Hereditary spherocytosis
Bite cells (degmacytes) and blister cells on smear	G6PD deficiency (acute oxidant haemolysis)
Heinz bodies on supravital stain (NMB or crystal violet)	G6PD deficiency or unstable haemoglobin
Echinocytes (uniform spiculated cells)	Pyruvate kinase deficiency
Sickle cells (drepanocytes) on smear	Sickle cell disease (HbSS, HbSC, HbS/β^0-thal)
African American adolescent with severe bone/back pain	SCD vaso-occlusive crisis
African American with new pulmonary infiltrate + fever + hypoxia	SCD acute chest syndrome
Sudden Hb drop with reticulocytes near zero in chronic haemolytic anaemia	Aplastic crisis (parvovirus B19)
Sudden splenomegaly + Hb drop + shock in young SCD child	Splenic sequestration crisis
Target cells with HbC crystals (rod-shaped)	HbCC disease
HbE common in Northeast India / Thailand / Cambodia	HbE / HbE-β-thalassaemia

Buzzword / Visual Cue	Most Likely Diagnosis
Cyanosis with normal pO_2; chocolate-brown blood; SpO_2 stuck at ~85%	Methaemoglobinaemia
Pulse oximetry FALSELY normal in suspected hypoxia (smoke inhalation)	Carbon monoxide poisoning
DAT positive for IgG only	Warm AIHA (or methyldopa-type DIIHA)
DAT positive for C3d only	Cold agglutinin disease (or PCH after lysis)
DAT NEGATIVE + intravascular haemolysis + venous thrombosis at unusual sites	Paroxysmal nocturnal haemoglobinuria (PNH)
Mycoplasma pneumonia + cold-induced haemolysis	Cold agglutinin disease (anti-I)
EBV / infectious mononucleosis + cold haemolysis	Cold agglutinin disease (anti-i)
Children + post-viral + dark urine + Donath–Landsteiner positive	Paroxysmal cold haemoglobinuria (PCH)
Methyldopa + AIHA + DAT-positive after weeks	Drug-induced AIHA — autoantibody type
High-dose IV penicillin + DAT-positive haemolysis	Drug-induced AIHA — hapten type
Quinidine + cytopenia (haemolysis or thrombocytopenia)	Drug-induced — immune complex (innocent bystander)
Schistocytes + thrombocytopenia + DAT-negative	MAHA — pursue ADAMTS13
Schistocytes + thrombocytopenia + neuro signs + ADAMTS13 <10%	TTP — start TPE immediately
Bloody diarrhoea + AKI + schistocytes in child	STEC-HUS
Schistocytes + DIC laboratory profile (low fibrinogen, high D-dimer)	DIC
Pregnant 3rd trimester + haemolysis + LFTs up + low platelets	HELLP syndrome
FLAER negative cells on flow cytometry	PNH
Eculizumab + meningococcal vaccination required	PNH or atypical HUS

Buzzword / Visual Cue	Most Likely Diagnosis
Donath–Landsteiner test (4 °C bind, 37 °C lyse)	PCH (anti-P specificity)

10.16 USMLE Vignettes

Ten vignettes covering the chapter's high-yield diagnoses. Read each stem before the answer.

VIGNETTE 1

Stem. A 16-year-old African American boy presents to the ED with 12 hours of severe pain in his lower back and bilateral thighs. He has had similar episodes before and takes hydroxyurea. Examination: tender extremities, no neurologic deficit, SpO_2 98% on room air. Hb 7.8 g/dL (baseline 8 g/dL), MCV 88 fL, reticulocytes 12%. Smear: sickle cells, target cells, Howell–Jolly bodies (functional asplenia).

VIGNETTE 2

Stem. A 24-year-old African American woman with HbSS presents with 24 hours of fever, pleuritic chest pain, and progressive dyspnea. Examination: temperature 38.7 °C, RR 28, SpO_2 86% on room air, crackles in the right lower lobe. Hb 6.4 g/dL (baseline 8), reticulocytes 14%. CXR shows a new right lower lobe infiltrate.

VIGNETTE 3

Stem. A 28-year-old man of Mediterranean descent presents with 2 days of fatigue, jaundice, and dark urine. He recently started TMP-SMX for a urinary tract infection. Examination: scleral icterus, mild splenomegaly. Hb 7.8 g/dL, reticulocytes 12%, indirect bilirubin 4.5 mg/dL, LDH markedly elevated, haptoglobin <10 mg/dL, urine dipstick positive for blood with no RBCs on microscopy (haemoglobinuria). Smear: bite cells and blister cells. DAT negative.

VIGNETTE 4

Stem. An 18-year-old woman is evaluated for chronic mild jaundice and splenomegaly. Her father had splenectomy as a child for similar symptoms. Hb 11.8 g/dL, MCV 84 fL, MCHC 38 g/dL, reticulocytes 8%, indirect bilirubin 2.4 mg/dL, LDH mildly elevated. Smear: numerous spherocytes. DAT NEGATIVE.

VIGNETTE 5

Stem. A 35-year-old man presents with 3 months of fatigue, episodic dark morning urine, and progressive abdominal pain over the last 2 weeks. Hb 7.6 g/dL, MCV 102 fL, reticulocytes 14%, LDH 1450 U/L (markedly elevated), haptoglobin undetectable. DAT NEGATIVE. Imaging: hepatic vein thrombosis (Budd–Chiari syndrome).

VIGNETTE 6

Stem. A 68-year-old woman with a 4-year history of CLL presents with 1 week of fatigue and jaundice. Examination: pallor, scleral icterus, cervical lymphadenopathy. Hb 6.9 g/dL, MCV 102 fL, reticulocytes 18%, indirect bilirubin 3.2 mg/dL, LDH elevated, haptoglobin undetectable. Smear: spherocytes and polychromasia. DAT POSITIVE for IgG.

VIGNETTE 7

Stem. A 32-year-old man presents with 2 weeks of cough and 3 days of dark urine and bluish discolouration of his fingertips after going outside in cold weather. He was recently treated for pneumonia. Examination: acrocyanosis of fingertips, no significant pallor. Hb 9.6 g/dL, reticulocytes 8%, LDH elevated, haptoglobin low. DAT POSITIVE for C3d only; IgG negative. Cold agglutinin titer 1:2048 at 4 °C with anti-I specificity. Mycoplasma pneumoniae IgM positive.

VIGNETTE 8

Stem. A 36-year-old previously healthy woman presents with 2 days of confusion and bruising. Examination: scattered petechiae and ecchymoses, no focal neurologic deficit, no hepatosplenomegaly. Hb 8.4 g/dL, platelets 14 $\times 10^9$/L, MCV 98 fL, reticulocytes 9%, LDH 1500 U/L, indirect bilirubin elevated, haptoglobin undetectable, creatinine 1.4 mg/dL. PT/APTT/fibrinogen normal. Smear: numerous schistocytes (3–5 per HPF). DAT negative.

VIGNETTE 9

Stem. A 4-year-old boy is brought to the ED with 5 days of bloody diarrhoea after attending a family barbecue. Today he has decreased urine output and pallor. Examination: lethargic, mildly dehydrated, no rash. Hb 7.8 g/dL, platelets 38 $\times 10^9$/L, creatinine 4.6 mg/dL (was normal 1 month ago), LDH elevated, schistocytes on smear. Stool culture grows E. coli O157:H7. ADAMTS13 activity normal.

VIGNETTE 10

Stem. A 26-year-old man presents with 6 months of intermittent jaundice, dark urine on rising, and recurrent abdominal pain. Examination: mild scleral icterus, normal abdomen. Hb 9.4 g/dL, MCV 100 fL, reticulocytes 12%, LDH 980 U/L, haptoglobin undetectable, indirect bilirubin 2.8 mg/dL. DAT NEGATIVE. Iron studies, B12, folate normal. Hb electrophoresis normal.

10.17 Closing Discriminators

Five closing distinctions worth carrying into the exam. Each compresses a recurring USMLE comparison.

HIGH-YIELD PEARL — Discriminator 1 — Hereditary spherocytosis vs warm AIHA (both have spherocytes)

DAT: NEGATIVE in HS; POSITIVE (IgG ± C3d) in warm AIHA. Single most useful test.

Family history: Often positive in HS (autosomal dominant in 75%); usually absent in AIHA.

MCHC: >36 g/dL characteristic of HS; usually normal in AIHA.

Onset: HS presents in childhood/early adulthood; AIHA can occur at any age, with adult onset more common.

HIGH-YIELD PEARL — Discriminator 2 — TTP vs HUS vs DIC

ADAMTS13: <10% defines TTP. Normal in HUS, DIC, HELLP.

Coagulation: Normal in TTP and HUS. Severely abnormal in DIC (long PT/APTT, low fibrinogen, very high D-dimer).

Renal: Mild in TTP. Severe in HUS (oliguria, dialysis). Variable in DIC.

Prodrome: Bloody diarrhoea points to STEC-HUS. Sepsis/cancer/obstetric trigger points to DIC. Pregnancy points to HELLP. Idiopathic/autoimmune-associated points to TTP.

HIGH-YIELD PEARL — Discriminator 3 — Aplastic vs sequestration crisis in SCD

Reticulocyte count: NEAR ZERO in aplastic crisis (parvovirus B19 → erythroid progenitor infection → no production). RAISED in sequestration crisis (marrow responds normally; cells are pooled in spleen).

Splenomegaly: Often dramatically enlarged spleen in sequestration; spleen size unchanged or small in aplastic crisis.

Treatment: Aplastic — transfusion support; isolate from pregnant healthcare workers; self-limited 7–10 days. Sequestration — emergency volume resuscitation + transfusion; recurrent → splenectomy.

HIGH-YIELD PEARL — Discriminator 4 — G6PD vs PK deficiency

Inheritance: G6PD = X-linked recessive. PK = autosomal recessive.

Haemolysis pattern: G6PD = episodic, triggered (oxidant drugs, infections, fava beans). PK = chronic, no trigger needed.

Smear: G6PD acute crisis — bite cells, blister cells, Heinz bodies on supravital stain. PK — echinocytes (uniform spiculated cells).

Splenectomy response: Not effective in G6PD. PARTIALLY effective in PK; paradoxical retic rise post-op. Mitapivat is a new oral PK activator (FDA-approved 2022).

IMG-TRAP — IMG-Trap recap — sickle cell demographics

The trap (#9): Black or African American patient with severe pain, anaemia, stroke, or unexplained hypoxia → SCD until proved otherwise. IMG candidates trained in non-tribal Indian regions see SCD infrequently and may underweight the demographic signal.

The rule: USMLE provides demographic information deliberately. African American + severe bone/back pain = vaso-occlusive crisis. African American + new pulmonary infiltrate + fever = ACS. African American child + sudden splenomegaly + Hb drop = sequestration. Universal newborn screening means by adulthood the diagnosis is established.

Why: US prevalence ~1 in 365 Black births; high enough that any unexplained anaemia, pain, or stroke in a Black US patient must include SCD at the top of the differential. Indian SCD is concentrated in tribal populations (Chhattisgarh, Odisha, Madhya Pradesh, Maharashtra, Gujarat) but uncommon elsewhere — different epidemiology, different prior.

10.18 Quick Recall — One-Page Compression

QUICK RECALL — ONE-PAGE COMPRESSION

1. The haemolysis triad. LDH up + indirect bilirubin up + haptoglobin down + reticulocytes up confirms haemolysis. Add haemoglobinuria + Rous test positive for chronic intravascular.

2. DAT branches the workup. Positive → immune (warm AIHA, cold AIHA, PCH, DIIHA). Negative → membrane / enzyme / haemoglobinopathy / mechanical / PNH.

3. HS. MCHC >36 g/dL flag. Spherocytes + DAT-negative. EMA binding test preferred over osmotic fragility. Treat with splenectomy if symptomatic; vaccinate first.

4. G6PD. X-linked. Bite cells + blister cells + Heinz bodies on supravital stain during acute haemolysis. NEVER test G6PD assay during crisis — false-normal due to reticulocyte enrichment. Test ≥3 months later.

5. G6PD + methaemoglobinaemia. Methylene blue is INEFFECTIVE in G6PD deficiency (NADPH-dependent step is the deficiency). Use ascorbic acid; severe → exchange transfusion.

6. PK deficiency. Autosomal recessive; chronic (not episodic) haemolysis; echinocytes; ATP depletion; paradoxical retic rise after splenectomy. Mitapivat oral PK activator (FDA-approved 2022).

7. SCD mutation. β-globin codon 6 GAG→GTG; Glu→Val. Hydrophobic valine in deoxygenated R→T transition fits hydrophobic pocket on adjacent HbS → polymer fibres → sickling.

8. Sickling modifiers. HbF (most potent — γ-chain cannot enter polymer; hydroxyurea induces it), HbA in trait, α-thal co-inheritance (lower MCHC). Voxelotor WITHDRAWN September 2024.

9. SCD demographics (IMG-Trap #9). African American patient + severe pain/anaemia/stroke = SCD until proved otherwise. US prevalence ~1 in 365 Black births.

10. SCD crises. VOC (most common; pain), ACS (most common cause of death; new infiltrate + hypoxia), aplastic (parvovirus; retics zero), sequestration (sudden splenomegaly + retics raised), stroke (emergency exchange transfusion).

11. SCD chronic mgmt. Hydroxyurea from 9 months. Penicillin prophylaxis through age 5. Pneumococcal/Hib/meningococcal vaccinations. Gene therapy approved Dec 2023 (Lyfgenia, Casgevy).

12. Methaemoglobinaemia. Cyanosis with normal pO_2; chocolate brown blood; SpO_2 stuck ~85%; co-oximetry needed. Treat with methylene blue (NOT in G6PD).

13. CO poisoning. Pulse ox FALSELY normal (CO-Hb mimics O_2-Hb). Treat with 100% O_2; hyperbaric for severe.

14. Warm AIHA. IgG. CLL most common cause. Spherocytes + DAT-positive. Steroids first; rituximab second-line; cyclosporine, MMF, or IVIG for refractory. No drug is FDA-approved specifically for warm AIHA.

15. Cold AIHA. IgM, anti-I (Mycoplasma) or anti-i (EBV). DAT C3d-only (IgM washes off at 37 °C). Cold avoidance + rituximab + sutimlimab (FDA 2022) for primary CAD.

16. PCH. Donath–Landsteiner antibody (biphasic IgG anti-P). Children post-viral. Diagnose by D-L test (4 °C bind + 37 °C lyse).

17. DIIHA mechanisms. Hapten (high-dose IV penicillin); immune complex (quinidine — "innocent bystander"); autoantibody (methyldopa, fludarabine — DAT remains positive after drug stopped).

18. PNH. PIGA somatic mutation; absent GPI anchor; absent CD55 + CD59; chronic intravascular haemolysis + venous thrombosis at unusual sites + cytopenias. DAT NEGATIVE. FLAER gold standard. Eculizumab + meningococcal vaccine.

19. MAHA. Schistocytes + thrombocytopenia + DAT-negative. ADAMTS13 is the discriminator: <10% = TTP; normal = HUS, DIC, HELLP.

20. TTP urgency. Start TPE IMMEDIATELY on suspicion — do not wait for ADAMTS13. Caplacizumab + rituximab adjuncts. NO platelet transfusions.

21. STEC-HUS. Bloody diarrhoea + AKI + schistocytes in child. Supportive care; NO antibiotics (increases toxin release). Eculizumab in severe.

End of Chapter 10. White cell disorders, leukocytosis, leukopenia, and bone marrow failure syndromes continue in Chapter 11.

Chapter 11 — White Cell Disorders and Reactive Conditions

Total WBC count alone is meaningless. The differential — which lineage is up or down — is the diagnostic branch point for every white cell abnormality.

11.1 Big Picture and Mechanism Hooks

BIG PICTURE

White cell disorders fall into two broad categories: quantitative (counts elevated or reduced) and qualitative (number normal but function defective). The quantitative axis splits further into leukocytosis (total WBC >11 × 10^9/L in adults) and leukopenia (total WBC <4 × 10^9/L), each with sub-categories defined by which lineage is affected. The single most important first step in evaluating any abnormal WBC is the differential count — total WBC without a differential is diagnostically meaningless. This chapter walks the lineage-based differential for leukocytosis, the severity-based approach to neutropenia, the bone marrow failure syndromes (aplastic anaemia, Fanconi anaemia), the reactive lymphadenopathy patterns, and the histiocytic disorders (LCH, HLH, Rosai–Dorfman) along with Castleman disease and Kikuchi–Fujimoto disease.

MECHANISM HOOK — Lineage as the branch point — five differentials, not one

Every leukocytosis collapses to the same first question: which cell type is elevated? The answer immediately narrows the differential to a manageable list. Neutrophilia points to bacterial infection, tissue necrosis, inflammation, corticosteroid effect, physiological stress, or — when extreme and unexplained — chronic myeloid leukaemia. Lymphocytosis points to viral infection (EBV, CMV, hepatitis), pertussis (often markedly elevated), or, in older adults with a monoclonal flow pattern, chronic lymphocytic leukaemia. Monocytosis points to chronic infections (tuberculosis, subacute bacterial endocarditis, brucellosis), inflammatory bowel disease, recovery from neutropenia, or chronic myelomonocytic leukaemia. Eosinophilia maps onto the NAACP framework — Neoplasm, Allergy, Adrenal insufficiency, Connective tissue disease, Parasites. Basophilia is unusual and, when persistent without identifiable cause, raises strong suspicion of chronic myeloid leukaemia (basophilia plus eosinophilia is a hallmark). The take-home is that the WBC differential is the fork in the road; once the elevated cell type is identified, the next test list essentially writes itself.

11.2 Approach to Leukocytosis

Leukocytosis is a total WBC count above 11 × 10^9/L in adults (higher cutoffs apply in neonates and infants — up to 30 × 10^9/L at birth, falling to adult values by adolescence). The first step is identifying the elevated lineage; the second is grading the magnitude and the morphology; the third is asking whether any feature suggests urgent exclusion of a clonal haematologic process.

Cell Type Elevated	Normal Count (×10⁹/L)	Definition of Excess	Common Causes	Causes Requiring Urgent Exclusion
Neutrophils	1.8–7.5	Neutrophilia: >7.5	Bacterial infection (most common); tissue necrosis; inflammation; corticosteroids; physiological (exercise, pregnancy); G-CSF therapy; CML	CML (BCR::ABL1 if WBC >30 with basophilia); leukemoid reaction; AML with maturation
Lymphocytes	1.0–4.0 (higher in children)	Lymphocytosis: >4.0 in adults	Viral infection (EBV, CMV, hepatitis); pertussis (very high counts); post-splenectomy	CLL (>5.0 × 10^9/L monoclonal B-cells on flow); ALL; mantle cell lymphoma; Sézary syndrome
Monocytes	0.2–1.0	Monocytosis: >1.0	Chronic infections (TB, SBE, brucellosis); inflammatory disorders (IBD, SLE, sarcoidosis); post-splenectomy recovery	CMML (monocytes ≥1.0 × 10^9/L and ≥10% of WBC for ≥3 months; check dysplasia and mutations); AML-M5
Eosinophils	0.05–0.5	Eosinophilia: >0.5; Hypereosinophilia: >1.5	Allergy/atopy; parasites; drugs; adrenal insufficiency; connective tissue disease (NAACP)	HES (>1.5 sustained ≥6 months + organ damage); CEL-NOS; FIP1L1-PDGFRA rearrangement (imatinib-responsive); AML-M4Eo; T-cell lymphoma–associated eosinophilia
Basophils	0.01–0.1	Basophilia: >0.1	CML (characteristic); allergy; hypothyroidism; polycythaemia vera	CML — persistent unexplained basophilia is highly suggestive; basophilia >20% suggests blast

Cell Type Elevated	Normal Count ($\times 10^9$/L)	Definition of Excess	Common Causes	Causes Requiring Urgent Exclusion
				phase; systemic mastocytosis (KIT D816V)

HIGH-YIELD PEARL — Leukocytosis without a differential is diagnostically meaningless

A WBC report of "22 × 10^9/L" tells the clinician almost nothing on its own. The same number means bacterial sepsis (predominantly neutrophils with toxic granulation, Döhle bodies, vacuoles, left shift), pertussis (marked lymphocytosis with normal lymphocyte morphology), CML (neutrophilia with full granulocytic spectrum from blasts to mature neutrophils plus basophilia and eosinophilia), or CLL (monoclonal mature lymphocytes with smudge cells), depending entirely on the differential and morphology. Always ask for the differential and the smear before interpreting an elevated WBC.

Paediatric variation: Normal WBC is higher in children. Lymphocyte predominance is normal until about age 4–6 (lymphocytes outnumber neutrophils — "lymphocyte cross-over"). Apparent "lymphocytosis" in a young child may be physiologic. Conversely, neutrophil predominance in a 1-year-old is abnormal and prompts evaluation.

11.3 Neutrophilia and Leukemoid Reaction vs CML

Neutrophilia is the most common form of leukocytosis. Mild-to-moderate neutrophilia (up to ~25 × 10^9/L) is almost always reactive: bacterial infection, tissue necrosis (myocardial infarction, pancreatitis, surgery), corticosteroid administration (demargination of the marginated pool), physiological stress (exercise, labour, seizures), or smoking. Marked neutrophilia (>50 × 10^9/L) raises the question of a leukemoid reaction or an underlying myeloproliferative neoplasm.

Leukemoid reaction

A leukemoid reaction is a reactive (non-clonal) leukocytosis with WBC count exceeding 50 × 10^9/L, morphologically resembling leukaemia. The most common cause is severe infection — particularly sepsis, pneumonia, or Clostridioides difficile colitis — followed by haemolytic anaemia and metastatic malignancy with marrow involvement. The peripheral blood shows a marked left shift (band forms, metamyelocytes, occasional myelocytes) but no blasts and no dysplasia. The neutrophils show toxic granulation, Döhle bodies, and cytoplasmic vacuolation — features of cytokine-driven activation, not malignancy. The classic discriminator from CML is the leukocyte alkaline phosphatase (LAP) score: markedly ELEVATED in leukemoid reaction; LOW or ZERO in CML.

HIGH-YIELD PEARL — Leukemoid reaction vs CML — three discriminators

Both: WBC >50 × 10^9/L; left shift; splenomegaly possible.

Leukemoid reaction: LAP score HIGH (markedly elevated, often >150); BCR::ABL1 NEGATIVE; basophilia and eosinophilia ABSENT; toxic granulation, Döhle bodies, vacuolation present; identifiable reactive cause (sepsis, severe infection, haemolysis, malignancy with marrow involvement, G-CSF therapy).

CML: LAP score LOW or ZERO (virtually diagnostic); BCR::ABL1 POSITIVE (t(9;22), Philadelphia chromosome); basophilia and eosinophilia CHARACTERISTIC (often >5%); splenomegaly often massive; no identifiable reactive cause; full granulocytic spectrum on smear (myeloblasts through mature neutrophils).

LAP score interpretation: Stain peripheral blood neutrophils with alkaline phosphatase; score 0–4 per cell × 100 cells. Normal: 20–100. CML: 0–10. Leukemoid reaction: >150. The LAP score has been largely replaced by BCR::ABL1 RT-PCR in modern practice but remains a high-yield USMLE concept.

11.4 Reactive Lymphocytosis — Infectious Mononucleosis and EBV

Reactive lymphocytosis is most often viral. The prototype is infectious mononucleosis (IM) caused by primary Epstein–Barr virus (EBV) infection — the classic teenage syndrome of fever, sore throat (exudative pharyngitis), generalised lymphadenopathy, splenomegaly, and fatigue.

MECHANISM HOOK — Atypical lymphocytes in IM are activated CD8 T-cells, NOT infected B-cells

EBV is transmitted through saliva ("the kissing disease") and infects B-lymphocytes by binding the CD21 receptor (complement receptor 2, CR2). Once inside the B-cell, EBV establishes latent infection and would, if unchecked, drive polyclonal B-cell proliferation. The host responds with a massive cytotoxic T-cell expansion: CD8+ T-cells recognise EBV antigens on infected B-cells and proliferate enormously to control the infection. These activated CD8 T-cells are what appear on the peripheral smear as "atypical lymphocytes" (Downey cells) — large, basophilic, cytoplasm-rich cells with irregular nuclear outlines and cytoplasm that appears indented or moulded around adjacent red cells. This is the testable point: the atypical lymphocytes are NOT the EBV-infected B-cells; they are the host immune response to those B-cells. Flow cytometry confirms it — the atypical lymphocytes are polyclonal CD3+ CD8+ T-cells, not monoclonal B-cells. Splenomegaly in IM reflects lymphoid hyperplasia of the same activated T-cells, and the splenic capsule becomes thinned and fragile — hence the four-to-six-week restriction on contact sports to avoid splenic rupture. Hepatomegaly with transaminase elevation is similarly common (IM-associated hepatitis). Most patients recover fully within a few weeks; a minority develop chronic active EBV. EBV is also the aetiologic agent of Burkitt lymphoma (endemic African form), nasopharyngeal carcinoma, primary CNS lymphoma in immunosuppressed patients, post-transplant lymphoproliferative disorder (PTLD), and a subset of classical Hodgkin lymphoma — chapters elsewhere in this volume cover those associations. The amoxicillin/ampicillin rash in IM deserves separate emphasis (see pearl below).

Clinical features and laboratory pattern

The classic clinical picture is a teenager or young adult with 1–2 weeks of fatigue and malaise, then high fever, severe exudative pharyngitis (often mistaken for streptococcal pharyngitis), tender posterior cervical lymphadenopathy, generalised lymphadenopathy, splenomegaly (up to 50% of patients), and hepatomegaly. The lymphadenopathy is typically symmetric and soft; the splenomegaly is mild to moderate. Rash is uncommon spontaneously but classic after amoxicillin or ampicillin (see pearl). Laboratory: lymphocytosis 10–20 × 10^9/L (predominantly atypical CD8 T-cells); atypical lymphocytes >10% of total lymphocytes; mild thrombocytopenia in ~50%; transaminase elevation in ~80% (rarely with clinical jaundice). Heterophile antibody (Monospot) — IgM antibodies that agglutinate horse or sheep red cells — is positive in ~85% of adults but only ~50% of children under age 4.

HIGH-YIELD PEARL — The amoxicillin/ampicillin rash in IM

The classical teaching is that 80–95% of patients with IM who receive amoxicillin or ampicillin develop a confluent maculopapular rash within 7–10 days. More recent studies (2013 onward) report a substantially lower rate of 30–70% — the discrepancy may reflect differences in antibiotic preparations, study populations, or definitions. Regardless of the exact figure, the association is real and clinically important. The rash is morbilliform, often pruritic, and can be alarming. It is NOT a true penicillin allergy — these patients can usually tolerate penicillins later in life. The mechanism is incompletely understood but appears to involve transient drug-specific T-cell activation in the setting of EBV-driven immune dysregulation. Document the event clearly in the medical record ("morbilliform rash with amoxicillin in setting of acute EBV — not consistent with true type I hypersensitivity") so the patient is not labelled penicillin-allergic for life. The exam point: a young patient with sore throat is treated empirically for strep with amoxicillin, develops a rash, and turns out to have IM. Diagnosis: EBV mononucleosis. The rash is reactive, not allergic.

Splenic rupture: The activated lymphocyte infiltrate weakens the splenic capsule. Spontaneous or minor-trauma rupture is rare but life-threatening. Standard advice: no contact sports, heavy lifting, or strenuous exertion for 4–6 weeks after diagnosis or until splenomegaly resolves on examination.

11.5 EBV Serology and Other Causes of Reactive Lymphocytosis

EBV serology — the EBNA IgG rule

EBV serology distinguishes acute primary infection from past infection (lifelong immunity). The four standard antibodies are viral capsid antigen (VCA) IgM, VCA IgG, early antigen-D (EA-D) IgG, and Epstein–Barr nuclear antigen (EBNA) IgG. The single most useful rule is that EBNA IgG appears LATE (6–12 weeks after primary infection) and persists for life — its absence in the setting of VCA IgG positivity confirms acute infection; its presence rules acute infection out.

Stage	VCA IgM	VCA IgG	EA-D IgG	EBNA IgG	Heterophile (Monospot)
Acute primary IM	POSITIVE	Positive (rising)	Positive	**NEGATIVE** Appears 6–12 weeks late.	Positive (~85% adults; ~50% children <4 yo)
Recent infection (convalescent)	Negative or low-titer	Positive	Positive (declining)	Becoming positive	May be negative
Past infection / lifelong immunity	NEGATIVE	POSITIVE (lifelong)	Negative or low-titer	POSITIVE (lifelong)	Negative
Reactivation (immunocompromised)	Variable	Positive	Positive (rising)	Positive	Variable

HIGH-YIELD PEARL — EBNA IgG positive + VCA IgM negative = past infection, NOT acute IM

This is the most testable point in EBV serology. EBNA IgG is the latest-appearing antibody and the only one that reliably distinguishes acute from past infection when both VCA IgG and a heterophile antibody have been documented. A patient with mononucleosis-like symptoms but a positive EBNA IgG has had EBV in the past — the current illness is something else (consider CMV, Toxoplasma, primary HIV, acute viral hepatitis). Conversely, a patient with classical IM symptoms, VCA IgM positive, and EBNA IgG negative has acute primary EBV infection — the EBNA IgG simply has not had time to develop yet.

Heterophile-negative mononucleosis

When the clinical picture suggests mononucleosis but the heterophile (Monospot) test is negative, the most common alternative aetiologies are CMV (next most common after EBV), Toxoplasma gondii, primary HIV infection, and acute viral hepatitis. The differential matters because management and counselling differ.

Aetiology	Distinguishing Features	Diagnosis
EBV (heterophile-negative IM)	Some patients (~10–15% adults; ~50% children <4 yo) are heterophile-negative despite acute EBV. Clinical picture identical.	EBV-specific serology (VCA IgM positive, EBNA IgG negative).
Cytomegaloviru	Most common cause of	CMV IgM positive; CMV PCR

Aetiology	Distinguishing Features	Diagnosis
s (CMV)	heterophile-negative mononucleosis in immunocompetent adults. Less prominent pharyngitis; more prominent fever and hepatitis; lymphadenopathy may be milder.	(viraemia) in immunocompromised.
Toxoplasma gondii	**Cervical lymphadenopathy (often posterior cervical or occipital).** Cat exposure (handling litter); undercooked meat. Mild systemic symptoms; rarely as severe as EBV. Important in pregnancy (congenital toxoplasmosis risk).	Toxoplasma IgM and IgG; PCR if available; lymph node biopsy may show characteristic features (Piringer–Kuchinka — clusters of epithelioid histiocytes within reactive germinal centres).
Primary HIV (acute retroviral syndrome)	Fever, lymphadenopathy, mucocutaneous ulcers, maculopapular rash, headache. Onset 2–4 weeks after exposure.	HIV-1/2 antigen/antibody combination test PLUS HIV RNA viral load (4th-generation Ag/Ab test may be negative very early; viral load is positive within days of symptom onset).
Acute viral hepatitis (HAV/HBV/HCV)	Prominent transaminase elevation; jaundice common; less prominent pharyngitis and lymphadenopathy.	Hepatitis A IgM, hepatitis B surface antigen + core IgM, hepatitis C antibody and RNA.
Pertussis (Bordetella pertussis)	**Marked lymphocytosis — sometimes 20–50 × 10^9/L or higher.** Lymphocytes are MORPHOLOGICALLY NORMAL (not atypical, distinguishing from EBV/CMV). Paroxysmal cough with inspiratory whoop; post-tussive vomiting; prolonged convalescent phase.	PCR of nasopharyngeal swab (preferred); culture; serology in convalescent phase. Treat with macrolide (azithromycin); contacts get prophylaxis.

11.6 Eosinophilia — The NAACP Differential

Eosinophilia is defined as an absolute eosinophil count above 0.5 × 10^9/L; hypereosinophilia is above 1.5 × 10^9/L. The differential is broad but collapses into the NAACP mnemonic: Neoplasm, Allergy, Adrenal insufficiency, Connective tissue disease, Parasites. Globally, parasitic infection is the most common cause of eosinophilia; in industrialised settings, allergy and atopy dominate.

Category	Examples	Clinical Clue
N — Neoplasm	Hypereosinophilic syndrome (HES); chronic eosinophilic leukaemia not otherwise specified (CEL-NOS); FIP1L1-PDGFRA-rearranged myeloid neoplasm; AML with t(16;16) or inv(16) (AML-M4Eo); T-cell lymphoma with paraneoplastic eosinophilia; Hodgkin lymphoma; metastatic carcinoma with marrow involvement	Persistent hypereosinophilia (>1.5 × 10^9/L for >6 months) plus organ damage (cardiac, pulmonary, neurologic, dermatologic) defines HES. FIP1L1-PDGFRA fusion is imatinib-responsive — always tested in unexplained hypereosinophilia.
A — Allergy / Atopy / Asthma	Allergic rhinitis; asthma; atopic dermatitis; food allergy; allergic bronchopulmonary aspergillosis (ABPA — eosinophilia + asthma + bronchiectasis + Aspergillus precipitins); eosinophilic oesophagitis; eosinophilic gastroenteritis	Most common cause of mild eosinophilia in industrialised countries. History of atopy; environmental triggers.
A — Adrenal insufficiency	Primary adrenal insufficiency (Addison disease); secondary adrenal insufficiency	**Loss of cortisol → loss of cortisol-mediated suppression of eosinophil margination → eosinophilia.** Look for hyponatraemia, hyperkalaemia, hypotension, hyperpigmentation. Eosinophilia is a subtle clue often missed.
C — Connective tissue / Collagen-vascular disease	Eosinophilic granulomatosis with polyangiitis (EGPA / Churg–Strauss — asthma + eosinophilia + vasculitis); rheumatoid arthritis; SLE; eosinophilic fasciitis (Shulman syndrome); IgG4-related disease	EGPA classic triad: late-onset asthma + hypereosinophilia + small/medium vessel vasculitis (mononeuritis multiplex, glomerulonephritis, pulmonary infiltrates). Anti-MPO ANCA in ~40%.
P — Parasites (helminths)	**Tissue-invasive helminths cause prominent eosinophilia.** Strongyloides stercoralis (chronic; hyperinfection in immunocompromised); hookworm (Necator, Ancylostoma); Schistosoma; filaria (Wuchereria, Brugia); Toxocara (visceral larva	Travel history; geographic exposure; food history (undercooked pork → Trichinella; freshwater swimming → Schistosoma); chronic eosinophilia of unknown cause should always trigger Strongyloides serology before steroids or chemotherapy (steroid-induced hyperinfection is fatal).

Category	Examples	Clinical Clue
	migrans); Trichinella; Ascaris (during migration). NOTE: protozoa (Plasmodium, Giardia, Entamoeba) do NOT typically cause eosinophilia — eosinophilia is essentially a helminth response.	
Drugs (separate but high-yield)	DRESS syndrome (anticonvulsants — phenytoin, carbamazepine, lamotrigine; allopurinol; sulfa antibiotics; vancomycin; minocycline); NSAIDs; β-lactams	**DRESS:** Drug Reaction with Eosinophilia and Systemic Symptoms. Fever + rash + eosinophilia + lymphadenopathy + hepatitis or other internal organ involvement, 2–8 weeks after starting offending drug. HHV-6 reactivation common. Stop the drug; supportive care; systemic steroids for severe organ involvement.

HIGH-YIELD PEARL — Strongyloides — test before steroids

Strongyloides stercoralis can persist asymptomatically for decades after initial exposure (autoinfection cycle). Corticosteroids or chemotherapy can trigger hyperinfection syndrome — massive larval dissemination to the lungs, brain, and bloodstream, often with gram-negative bacteraemia from gut translocation. Mortality approaches 80–90%. Any patient with eosinophilia of unknown cause AND any history of travel or residence in an endemic area (tropical/subtropical regions, including the southeastern United States) should have Strongyloides serology drawn before high-dose corticosteroids or chemotherapy. Empiric ivermectin is given if serology is positive or strongly suspected. This is a high-yield USMLE point in any vignette pairing eosinophilia with planned immunosuppression.

FIP1L1-PDGFRA: An interstitial deletion on chromosome 4q12 fuses FIP1L1 to PDGFRA, creating a constitutively active tyrosine kinase. The resulting myeloid neoplasm presents as hypereosinophilia with cardiac (endomyocardial fibrosis), pulmonary, and dermatologic involvement, classically in middle-aged men. Imatinib produces dramatic, sustained responses at low doses — testing for FIP1L1-PDGFRA in unexplained hypereosinophilia is essential because the treatment changes from supportive care to a single oral tyrosine kinase inhibitor.

11.7 Monocytosis and Basophilia

Monocytosis

Monocytosis is defined as an absolute monocyte count above $1.0 \times 10^9/L$. Reactive monocytosis accompanies chronic infections — tuberculosis, subacute bacterial endocarditis, brucellosis, syphilis, and recovery from severe neutropenia (the marrow rebounds with a monocyte burst before normal neutrophil production resumes). Inflammatory disorders (inflammatory bowel disease, sarcoidosis, SLE) and post-splenectomy states also produce monocytosis. The clonal differential is dominated by chronic myelomonocytic leukaemia (CMML), defined by persistent monocytosis (≥1.0 × 10^9/L AND ≥10% of WBC for ≥3 months) plus dysplasia or characteristic mutations (TET2, SRSF2, ASXL1). Acute monoblastic and monocytic leukaemias (AML-M5) present with markedly elevated monocyte and promonocyte counts plus blasts.

Basophilia

Basophilia is defined as an absolute basophil count above 0.1 × 10^9/L. It is uncommon and, when persistent without an obvious reactive cause, is highly suggestive of a myeloproliferative neoplasm — most often chronic myeloid leukaemia. Basophilia plus eosinophilia in an unexplained leukocytosis is a near-pathognomonic CML pattern; basophilia exceeding 20% of WBC indicates accelerated or blast phase. Reactive basophilia occurs in allergy (especially urticaria), hypothyroidism, polycythaemia vera (basophilia is part of the PV pattern), and chronic inflammation.

HIGH-YIELD PEARL — Basophilia + eosinophilia + neutrophilia → think CML

The combination of basophilia plus eosinophilia plus neutrophilia (with or without thrombocytosis) in an unexplained leukocytosis is one of the most specific peripheral blood patterns in haematology. It almost always means CML. Confirmatory testing is BCR::ABL1 RT-PCR on peripheral blood, which detects the fusion transcript directly. The Philadelphia chromosome — t(9;22)(q34;q11) — is the cytogenetic correlate. Once confirmed, first-line therapy is a tyrosine kinase inhibitor (imatinib, dasatinib, nilotinib, or bosutinib), with response monitored by quantitative BCR::ABL1 transcript levels on the International Scale (chapter on chronic leukaemias covers in detail).

Persistent unexplained monocytosis: Always check duration. Reactive monocytosis is transient and tied to an identifiable cause. Persistent monocytosis (≥3 months) without obvious explanation, especially in older adults with cytopenias or dysplastic features, requires bone marrow examination to evaluate for CMML.

11.8 Approach to Leukopenia and Neutropenia

Leukopenia is a total WBC count below 4 × 10^9/L. Like leukocytosis, the diagnostic value comes from the differential — usually neutropenia, sometimes lymphopenia, occasionally both. Neutropenia is the more clinically urgent reduction because neutrophils are the primary defence against pyogenic bacteria and invasive fungi; severe neutropenia carries an immediate infection risk that drives every management decision.

Severity grading and clinical implications

Grade	ANC (×10^9/L)	Infection Risk	Management
Mild neutropenia	1.0–1.5	Minimal increase	Investigate cause; no urgent intervention.

Grade	ANC ($\times 10^9$/L)	Infection Risk	Management
Moderate neutropenia	0.5–1.0	Modest increase, especially with skin or mucosal breaks	Investigate cause; avoid live vaccines; routine infection precautions.
Severe neutropenia	<0.5	MARKEDLY elevated — pyogenic bacteria and invasive fungi	Neutropenic precautions; G-CSF if appropriate; emergent broad-spectrum antibiotics on first sign of fever.
Agranulocytosis	<0.1	**Life-threatening.** Sepsis from gut-derived gram-negatives and oral streptococci common; mucositis sources; high mortality without prompt antibiotic coverage.	Reverse isolation; emergent broad-spectrum coverage; G-CSF; identify and stop offending drug if possible; SCT consideration if persistent.

Causes of neutropenia

Category	Examples	Clinical Clue
Drug-induced (most common in adults)	**Cytotoxic chemotherapy** (predictable, dose-dependent). **Idiosyncratic (unpredictable, dose-independent):** Methimazole, propylthiouracil (PTU), clozapine (mandatory ANC monitoring), ticlopidine, anticonvulsants (carbamazepine, phenytoin, valproate), sulfonamides, β-lactams (high-dose IV), vancomycin, linezolid, dapsone, NSAIDs.	Time course: chemotherapy nadir typically 7–14 days post-dose. Idiosyncratic onset 2 weeks to 6 months after starting drug. Resolution within days to weeks of stopping the drug.
Marrow failure	Aplastic anaemia; myelodysplastic syndrome; acute leukaemia (marrow infiltration with blasts crowding out normal cells); marrow fibrosis (myelofibrosis, granulomatous infiltration)	Cytopenias usually multilineage. Bone marrow examination required.
Nutritional	Vitamin B12 deficiency; folate deficiency; copper deficiency (rare; bariatric surgery,	Macrocytic anaemia, hypersegmented neutrophils on smear, low retics.

Category	Examples	Clinical Clue
	parenteral nutrition without copper)	
Hypersplenism	Cirrhosis with portal hypertension; lymphoma with splenic involvement; Felty syndrome (rheumatoid arthritis + splenomegaly + neutropenia)	Cytopenias proportional to splenic enlargement; splenectomy or treatment of underlying cause restores counts.
Autoimmune	Felty syndrome; SLE; primary autoimmune neutropenia (children); large granular lymphocyte (LGL) leukaemia (T-cell or NK-cell clonal expansion suppressing myelopoiesis)	Anti-neutrophil antibodies; LGL leukaemia confirmed by clonal TCR rearrangement and STAT3 mutations.
Infection	HIV (direct marrow effect plus immune-mediated); EBV, CMV, hepatitis B/C, parvovirus B19; severe sepsis (acute neutropenia with fall from very high counts during cytokine storm); typhoid, brucellosis, malaria, miliary TB	Viral marker panel including HIV, hepatitis serologies; CMV/EBV serology if clinical context fits.
Constitutional / inherited	**Benign ethnic neutropenia (BEN)** Common in individuals of African, Middle Eastern, or West Indian ancestry — ANC may be persistently 1.0–1.5 × 10^9/L without clinical consequence. Linked to the DARC/ACKR1 −46 C/C genotype (the same polymorphism that confers Plasmodium vivax resistance). NOT a disease — does NOT require evaluation if isolated and stable.	Persistent mild-moderate neutropenia in a healthy patient of relevant ancestry, no signs of infection, no other cytopenias = BEN. Do not over-investigate.
Congenital	Severe congenital neutropenia (Kostmann syndrome — ELANE, HAX1 mutations); cyclic neutropenia (ELANE); Shwachman–Diamond syndrome (SBDS); Wiskott–Aldrich; chronic granulomatous disease (functional, not quantitative)	Recurrent severe infections from infancy; family history; specific genetic testing.

HIGH-YIELD PEARL — Benign ethnic neutropenia — recognise and do not over-investigate

Approximately 25–50% of individuals of African or West Indian ancestry have an absolute neutrophil count persistently in the 1.0–1.5 × 10^9/L range — sometimes lower — without any clinical infection susceptibility. This is benign ethnic neutropenia (BEN), linked to the Duffy-null (DARC/ACKR1 -46 C/C) genotype that also confers protection against Plasmodium vivax malaria. The key features: persistent (not progressive), isolated to neutrophils (other lineages normal), no recurrent infections, no marrow abnormality, often documented from childhood. Misclassifying BEN as pathologic neutropenia leads to unnecessary bone marrow biopsy, medication discontinuation, and treatment delays for legitimate therapies (chemotherapy, clozapine). On USMLE, a healthy Black patient with isolated mild neutropenia and no infection history is BEN — answer choice will be "reassurance and no further workup," not bone marrow biopsy.

ANC reference ranges: The lower limit of "normal" was traditionally set at 1.5 × 10^9/L based predominantly on White populations. Some laboratories now report population-adjusted reference ranges. Clinically, an ANC of 1.0–1.5 in a healthy individual of African ancestry without infection history requires no further evaluation; one of 1.0–1.5 in any patient with a known offending drug or recent illness does.

11.9 Febrile Neutropenia — A Medical Emergency

Fever in a neutropenic patient is a medical emergency. Untreated febrile neutropenia carries mortality of 30–70% from gram-negative sepsis (most often E. coli, Klebsiella, Pseudomonas) and oral viridans streptococci translocating through mucositis-damaged barriers. Empiric broad-spectrum antibiotics started within one hour of presentation reduce mortality to single digits. The exam-favoured definition and management are below.

STEP 2 BRIDGE — Febrile neutropenia — definition, workup, empiric therapy

Definition: ANC <0.5 × 10^9/L (or expected to fall below 0.5 within 48 hours) AND a single oral temperature ≥38.3 °C (101 °F) OR sustained temperature ≥38.0 °C (100.4 °F) for one hour. Some patients (steroid-treated, elderly) may not mount fever — hypothermia or haemodynamic deterioration substitutes.

Initial workup (parallel with antibiotics, not before): Two sets of blood cultures (peripheral plus each central venous catheter lumen if present); CBC with differential; comprehensive metabolic panel; lactate; urinalysis and culture; chest radiograph; targeted cultures from any symptomatic site (sputum, stool with C. difficile if diarrhoea, lumbar puncture if meningismus, swabs of skin/perirectal lesions). Physical exam attending to oral cavity, perianal area, central line sites, and skin.

Empiric antibiotics — within ONE HOUR: Anti-pseudomonal β-lactam monotherapy is standard: cefepime 2 g IV q8h, OR piperacillin-tazobactam 4.5 g IV q6h, OR meropenem 1 g IV q8h (reserved for prior resistant organisms or severe sepsis). Do NOT delay antibiotics for cultures or for antibiotic level monitoring.

Add vancomycin (or linezolid/daptomycin) if: Haemodynamic instability or sepsis; suspected catheter-related infection; known MRSA colonisation or prior MRSA infection; severe mucositis (high oral viridans streptococci risk); skin or soft tissue infection. Vancomycin is NOT routinely added for all febrile neutropenia — it is reserved for the indications above and discontinued at 48 hours if cultures are negative for gram-positive resistant organisms.

Risk stratification (MASCC score): Multinational Association for Supportive Care in Cancer score predicts low-risk febrile neutropenia (anticipated short duration, no comorbidities, haemodynamically stable, solid tumour not haematologic). Score ≥21 = low risk; outpatient management with oral ciprofloxacin + amoxicillin-clavulanate is acceptable in selected patients with reliable follow-up.

Antifungal coverage: Add empiric antifungal (typically caspofungin or liposomal amphotericin B) if fever persists ≥4–7 days on broad-spectrum antibacterial therapy without identified source — invasive Aspergillus and Candida become major concerns in prolonged neutropenia.

G-CSF (filgrastim, pegfilgrastim): Primary prophylaxis indicated for chemotherapy regimens with febrile neutropenia risk ≥20%. Therapeutic G-CSF in established febrile neutropenia shortens neutrophil recovery but does not reduce mortality — used selectively in high-risk patients (prolonged neutropenia anticipated, sepsis, fungal pneumonia).

11.10 Aplastic Anaemia — Pathogenesis and Diagnosis

Aplastic anaemia is pancytopenia with a hypocellular bone marrow and no abnormal infiltrate — a stem cell failure syndrome. The presentation is usually subacute over weeks to months: fatigue and pallor (from anaemia), bruising and bleeding (from thrombocytopenia), and recurrent or severe infection (from neutropenia). The peripheral smear shows reduced cells of all three lineages without dysplasia, blasts, or fragments. The reticulocyte count is markedly reduced — a key feature distinguishing aplastic anaemia from peripheral destruction syndromes that have rising reticulocytes.

Pathogenesis — autoimmune in 80%

The majority (~80%) of acquired aplastic anaemia is immune-mediated. Autoreactive cytotoxic CD8+ T-cells (with a Th1 phenotype) inappropriately attack haematopoietic stem cells. The cytokines they secrete — interferon-γ and tumour necrosis factor-α — induce HSC apoptosis through the Fas/FasL pathway. The evidence for this autoimmune model is strong: most cases respond to immunosuppressive therapy with anti-thymocyte globulin and cyclosporine; HLA-DR2 and HLA-B14 associations exist; and PNH clones are detectable in ~50% of patients (because GPI-deficient stem cells are relatively resistant to the immune attack and expand by selection).

Causes

Category	Specific Causes	Comment
Idiopathic	—	No identifiable trigger after

Category	Specific Causes	Comment
(most common ~70%)		thorough workup.
Drugs	Chloramphenicol (classic, idiosyncratic — distinct from dose-dependent reversible suppression); benzene; gold salts; carbamazepine, felbamate; sulfonamides; methimazole, PTU; NSAIDs (indomethacin, phenylbutazone)	Idiosyncratic reactions are dose-INdependent and may appear weeks to months after exposure.
Viruses	Hepatitis-associated aplastic anaemia (HAAA — follows acute seronegative hepatitis; not A, B, or C; presumed novel virus; presents 2–3 months after hepatitis with severe AA); EBV; HHV-6; HIV; parvovirus B19	Parvovirus B19 typically causes pure red cell aplasia (single-lineage suppression of erythroid progenitors via P antigen) — full aplastic anaemia is less common.
Pregnancy	Rare; usually resolves after delivery	Recurs in subsequent pregnancies in some cases.
Thymoma	Associated with pure red cell aplasia more than full AA	Thymectomy may resolve; immune-mediated mechanism.
PNH evolution	Established PNH may evolve to aplastic anaemia; aplastic anaemia may have a small PNH clone that expands	Bidirectional relationship; FLAER flow cytometry indicated in any suspected AA.
Inherited bone marrow failure syndromes	Fanconi anaemia (most common); dyskeratosis congenita (telomere maintenance defects); Shwachman–Diamond syndrome; Diamond–Blackfan anaemia (pure red cell)	Always considered in young patients before initiating therapy — see Fanconi pearl below.

Severity grading — Camitta criteria

Severity	Criteria	Management Implication
Non-severe (NSAA)	Hypocellular marrow + cytopenia not meeting severe criteria below	Observation if asymptomatic; immunosuppressive therapy if transfusion-dependent.
Severe (SAA)	**Bone marrow cellularity <25% (or <50% with <30% haematopoietic cells) PLUS at**	Allogeneic HSCT first-line if matched sibling donor available and patient ≤40–50 years;

Severity	Criteria	Management Implication
	least 2 of the following 3 peripheral blood criteria: • Reticulocytes <60 × 10^9/L (<60,000/µL) — modern Delphi consensus 2024; some guidelines still use <20 × 10^9/L • ANC <0.5 × 10^9/L • Platelets <20 × 10^9/L	immunosuppressive therapy (ATG + cyclosporine + eltrombopag) otherwise.
Very severe (VSAA)	Same as SAA but ANC <0.2 × 10^9/L	Highest urgency; very high infection mortality without prompt treatment.

Workup — exclude the look-alikes

Aplastic anaemia is a diagnosis of exclusion. Pancytopenia with a hypocellular marrow has several causes that require different management. The complete workup includes: bone marrow aspirate AND trephine biopsy (cellularity, morphology, blast count); cytogenetics and a myeloid mutation panel (rule out hypocellular MDS or aleukaemic AML); FLAER flow cytometry on granulocytes and monocytes (rule out PNH); chromosome breakage testing (DEB or MMC) in patients under ~50 years to rule out Fanconi anaemia; viral serologies (hepatitis A/B/C, EBV, CMV, HIV, parvovirus B19); telomere length analysis if clinical suspicion of dyskeratosis congenita.

HIGH-YIELD PEARL — Always test for Fanconi anaemia before SCT conditioning in young patients

Fanconi anaemia (FA) is an autosomal recessive (rarely X-linked) inherited bone marrow failure syndrome caused by mutations in genes encoding the FA-BRCA DNA repair pathway. At least 22 complementation groups are described; FANCA mutations account for ~65%. The pathway repairs interstrand DNA crosslinks (ICLs); when defective, ICLs accumulate, replication stalls, and HSCs progressively die. Median age at marrow failure is 7–9 years, but presentation can extend into adulthood.

Clinical features: Progressive pancytopenia from ages 5–10; congenital anomalies in ~75% (radial ray defects, thumb hypoplasia or absent thumbs, café-au-lait macules, short stature, microcephaly, renal anomalies, hypogonadism); markedly elevated risk of acute myeloid leukaemia and squamous cell carcinomas (head/neck, oesophagus, anogenital). Some patients have minimal physical findings — silent FA is real and dangerous.

Diagnosis: Chromosome breakage testing — DEB (diepoxybutane) or MMC (mitomycin C) chromosome fragility test. FA cells show characteristic excessive chromosomal breakage when exposed to these crosslinking agents. Molecular confirmation by sequencing of FANC genes.

Why testing matters before SCT: Standard alkylating-agent conditioning regimens (cyclophosphamide, busulfan) cause CATASTROPHIC toxicity in undiagnosed FA patients because their cells cannot repair the induced DNA damage. A reduced-intensity conditioning regimen (low-dose cyclophosphamide + fludarabine ± low-dose total body irradiation) is mandatory. Failure to diagnose FA before SCT is among the most consequential errors in paediatric haematology — exam-favoured point: pancytopenia in a young patient → DEB test BEFORE any SCT planning.

HIGH-YIELD PEARL — Parvovirus B19 — pure red cell aplasia, not pancytopenia

Parvovirus B19 has a unique tropism: it infects erythroid progenitors via the P antigen (globoside) receptor. The virus replicates inside the progenitor and lyses it. The result is selective erythroid aplasia — reticulocytopenia with falling haemoglobin, but normal white cells and platelets. In healthy individuals, this is clinically silent (the slight anaemia goes unnoticed). In patients with chronic haemolytic anaemia (sickle cell disease, hereditary spherocytosis, thalassaemia — anyone running a baseline reticulocyte count of 5–15%), the temporary halt of red cell production produces a sudden severe drop in haemoglobin known as APLASTIC CRISIS. The reticulocyte count falls to near zero. The picture is distinct from full aplastic anaemia — only the red cell line is affected.

Diagnosis: Parvovirus B19 IgM and PCR. Bone marrow shows giant pronormoblasts with viral inclusions (intranuclear "lantern" inclusions). Self-limited 7–10 days. Supportive transfusion. In immunocompromised patients (HIV, transplant), persistent infection causes chronic pure red cell aplasia — treated with IVIG.

11.11 Aplastic Anaemia Management

STEP 2 BRIDGE — Severe aplastic anaemia — first-line algorithm

Branch point: Patient age and donor availability. Allogeneic HSCT from an HLA-matched sibling donor offers the best long-term outcome (overall survival 80–90% in young patients) and is first-line for patients younger than 40–50 years with an available donor. Patients older than 50 or without a matched donor receive immunosuppressive therapy.

Allogeneic HSCT (matched sibling donor, age ≤40–50): Conditioning: cyclophosphamide + ATG (or fludarabine-based reduced-intensity if older). Outcomes: 80–90% long-term survival; lower relapse rate than IST; no risk of clonal evolution to MDS/AML. Risks: graft-versus-host disease (acute and chronic), infection during cytopenic phase, infertility.

Immunosuppressive therapy (IST) — first-line if no matched donor: Horse anti-thymocyte globulin (ATG) PLUS cyclosporine PLUS eltrombopag (since 2018, eltrombopag is part of the first-line IST combination — adds ~30% absolute response over ATG + CsA alone). Horse ATG is preferred over rabbit ATG (better outcomes in randomised trials). Response rate 60–70% at 6 months; relapse in ~30% requiring a second course or alternative donor SCT. Long-term risk: clonal evolution to MDS or AML in 10–20% over 10–15 years.

Eltrombopag — mechanism and approval: Eltrombopag is an oral thrombopoietin (TPO) receptor agonist that binds the TPO receptor and stimulates HSC proliferation and differentiation. Originally FDA-approved 2008 for chronic ITP, expanded indication for severe aplastic anaemia refractory to immunosuppression in 2014, and added to first-line IST combination in 2018. Improves trilineage response rates.

Salvage and alternative options: Patients who fail first-line IST may receive a second course of ATG (rabbit if horse failed first); matched unrelated donor or haploidentical SCT; eltrombopag monotherapy; or experimental therapies. AlloHSCT remains the only curative option in patients with severe disease who fail IST.

Supportive care (universal): Transfusion support — irradiated, leukoreduced red cells and platelets; CMV-negative blood products in transplant candidates; iron chelation if heavily transfused. Antimicrobial prophylaxis during severe neutropenia (fluoroquinolone for bacteria, posaconazole or voriconazole for fungi, acyclovir if HSV-positive). Avoid live vaccines on IST. Pregnancy avoidance during active disease and IST.

What NOT to do: Do NOT give corticosteroid monotherapy (ineffective for aplastic anaemia and toxic). Do NOT give G-CSF as primary therapy (does not restore stem cell function). Do NOT give androgens (danazol) as first-line in severe disease (used historically and in non-severe AA only).

11.12 Reactive Lymphadenopathy Patterns

Lymphadenopathy is among the most common clinical findings in general medicine. The diagnostic approach distinguishes reactive (benign, self-limiting) from neoplastic (lymphoma, leukaemia) causes and from infiltrative or granulomatous aetiologies. The clinical features that drive workup are age, duration (under 4 weeks favours reactive; over 6–8 weeks requires investigation), anatomic distribution (localised vs generalised), associated systemic features (fever, night sweats, unintentional weight loss — "B symptoms" suggesting lymphoma), and the character of the node (tender suggests reactive; rubbery, non-tender, matted suggests lymphoma; rock-hard suggests metastatic carcinoma).

Histologic patterns

Pattern	Common Causes	Key Histologic Features
Follicular hyperplasia	Early EBV/HIV; syphilis (luetic lymphadenitis); rheumatoid arthritis; SLE; Castleman disease (HHV-8 MCD)	**Expanded reactive germinal centres with intact mantle zones.** Germinal centres show polarity (light and dark zones); tingible body macrophages produce a "starry sky" appearance from phagocytosed apoptotic debris. CD20-positive B-cells. BCL2 NEGATIVE in germinal centres — the critical distinguisher from follicular lymphoma, where neoplastic follicles are BCL2 POSITIVE.

Pattern	Common Causes	Key Histologic Features
Paracortical (interfollicular) hyperplasia	Viral infections (EBV, CMV, HSV); drug reactions (phenytoin classic); dermatopathic lymphadenitis (chronic skin disease draining to regional nodes)	Expansion of T-cell zones with interdigitating dendritic cells, immunoblasts, and prominent high endothelial venules. Pigment-laden macrophages in dermatopathic pattern.
Sinus hyperplasia	Reactive sinus histiocytosis; nodes draining inflammatory or neoplastic sites; Whipple disease; Rosai–Dorfman (when extreme)	Expanded subcapsular and medullary sinuses filled with macrophages. Rosai–Dorfman shows characteristic emperipolesis.
Necrotising lymphadenitis	Kikuchi–Fujimoto disease; SLE lymphadenitis; cat-scratch disease (Bartonella henselae); tularaemia; Yersinia pseudotuberculosis	Areas of necrosis with karyorrhectic debris. Cat-scratch and tularaemia show stellate microabscesses with neutrophils. Kikuchi shows necrosis WITHOUT neutrophils — the distinguishing feature.
Granulomatous lymphadenitis	Mycobacterial infection (TB and atypical); sarcoidosis; fungal (histoplasmosis, coccidioidomycosis, blastomycosis); Brucella; cat-scratch (late stage)	Caseating granulomas suggest tuberculosis or fungal infection (acid-fast bacilli or fungal stains required). Non-caseating granulomas suggest sarcoidosis, Brucella, or early Crohn disease.

HIGH-YIELD PEARL — BCL2 separates reactive follicular hyperplasia from follicular lymphoma

Reactive follicular hyperplasia: Germinal centre B-cells are CD20+, CD10+, BCL6+, and BCL2 NEGATIVE. The germinal centre is a tightly regulated structure where BCL2 is downregulated to allow apoptosis of B-cells that fail antigen affinity selection.

Follicular lymphoma: Neoplastic follicles carry the t(14;18) translocation that places BCL2 under control of the IGH enhancer, producing constitutive BCL2 expression. The neoplastic germinal-centre B-cells are CD20+, CD10+, BCL6+, and BCL2 POSITIVE.

The IHC algorithm in any follicular lymphoid proliferation: CD20 confirms B-cell origin; CD10 and BCL6 confirm germinal-centre phenotype; BCL2 distinguishes reactive (negative) from neoplastic (positive). Positive BCL2 staining within architecturally normal-looking germinal centres establishes follicular lymphoma even before flow cytometry or molecular studies return.

11.13 Langerhans Cell Histiocytosis

Langerhans cell histiocytosis (LCH) is a clonal proliferation of cells with the phenotype of dendritic Langerhans cells. Modern molecular pathology has reclassified LCH as a myeloid neoplasm with characteristic MAPK pathway mutations rather than a true reactive condition — but its inclusion in this chapter reflects how it presents clinically and morphologically alongside the histiocytic disorders. The clinical spectrum is wide: from a solitary lytic bone lesion (eosinophilic granuloma) to disseminated multisystem disease (historically called Letterer–Siwe disease) involving liver, spleen, bone marrow, lung, and skin.

Clinical presentations

Single-system LCH most commonly involves bone — solitary lytic lesions of the skull (classic), vertebra (vertebra plana), or long bones. Vertebral collapse is a typical paediatric presentation. Skin involvement in infants produces a seborrheic dermatitis–like rash on the scalp (often misdiagnosed as cradle cap), behind the ears, and in skin folds. Pulmonary LCH in adults occurs almost exclusively in cigarette smokers and presents with cystic lung disease and spontaneous pneumothorax — smoking cessation alone produces remission in most cases. Multisystem LCH involves the high-risk organs (liver, spleen, bone marrow) with cytopenias, hepatosplenomegaly, and constitutional symptoms; the classic central diabetes insipidus arises from posterior pituitary involvement at the hypothalamic stalk.

Morphology and immunophenotype

LCH cells are large, oval to kidney-shaped, with prominent nuclear grooves and folds — the so-called "coffee-bean" nucleus. Cytoplasm is abundant and pale eosinophilic. The background is characteristically rich in eosinophils, with admixed lymphocytes, plasma cells, and multinucleate giant cells. The triad of immunophenotypic markers is CD1a+ (surface), langerin (CD207)+ (cytoplasmic), and S100+. CD207 (langerin) is the protein that forms Birbeck granules — the racquet-shaped intracytoplasmic organelles visible only on electron microscopy that historically defined Langerhans cells. CD207 IHC has replaced electron microscopy in routine diagnosis. BRAF V600E mutations are detected in approximately 50% of LCH cases and can be confirmed by VE1 immunohistochemistry or molecular testing; remaining cases carry MAP2K1 mutations or other MAPK pathway alterations.

HIGH-YIELD PEARL — LCH — the immunophenotype triad and BRAF V600E

Diagnostic triad: CD1a+ (surface), CD207 (langerin)+ (cytoplasmic, Birbeck granule protein), S100+. All three positive confirms LCH.

Coffee-bean nucleus: Nuclear grooves and folds give the characteristic coffee-bean appearance. Eosinophil-rich background with multinucleate giant cells completes the picture.

Birbeck granules: Tennis-racquet or rod-shaped intracytoplasmic organelles on electron microscopy — pathognomonic of Langerhans cells, formed by langerin endocytosis. Largely supplanted by CD207 IHC in routine diagnostic practice but remains a high-yield exam concept.

BRAF V600E and targeted therapy: Approximately 50% of LCH cases carry BRAF V600E. Vemurafenib and dabrafenib (BRAF inhibitors) produce dramatic responses in BRAF-mutated multisystem LCH and have transformed treatment of refractory disease. Universal BRAF testing is now standard.

Distinction from Rosai–Dorfman: Rosai–Dorfman histiocytes are S100+, CD68+, but CD1a NEGATIVE and CD207 NEGATIVE. The CD1a/CD207 status separates the two definitively.

11.14 Haemophagocytic Lymphohistiocytosis

Haemophagocytic lymphohistiocytosis (HLH) is a life-threatening hyperinflammatory syndrome characterised by uncontrolled activation of macrophages and cytotoxic T-cells. The cytokine storm — extreme elevations of ferritin, IFN-γ, IL-18, IL-6, and soluble IL-2 receptor (sCD25) — produces multiorgan failure with high mortality if untreated. Recognition is delayed in many cases because the presentation overlaps with sepsis, viral infection, and lymphoma.

Pathogenesis

Primary (familial) HLH results from inherited defects in the cytolytic granule pathway: mutations in PRF1 (perforin), UNC13D (Munc13-4), STX11 (syntaxin 11), and STXBP2 (Munc18-2), among others. These genes encode proteins required for cytotoxic T-cells and NK cells to kill antigen-presenting target cells. When killing fails, the antigen-bearing cell persists, T-cells continue to be activated, and the resulting cytokine storm activates macrophages systemically. Familial HLH typically presents in infants and young children. Secondary (acquired) HLH is triggered by an external stimulus in a previously normal immune system: infections (Epstein–Barr virus is the most common trigger; also CMV, other herpesviruses, dengue, leishmania, mycobacteria), haematologic malignancies (T-cell lymphoma is particularly associated — AITL and extranodal NK/T-cell lymphoma; aggressive B-cell lymphomas), and autoimmune disease (where it is termed macrophage activation syndrome, MAS, in systemic juvenile idiopathic arthritis and SLE).

HLH-2004 diagnostic criteria

Diagnosis requires either molecular confirmation of an HLH-associated mutation OR fulfilment of 5 of the following 8 clinical/laboratory criteria:

- **Fever** ≥38.5 °C
- **Splenomegaly**
- **Cytopenias** in ≥2 of 3 lineages (haemoglobin <9 g/dL; platelets $<100 \times 10^9$/L; neutrophils $<1.0 \times 10^9$/L)
- **Hypertriglyceridaemia** (fasting ≥3 mmol/L or 265 mg/dL) AND/OR **hypofibrinogenaemia** (≤1.5 g/L)
- **Haemophagocytosis** in bone marrow, spleen, liver, or lymph node — visualised as macrophages engulfing red cells, platelets, and nucleated cells
- Low or absent NK cell activity on functional assay
- **Ferritin** ≥500 µg/L (≥10,000 µg/L has ~90% positive predictive value for HLH in the right clinical context)
- **Elevated soluble IL-2 receptor** (soluble CD25) ≥2400 U/mL

HIGH-YIELD PEARL — Ferritin >10,000 in a febrile cytopenic patient — think HLH
Ferritin is the single most clinically useful marker of HLH. Levels above 10,000 µg/L carry approximately 90% positive predictive value for HLH in the appropriate clinical context (febrile cytopenic patient with splenomegaly), and levels above 50,000 are nearly specific. Ferritin is also rapidly available — most hospital laboratories report it within hours, far faster than NK cell activity or soluble IL-2 receptor. Any patient with unexplained fever, cytopenias, splenomegaly, and ferritin above 10,000 warrants immediate haematology consultation and consideration of HLH-directed therapy.

Haemophagocytosis is neither sensitive nor specific alone: The bone marrow finding of macrophages engulfing blood cells is named for the disease but is unreliable as a single diagnostic criterion. Haemophagocytosis can be absent in confirmed HLH (especially early) and can be present without HLH (in sepsis, haematopoietic stem cell transplant, transfusion). Diagnosis requires the full HLH-2004 constellation, not the marrow finding alone.

EBV-driven HLH: EBV is the single most common infectious trigger of secondary HLH. The presentation overlaps with severe infectious mononucleosis but with cytopenias, ferritin elevation, and progressive organ failure. EBV-driven HLH carries high mortality and often requires etoposide-based therapy beyond simple antiviral measures (which are largely ineffective for EBV).

Treatment

The HLH-94/HLH-2004 protocol — dexamethasone PLUS etoposide PLUS cyclosporine — is standard initial therapy for primary HLH and severe secondary HLH. Etoposide (a topoisomerase II inhibitor) is the active agent against the activated macrophage and T-cell compartment. Emapalumab (anti-IFN-γ monoclonal antibody) was FDA-approved in November 2018 for primary refractory or progressive HLH and represents the first targeted therapy. Allogeneic HSCT is the only curative option for primary (familial) HLH — without transplant, primary HLH is uniformly fatal. For secondary HLH, treatment of the underlying trigger is essential alongside immunosuppression: rituximab and antiviral measures for EBV-driven disease (with the caveat that rituximab is more effective than antivirals); chemotherapy for lymphoma-associated HLH; high-dose corticosteroids and disease-targeted therapy for autoimmune-associated MAS.

11.15 Rosai–Dorfman Disease

Rosai–Dorfman disease (RDD) — also called sinus histiocytosis with massive lymphadenopathy — is a rare non-Langerhans histiocytic disorder. It typically affects children and young adults and presents with massive, painless, bilateral cervical lymphadenopathy. Systemic features (fever, elevated ESR, leukocytosis, polyclonal hypergammaglobulinaemia) are common. Extranodal disease (skin, sinuses, soft tissue, central nervous system) occurs in up to 40% of cases.

Histology and immunophenotype

The lymph node shows markedly dilated sinuses stuffed with large pale histiocytes — at low magnification, the sinuses appear expanded and clear. The hallmark feature is emperipolesis: viable lymphocytes, plasma cells, and red cells engulfed within the cytoplasm of the histiocytes. The engulfed cells remain morphologically intact (distinct from phagocytosis, where the ingested cell is digested). The immunophenotype distinguishes RDD from LCH:

Marker	Rosai-Dorfman Disease	Langerhans Cell Histiocytosis
S100	POSITIVE (strongly)	POSITIVE
CD68	POSITIVE	Variable
CD1a	**NEGATIVE**	POSITIVE
CD207 (langerin)	**NEGATIVE**	POSITIVE
Birbeck granules on EM	Absent	Present (pathognomonic)
Hallmark histologic finding	**Emperipolesis** Intact lymphocytes within histiocyte cytoplasm.	**Coffee-bean nucleus** Nuclear grooves; eosinophil-rich background.
Mutations	SLC29A3 (familial); KRAS, MAP2K1 (sporadic)	BRAF V600E ~50%; MAP2K1 in others

Most cases of RDD are self-limited, with spontaneous regression over months to years. Symptomatic or mass-effect disease is treated with corticosteroids; refractory cases may require sirolimus, methotrexate, or surgical excision. The prognosis is generally favourable, in marked contrast to LCH multisystem disease.

11.16 Castleman Disease

Castleman disease is a heterogeneous lymphoproliferative disorder. Two histologic types and two clinical forms produce a 2 × 2 matrix that drives diagnosis and management.

Histologic types and clinical forms

Form	Histology	Demographics	Treatment
Unicentric Castleman disease (UCD)	**Hyaline-vascular (HV) type — ~80–90% of unicentric cases.** Unicentric disease is the most common form of Castleman overall (>70%). Single enlarged	Young to middle-aged adults; no sex predilection; usually asymptomatic — mass found incidentally	Surgical excision is curative. No systemic therapy required.

Form	Histology	Demographics	Treatment
	lymph node (mediastinum, neck, abdomen). Regressed germinal centres with central hyalinised blood vessel penetrating the follicle in a "lollipop" pattern. Mantle zones expanded with concentric lymphocytes ("onion-skin"). Plasma cells sparse.		
Idiopathic multicentric Castleman disease (iMCD)	**Plasma cell or mixed type.** Multicentric lymphadenopathy with sheets of mature plasma cells in interfollicular zones. Germinal centres typically reactive rather than regressed. HHV-8 NEGATIVE. Polyclonal lymphoplasmacytosis.	Adults, any age; multiple peripheral nodes plus systemic features (fever, weight loss, organomegaly, anaemia, polyclonal hypergammaglobulinaemia)	Driven by IL-6 excess. Siltuximab (anti–IL-6 monoclonal antibody) is first-line — FDA-approved 2014 for iMCD. Tocilizumab (anti–IL-6 receptor) is an alternative.
HHV-8-associated MCD	**Plasma cell type with HHV-8-positive plasmablasts.** Localised in the mantle zones; co-express IgM-λ. HHV-8 LANA-1 positive by IHC.	**HIV-positive patients overwhelmingly.** Coexists with Kaposi sarcoma in many cases. Episodic flares of fever and cytokine storm.	Rituximab is first-line (depletes HHV-8-infected B-cells). Antiviral therapy (valganciclovir) and HIV antiretroviral therapy adjunctive. Siltuximab not effective in HHV-8-driven disease.

HIGH-YIELD PEARL — Castleman highlights — lollipop, IL-6, HHV-8, POEMS

Lollipop sign: The hallmark histologic feature of hyaline-vascular Castleman is a regressed germinal centre penetrated by a hyalinised blood vessel — the "lollipop" or twinning pattern. Mantle zones are expanded in concentric onion-skin rings. Pathognomonic in the right clinical context.

IL-6 in iMCD: Idiopathic multicentric Castleman disease is driven by excess IL-6 production. The cytokine produces all the systemic features (fever, anaemia of inflammation, hypergammaglobulinaemia, elevated CRP, hepcidin elevation). Siltuximab (anti–IL-6) is FDA-approved for iMCD; tocilizumab (anti–IL-6 receptor) is an effective alternative.

HHV-8 family of diseases: HHV-8 (also called Kaposi sarcoma–associated herpesvirus, KSHV) causes three distinct B-cell lymphoproliferative disorders plus Kaposi sarcoma: (1) HHV-8-associated multicentric Castleman disease; (2) primary effusion lymphoma (PEL — body-cavity effusion lymphoma in HIV); (3) Kaposi sarcoma; and (4) HHV-8-positive germinotropic lymphoproliferative disorder. All occur predominantly in HIV-positive or otherwise immunosuppressed patients.

POEMS syndrome and Castleman: POEMS — Polyneuropathy, Organomegaly, Endocrinopathy, M-protein, Skin changes — is a plasma cell disorder that can coexist with Castleman disease (especially the multicentric form). The clinical presentation can resemble multiple myeloma but with prominent neuropathy and Castleman histology in lymph nodes.

11.17 Kikuchi–Fujimoto Disease

Kikuchi–Fujimoto disease (KFD) — also called histiocytic necrotising lymphadenitis — is a self-limiting cause of cervical lymphadenopathy that disproportionately affects young women of Asian descent, although it is reported worldwide. The aetiology is unknown; viral triggers (EBV, HHV-6, parvovirus B19) and autoimmune mechanisms have both been implicated. The condition resolves spontaneously over 1–4 months in the great majority of cases.

Clinical presentation

Tender cervical (especially posterior cervical) lymphadenopathy is the dominant feature, often unilateral. Low-grade fever, fatigue, night sweats, and arthralgia accompany the lymphadenopathy in ~50% of patients. Leukopenia with mild lymphopenia is common — atypical for a primary infection — and may mimic SLE. Skin involvement (rash on the face, trunk) occurs in a minority. The differential diagnosis prioritises lymphoma (especially Hodgkin or T-cell lymphoma in young patients), tuberculous lymphadenitis (high prevalence in endemic regions), and SLE lymphadenitis (which can be histologically similar).

Histology — the key distinguisher

The diagnostic features are well-circumscribed paracortical zones of necrosis with abundant karyorrhectic debris, surrounded by a striking population of crescentic histiocytes (plasmacytoid monocytes and dendritic cells) with engulfed nuclear material. Three negative findings clinch the diagnosis: ABSENCE of neutrophils within the necrotic foci (distinguishing from suppurative lymphadenitis from cat-scratch, tularaemia, or Yersinia); ABSENCE of plasma cells (distinguishing from many infectious lymphadenitides); and ABSENCE of granulomas (distinguishing from tuberculosis or sarcoidosis). The histiocytes express CD68 and myeloperoxidase; the surrounding lymphocytes are predominantly CD8+ T-cells.

HIGH-YIELD PEARL — Kikuchi — necrotising lymphadenitis WITHOUT neutrophils

The single best discriminator: Necrosis with karyorrhectic debris but NO neutrophils. Suppurative necrotising lymphadenitis (cat-scratch disease, tularaemia, Yersinia, lymphogranuloma venereum) shows necrosis with abundant neutrophils. The absence of neutrophils plus the presence of crescentic histiocytes is essentially specific for Kikuchi.

Demographics on USMLE: Young Asian woman with tender cervical lymphadenopathy, low-grade fever, mild leukopenia, and lymph node biopsy showing necrosis without neutrophils = Kikuchi–Fujimoto. Self-limited; reassurance and follow-up; no specific treatment needed in most cases (NSAIDs for symptoms; corticosteroids for severe systemic disease).

SLE follow-up: Approximately 10–30% of patients with Kikuchi–Fujimoto disease subsequently develop systemic lupus erythematosus. The histologic features overlap substantially (SLE lymphadenitis can be nearly indistinguishable from Kikuchi). All Kikuchi patients should have ANA and anti-dsDNA testing at diagnosis and periodic clinical follow-up for at least 1–2 years to evaluate for emerging SLE.

11.18 Buzzwords and Visual Cues

Single-phrase USMLE cues mapped to the most likely diagnosis. The cue often arrives at the answer faster than working through the differential.

Buzzword / Visual Cue	Most Likely Diagnosis
Atypical lymphocytes (Downey cells) on smear	Infectious mononucleosis (EBV)
Heterophile antibody (Monospot) positive	EBV mononucleosis
Ampicillin/amoxicillin rash in young patient with sore throat	Acute EBV mononucleosis (reactive rash, not true penicillin allergy)
VCA IgM positive + EBNA IgG negative	Acute primary EBV infection
VCA IgM negative + EBNA IgG positive	Past EBV infection / lifelong immunity (NOT acute)
Heterophile-negative mononucleosis in immunocompetent adult	CMV (most common); also Toxoplasma, primary HIV, hepatitis
Cervical lymphadenopathy + cat exposure	Toxoplasma gondii
Paroxysmal cough with inspiratory whoop + marked lymphocytosis with normal morphology	Pertussis (Bordetella pertussis)
WBC >50 × 10^9/L + left shift + LAP score HIGH	Leukemoid reaction
WBC >50 × 10^9/L + basophilia + eosinophilia + LAP score LOW	CML (BCR::ABL1)
Basophilia + eosinophilia + neutrophilia in unexplained leukocytosis	CML

Buzzword / Visual Cue	Most Likely Diagnosis
Persistent monocytosis ≥1 × 10^9/L AND ≥10% of WBC for ≥3 months + dysplasia	Chronic myelomonocytic leukaemia (CMML)
Asthma + eosinophilia + small/medium vessel vasculitis	Eosinophilic granulomatosis with polyangiitis (EGPA / Churg–Strauss)
Hypereosinophilia + cardiac (endomyocardial fibrosis) + neurologic features	Hypereosinophilic syndrome / FIP1L1-PDGFRA myeloid neoplasm
Travel to tropics + eosinophilia + planned immunosuppression	Strongyloides — test serology and treat with ivermectin BEFORE steroids
Black or West Indian patient with isolated mild neutropenia, no infections	Benign ethnic neutropenia (DARC/ACKR1 –46 C/C)
RA + splenomegaly + neutropenia	Felty syndrome
ANC <0.5 + fever ≥38.3 °C	Febrile neutropenia — empiric antipseudomonal β-lactam within 1 hour
Pancytopenia + hypocellular marrow + reticulocytes near zero	Aplastic anaemia
Pancytopenia + radial ray defects + café-au-lait + young patient	Fanconi anaemia — order DEB chromosome breakage test
Parvovirus B19 + chronic haemolytic anaemia (sickle, HS, thalassaemia)	Aplastic crisis (pure red cell aplasia)
Giant pronormoblasts with intranuclear "lantern" inclusions in marrow	Parvovirus B19 infection
Ferritin >10,000 μg/L + fever + cytopenias + splenomegaly	Haemophagocytic lymphohistiocytosis (HLH)
Haemophagocytosis on marrow biopsy + EBV-positive	EBV-driven secondary HLH
Coffee-bean nucleus + eosinophil-rich background + CD1a+ + langerin+	Langerhans cell histiocytosis
Birbeck granules on electron microscopy	LCH (pathognomonic)
BRAF V600E in histiocytic disorder	LCH (~50% of cases) — vemurafenib responsive
Lytic skull lesion in child + eosinophil-rich infiltrate	LCH — eosinophilic granuloma
Vertebra plana in child	LCH (single-system bone)

Buzzword / Visual Cue	Most Likely Diagnosis
Diabetes insipidus + lytic bone lesions in child	LCH with hypothalamic-pituitary involvement
Massive painless cervical lymphadenopathy + emperipolesis	Rosai–Dorfman disease
S100+, CD68+, CD1a NEGATIVE, CD207 NEGATIVE in histiocytic disorder	Rosai–Dorfman (NOT LCH)
Mediastinal mass + germinal centre with hyalinised vessel "lollipop" pattern	Unicentric Castleman disease (hyaline-vascular type)
Multicentric lymphadenopathy + IL-6 elevation + B symptoms (HIV-negative)	Idiopathic multicentric Castleman disease — siltuximab
Multicentric Castleman + HIV-positive + Kaposi sarcoma coexists	HHV-8-associated MCD — rituximab
Young Asian woman + tender cervical LAD + necrotising lymphadenitis WITHOUT neutrophils	Kikuchi–Fujimoto disease
Crescentic histiocytes + karyorrhectic debris + no neutrophils + no plasma cells	Kikuchi–Fujimoto
BCL2 NEGATIVE in germinal centres (with intact mantle zones)	Reactive follicular hyperplasia (NOT follicular lymphoma)
BCL2 POSITIVE in germinal centres	Follicular lymphoma (t(14;18))

11.19 USMLE Vignettes

Eight vignettes covering the chapter's high-yield diagnoses. Read each stem before the answer.

VIGNETTE 1

Stem. A 17-year-old girl presents with 1 week of severe sore throat, fatigue, and fever. She was given amoxicillin 4 days ago for presumed streptococcal pharyngitis and developed a confluent maculopapular rash on her trunk yesterday. Examination: temperature 38.5 °C, exudative pharyngitis, tender posterior cervical and axillary lymphadenopathy, splenomegaly. CBC: WBC 14 × 10^9/L with 60% lymphocytes (many atypical, large basophilic, irregular nuclei), platelets 130 × 10^9/L. AST 95 U/L. Heterophile antibody positive.

VIGNETTE 2

Stem. A 6-year-old boy presents with 3 weeks of progressive cough. The cough comes in violent paroxysms followed by an inspiratory whoop, often ending in vomiting. He is well between paroxysms and afebrile. CBC: WBC 32 × 10^9/L with 80% lymphocytes — all morphologically NORMAL (no atypical forms). Vaccinations are not up to date.

VIGNETTE 3

Stem. A 28-year-old previously healthy woman presents with fever (39.2 °C), productive cough, and right-sided pleuritic chest pain. CXR shows right lower lobe consolidation. CBC: WBC 65 × 10^9/L (markedly elevated), 75% neutrophils with toxic granulation, Döhle bodies, and cytoplasmic vacuolation, 12% bands, 4% metamyelocytes, 1% myelocytes; 0% blasts; basophils 1%; eosinophils 1%. Haemoglobin 12.0 g/dL, platelets 380 × 10^9/L. LAP score 280. Spleen tip palpable.

VIGNETTE 4

Stem. A 52-year-old woman emigrated from rural Brazil 8 years ago. She presents with newly diagnosed minimal-change disease and is about to start prednisone 60 mg daily. Routine pre-treatment labs reveal eosinophil count 1.8 × 10^9/L. She has no respiratory symptoms, no rash, and no travel since immigration.

VIGNETTE 5

Stem. A 9-year-old boy presents with progressive fatigue, easy bruising, and recurrent epistaxis over 4 months. Examination: pallor, scattered petechiae and ecchymoses, multiple café-au-lait macules on the trunk, short stature, and absent left thumb ("thumb hypoplasia"). CBC: haemoglobin 6.4 g/dL, MCV 102 fL, WBC 2.1 × 10^9/L (ANC 0.4), platelets 18 × 10^9/L, reticulocytes <10 × 10^9/L. Bone marrow biopsy: hypocellular (10%) with no blasts, dysplasia, or infiltrate.

VIGNETTE 6

Stem. A 4-year-old girl presents with 10 days of high fever, increasing fatigue, and abdominal distension. Examination: temperature 39.4 °C, hepatosplenomegaly (spleen 6 cm below costal margin). Hb 7.2 g/dL, WBC 1.8 × 10^9/L (ANC 0.5), platelets 38 × 10^9/L. Triglycerides 380 mg/dL, fibrinogen 1.2 g/L, ferritin 24,000 µg/L, AST 280 U/L. Bone marrow biopsy: macrophages engulfing red cells, platelets, and nucleated cells. EBV PCR positive (10^5 copies/mL).

VIGNETTE 7

Stem. A 5-year-old boy presents with a 6-week history of localised scalp tenderness over the right parietal region and recent onset of polyuria and polydipsia. Skull X-ray shows a lytic, punched-out lesion with sharp margins. Lesion biopsy: large cells with grooved, kidney-shaped "coffee-bean" nuclei and pale eosinophilic cytoplasm, embedded in an eosinophil-rich background. Immunohistochemistry: CD1a+, CD207 (langerin)+, S100+, BRAF V600E mutation detected.

VIGNETTE 8

Stem. A 24-year-old Korean-American woman presents with 3 weeks of tender right cervical lymphadenopathy and low-grade fever (37.8 °C), fatigue, and night sweats. Examination: 2.5 cm tender posterior cervical lymph node; no hepatosplenomegaly; faint malar erythema. CBC: WBC 3.2 × 10^9/L, lymphocytes 0.9 × 10^9/L, haemoglobin 12.4 g/dL, platelets 195 × 10^9/L. ANA 1:160 (titer borderline). Excisional lymph node biopsy: paracortical zones of necrosis with abundant karyorrhectic debris and crescentic histiocytes (CD68+); striking absence of neutrophils and plasma cells;

surrounding T-cells predominantly CD8+.

11.20 Closing Discriminators

Five closing distinctions worth carrying into the exam. Each compresses a recurring USMLE comparison.

HIGH-YIELD PEARL — Discriminator 1 — Leukemoid reaction vs CML

LAP score: HIGH (markedly elevated, often >150) in leukemoid reaction. LOW or ZERO in CML.

Basophilia and eosinophilia: ABSENT in leukemoid reaction. CHARACTERISTIC in CML (basophilia >5% is highly suggestive).

Identifiable trigger: Severe infection, haemolysis, malignancy with marrow involvement, or G-CSF in leukemoid reaction. Absent in CML.

Confirmation: BCR::ABL1 RT-PCR is positive in CML, negative in leukemoid reaction.

HIGH-YIELD PEARL — Discriminator 2 — LCH vs Rosai–Dorfman disease

Both: S100 POSITIVE; histiocytic disorder; lymphadenopathy possible; CD68 POSITIVE.

LCH only: CD1a POSITIVE; CD207 (langerin) POSITIVE; Birbeck granules on EM; coffee-bean nucleus; eosinophil-rich background; BRAF V600E in ~50%.

Rosai–Dorfman only: CD1a NEGATIVE; CD207 NEGATIVE; emperipolesis (intact lymphocytes within histiocyte cytoplasm); massive painless cervical lymphadenopathy; usually self-limited benign course.

HIGH-YIELD PEARL — Discriminator 3 — Necrotising lymphadenitis with vs without neutrophils

Necrosis WITH neutrophils (suppurative): Cat-scratch disease (Bartonella henselae) — stellate microabscesses; tularaemia (Francisella tularensis); Yersinia pseudotuberculosis; lymphogranuloma venereum (Chlamydia trachomatis L1–L3).

Necrosis WITHOUT neutrophils: Kikuchi–Fujimoto disease (crescentic histiocytes; young Asian women); SLE lymphadenitis (often very similar histologically — clinical context separates).

Granulomatous necrosis: Tuberculosis (caseating); fungal infection; cat-scratch (late stage).

HIGH-YIELD PEARL — Discriminator 4 — Reactive follicular hyperplasia vs follicular lymphoma

BCL2 IHC is the single most useful test: NEGATIVE in reactive germinal centres; POSITIVE in neoplastic germinal centres of follicular lymphoma.

Architecture: Reactive — preserved nodal architecture; mantle zones intact; germinal centres show polarity (light and dark zones); tingible body macrophages produce starry-sky pattern. Follicular lymphoma — effaced architecture; back-to-back follicles; loss of mantle zones; loss of polarity; no tingible body macrophages.

Molecular: t(14;18) IGH/BCL2 translocation in 80–90% of follicular lymphoma.

HIGH-YIELD PEARL — Discriminator 5 — Aplastic anaemia vs hypocellular MDS

Both: Pancytopenia; hypocellular bone marrow.

Aplastic anaemia: No dysplasia; no blasts; cytogenetics typically normal; mutations rare. Reticulocytes very low. Treatment is immunosuppressive therapy or HSCT.

Hypocellular MDS: Dysplasia present in at least one lineage (assess on aspirate smear); cytogenetic abnormalities common (-5/del(5q), -7/del(7q), +8, complex karyotype); mutations in TET2, SF3B1, ASXL1, RUNX1, etc. Different prognosis and treatment (azacitidine, decitabine, supportive care).

Why it matters: Aplastic anaemia responds to immunosuppression; MDS does not — and immunosuppression in undiagnosed MDS may accelerate progression. Always send full cytogenetics and a myeloid mutation panel on initial workup.

11.21 Quick Recall — One-Page Compression

QUICK RECALL — ONE-PAGE COMPRESSION

1. Differential is everything. Total WBC alone is meaningless. Identify the elevated lineage first; the differential narrows immediately.

2. Lineage map. Neutrophils: bacterial, inflammation, steroids, CML. Lymphocytes: viral (EBV, CMV), pertussis, CLL. Monocytes: TB, SBE, IBD, CMML. Eosinophils: NAACP. Basophils: CML, allergy.

3. Leukemoid vs CML. LAP score HIGH = leukemoid; LOW/ZERO = CML. Basophilia + eosinophilia + neutrophilia → CML. BCR::ABL1 confirms.

4. IM atypical lymphs. Activated CD8 T-cells, NOT EBV-infected B-cells. Heterophile positive ~85% adults; ampicillin rash in a high proportion (classically 80–95%, modern estimates 30–70%); no contact sports 4–6 weeks (splenic rupture).

5. EBV serology rule. VCA IgM+/EBNA IgG− = acute IM. VCA IgM−/EBNA IgG+ = past infection. EBNA IgG appears 6–12 weeks after primary infection.

6. Heterophile-negative mono. CMV (most common), Toxoplasma, primary HIV, acute hepatitis. Always include HIV in differential — primary HIV requires Ag/Ab plus viral load.

7. Pertussis. Marked lymphocytosis with NORMAL morphology (not atypical). Paroxysmal cough + whoop + post-tussive emesis. Azithromycin.

8. NAACP eosinophilia. Neoplasm (HES, FIP1L1-PDGFRA = imatinib), Allergy/atopy, Adrenal insufficiency, Connective tissue (EGPA), Parasites (helminths).

9. Strongyloides + steroids. Always test serology in any eosinophilia + travel history before high-dose corticosteroids or chemotherapy. Hyperinfection mortality 80–90%.

10. Benign ethnic neutropenia. DARC/ACKR1 −46 C/C in African ancestry. Persistent isolated mild-moderate neutropenia, no infections — reassure, no workup.

11. Felty syndrome. RA + splenomegaly + neutropenia. Increased infection risk; LGL leukaemia in differential.

12. Febrile neutropenia. ANC <0.5 + fever ≥38.3 °C → empiric anti-pseudomonal β-lactam (cefepime, pip-tazo, meropenem) within 1 hour. Add vancomycin only for specific indications.

13. Aplastic anaemia. Pancytopenia + hypocellular marrow + low retics; 80% autoimmune (CD8 T-cell mediated); Camitta criteria (cellularity <25% + 2 of 3 cytopenias) define severe.

14. AA management. Matched sibling donor + age ≤40–50 → alloHSCT first-line. No donor → IST = ATG (horse) + cyclosporine + eltrombopag. Eltrombopag added to first-line in 2018.

15. Fanconi anaemia. Autosomal recessive; FA-BRCA DNA repair pathway; pancytopenia + congenital anomalies (radial ray, café-au-lait); DEB/MMC chromosome breakage test; reduced-intensity HSCT conditioning mandatory.

16. Parvovirus B19. Pure red cell aplasia via P antigen receptor on erythroid progenitors. In chronic haemolytic anaemia → APLASTIC CRISIS. Giant pronormoblasts with intranuclear lantern inclusions.

17. LCH. CD1a+, CD207 (langerin)+, S100+ triad. Coffee-bean nucleus. Eosinophil-rich background. Birbeck granules on EM. BRAF V600E in ~50%.

18. HLH. 5 of 8 HLH-2004 criteria. Ferritin >10,000 ~90% PPV. EBV most common trigger. Treat with dexamethasone + etoposide + cyclosporine. Emapalumab (anti-IFN-γ, FDA 2018) for refractory.

19. Rosai–Dorfman. S100+, CD68+, CD1a NEGATIVE, CD207 NEGATIVE. Massive painless cervical LAD with emperipolesis (intact lymphocytes in histiocyte cytoplasm).

20. Castleman. HV unicentric ~90% — "lollipop" sign — surgical excision curative. iMCD — IL-6 driven — siltuximab. HHV-8 MCD — HIV+ — rituximab.

21. Kikuchi–Fujimoto. Necrotising lymphadenitis WITHOUT neutrophils. Young Asian women. Crescentic histiocytes. Self-limited 1–4 months. ~10–30% develop SLE — follow up with ANA.

22. BCL2 in germinal centres. NEGATIVE = reactive follicular hyperplasia. POSITIVE = follicular lymphoma (t(14;18)).

End of Chapter 11. Acute leukaemias (AML and ALL) continue in Chapter 12, the haematology block pilot.

CHAPTER 12

Chapter 12 — Acute Leukaemias: AML and ALL

BIG PICTURE

Acute leukaemias are clonal expansions of immature haematopoietic precursors that crowd out normal marrow function. The diagnostic question on the USMLE is rarely "is this a leukaemia" — it is "which lineage, which genetic driver, and what does that driver predict?" AML and ALL share a final common pathway of marrow failure and blast accumulation, but they diverge sharply in age, cytogenetics, treatment, and the buzzwords examiners use to flag them. Master the divergence and the chapter is yours.

MECHANISM HOOK — Why AML happens

AML is the product of two collaborating mutational classes acting on a single myeloid progenitor. Class I mutations (FLT3-ITD, KIT, RAS, BCR::ABL1) drive proliferation by activating tyrosine kinase or RAS signalling — they push the cell to divide. Class II mutations (PML::RARA, RUNX1::RUNX1T1, CBFB::MYH11, NPM1, CEBPA, KMT2A rearrangements) block differentiation by disrupting transcription factors that drive granulocytic and monocytic maturation — they prevent the cell from growing up. A proliferating cell that cannot mature is, by definition, an accumulating blast. The "two-hit" model explains why a single lesion is rarely enough: t(8;21) alone produces preleukaemic clones in healthy newborns and is detectable years before overt AML, but the disease emerges only when a cooperating signalling mutation is acquired. WHO 2022 reorganises AML around this biology — the recurrent genetic abnormality (the Class II event) defines the disease, and cooperating Class I mutations modulate prognosis.

12.1 AML — Definition, Pathogenesis, and WHO 2022 Classification

Acute myeloid leukaemia is a clonal malignancy of myeloid progenitors in which the differentiation block produces an accumulation of immature myeloid blasts in marrow and blood. The historical diagnostic threshold — twenty percent or more myeloid blasts in marrow or peripheral blood — remains the default, but WHO 2022 has eliminated the blast threshold for most genetically defined entities. AML with PML::RARA, RUNX1::RUNX1T1, CBFB::MYH11, NPM1 mutation, KMT2A rearrangement, MECOM rearrangement, NUP98 rearrangement, DEK::NUP214, and RBM15::MRTFA are now diagnosable at any blast count. The two genetic categories that still require ≥20% blasts are AML with BCR::ABL1 (to distinguish from CML in blast phase) and AML with CEBPA bZIP mutation. The conceptual move is decisive: the lesion is the disease, and the blast count is a residual descriptor. The concurrent ICC 2022 classification (Arber et al., Blood 2022) takes the opposite stance: ICC 2022 retains the ≥20% blast threshold across all AML categories, recognising the defining genetic lesions but not allowing them to override the morphological count. The two 2022 classifications therefore diverge most sharply at the low-blast end of the AML spectrum, and either may be cited in vignette stems.

Incidence is approximately 4 per 100,000 per year in the United States, with a median age at diagnosis near 68. AML is the most common acute leukaemia in adults but is uncommon in children, where ALL dominates. Therapy-related AML — arising after alkylating agents, topoisomerase II inhibitors, or radiation — is now grouped under AML, myelodysplasia-related (AML-MR) when no AML-defining fusion is present.

WHO 2022 categories at a glance

WHO 2022 entity	Defining feature	Blast threshold	Prognosis
AML with PML::RARA (APL)	t(15;17); HLA-DR negative; CD34 typically negative; CD117 bright; faggot cells	Any	Favourable with ATRA + arsenic; DIC and differentiation syndrome are the lethal complications
AML with RUNX1::RUNX1T1	t(8;21); aberrant CD19 on myeloid blasts; bright MPO; dyserythropoiesis common	Any	Favourable; >90% complete remission with standard induction
AML with CBFB::MYH11	inv(16) or t(16;16); abnormal marrow eosinophils with basophilic granules	Any	Favourable
AML with NPM1 mutation	Cytoplasmic NPM1 staining; CD34 typically negative; HLA-DR negative; cup-like nuclear invaginations	Any	Favourable only if FLT3-ITD is absent; intermediate when FLT3-ITD coexists
AML with KMT2A rearrangement	11q23 rearrangement; monocytic differentiation common; gum hypertrophy and skin lesions	Any	Adverse — except t(9;11)/MLLT3::KMT2A which is intermediate; menin inhibitors revumenib (KMT2A-r, NPM1) and ziftomenib (NPM1) now FDA-approved
AML with DEK::NUP214	t(6;9); marrow basophilia; FLT3-ITD frequently co-mutated	Any	Adverse
AML with BCR::ABL1	Ph-positive AML; must exclude CML in blast phase	≥20%	Adverse; TKI added to induction
AML with CEBPA bZIP mutation	In-frame bZIP domain mutation (single or biallelic)	≥20%	Favourable
AML, myelodysplasia-related	Prior MDS, MDS-related cytogenetics (−7, del(5q), complex), or MDS-related mutations (ASXL1, BCOR, EZH2, SF3B1, SRSF2, STAG2, U2AF1, ZRSR2)	≥20%	Adverse; subsumes most therapy-related AML without a defining fusion

WHO 2022 entity	Defining feature	Blast threshold	Prognosis
AML, NOS	No defining genetic abnormality; classified by differentiation (FAB-equivalent)	≥20%	Variable; depends on cytogenetics and cooperating mutations

Table 12.1. WHO 2022 categories of AML. Most genetically defined entities no longer require the 20% blast threshold; BCR::ABL1 and CEBPA bZIP are the surviving exceptions. ICC 2022 (the parallel international consensus, Arber et al., Blood 2022) keeps ≥20% blasts as the universal AML threshold across every category.

12.2 AML — Morphology, Cytochemistry, and Flow Cytometry

A myeloid blast on the smear is a medium-to-large cell with a high nuclear-to-cytoplasmic ratio, fine open chromatin, prominent nucleoli, and pale-blue cytoplasm that may contain primary azurophilic granules. The single most important morphological finding in AML is the Auer rod — a needle-shaped or rod-shaped reddish cytoplasmic inclusion formed by abnormal fusion of azurophilic granules. Auer rods are pathognomonic of myeloid lineage. Their presence excludes ALL. A bundle of Auer rods within a single cell — a "faggot cell" — is essentially diagnostic of acute promyelocytic leukaemia and demands ATRA before molecular confirmation arrives.

Cytochemistry remains useful where flow cytometry is unavailable and as a confirmatory layer in any laboratory. Myeloperoxidase (MPO) shows brown-black cytoplasmic granular positivity in myeloblasts and is the cytochemical gold standard for myeloid lineage. Sudan Black B parallels MPO and stains lipid in granules. Non-specific esterase (NSE) shows brick-red cytoplasmic positivity in monoblasts and promonocytes that is abolished by sodium fluoride — the defining stain for monocytic differentiation (FAB M4 and M5). Periodic acid-Schiff (PAS) shows coarse, chunky "block" positivity in B-lymphoblasts and in the dyserythropoietic precursors of erythroleukaemia. Terminal deoxynucleotidyl transferase (TdT) is a nuclear DNA polymerase expressed by lymphoid precursors; its presence flags ALL or mixed-phenotype acute leukaemia rather than typical AML.

Flow cytometry establishes lineage, identifies aberrant marker combinations, and provides a leukaemia-associated immunophenotype (LAIP) for measurable residual disease (MRD) monitoring. The myeloid panel includes CD13, CD33, CD117, MPO (intracellular), and CD34. Monocytic differentiation is captured by CD14, CD64, and CD11b. Megakaryocytic blasts express CD41 and CD61. Aberrant lymphoid antigens are common and informative — CD19 on a myeloid blast is the immunophenotypic signature of AML with t(8;21), and CD7 is a frequent aberrant marker on AML with adverse cytogenetics.

FAB subtypes within AML, NOS

FAB	Morphology	Flow	Clinical clue
M0 — minimal differentiation	Agranular blasts; no Auer rods; MPO negative by cytochemistry	CD34+, CD117+, HLA-DR+; intracellular MPO positive	Aggressive; lineage proven by flow MPO or ultrastructure

FAB	Morphology	Flow	Clinical clue
M1 — without maturation	Blasts ≥90% of non-erythroid; MPO+ ≥3%; few/no Auer rods	CD34+, CD117+, MPO+; absent CD15, CD11b	No maturing granulocytes
M2 — with maturation	Blasts 20–89%; Auer rods common; visible maturing granulocytes	CD13+, CD33+, MPO+, CD15+; CD19 if t(8;21)	Classic morphology of t(8;21)/RUNX1::RUNX1T1
M3 — APL (PML::RARA)	Hypergranular promyelocytes; bundles of Auer rods (faggot cells); bilobed/reniform nucleus in microgranular variant	CD117 bright, CD33 bright; HLA-DR negative; CD34 typically negative	DIC at presentation; ATRA on morphology — do not wait for molecular confirmation
M4 — myelomonocytic	Both granulocytic and monocytic populations; MPO+ and NSE+ subsets	CD13+, CD33+, CD14+, CD64+	Gum hypertrophy; M4 with eosinophilia → inv(16)
M5 — monocytic	Monoblasts and promonocytes >80% of non-erythroid; NSE+, MPO−	CD14 bright, CD64+, CD11b+; CD34 typically negative	Highest rate of gum infiltration, skin lesions, and CNS disease; t(9;11)/MLLT3::KMT2A common
M6 — erythroid	Erythroid predominance; dysplastic precursors; PAS-positive	CD71+, glycophorin A+ on erythroid component	Most cases now classified as AML-MR under WHO 2022
M7 — megakaryoblastic	Blasts with cytoplasmic blebs; marrow fibrosis common	CD41+, CD61+, CD42b+; MPO−	Down syndrome–associated AMKL in young children

Table 12.2. FAB subtypes within AML, NOS. The FAB scheme retains diagnostic utility within the NOS category and remains a vocabulary item examiners use freely.

HIGH-YIELD PEARL — CD19 on a myeloid blast

CD19 is the canonical pan-B marker, but its expression on otherwise myeloid blasts (CD13+, CD33+, MPO+, CD117+) is the immunophenotypic fingerprint of AML with RUNX1::RUNX1T1, t(8;21). The mechanism is direct: the RUNX1::RUNX1T1 fusion protein dysregulates a B-cell transcriptional program in myeloid cells. CD19 here does not make this MPAL — myeloid lineage is established by MPO, and a defining genetic abnormality (RUNX1::RUNX1T1) takes precedence over phenotype. On the USMLE, "CD19 on AML" → t(8;21) → favourable prognosis.

12.3 Acute Promyelocytic Leukaemia — The Haematological Emergency

APL is the AML the examiner wants you to recognise fastest. It is simultaneously the most curable acute leukaemia (long-term remission rates above 90% with ATRA plus arsenic trioxide) and the deadliest if mismanaged in the first 24 hours, because the abnormal promyelocytes release tissue factor and cancer procoagulant that drive a fulminant disseminated intravascular coagulation. Patients die from intracranial or pulmonary haemorrhage before chemotherapy can act. The therapeutic answer is mechanistic: the PML::RARA fusion protein binds the retinoic acid receptor in a high-affinity complex that blocks granulocytic differentiation. Pharmacological doses of all-trans retinoic acid (ATRA) overcome this block and force the malignant promyelocytes to mature into neutrophils. Arsenic trioxide degrades the PML::RARA protein outright. The combination cures most patients without conventional cytotoxic chemotherapy.

Recognition is on the smear. Hypergranular promyelocytes have heavy red-purple cytoplasmic granules that may obscure the nuclear contour, the nucleus is round to reniform with frequent indentations, and bundles of Auer rods within a single cell — faggot cells — are essentially diagnostic. The microgranular variant (M3v) lacks visible granules on light microscopy (granules are submicroscopic), shows a strikingly bilobed or reniform "butterfly" nucleus, and tends to present with a high white blood cell count and an even higher early haemorrhage risk. Both variants share the same molecular lesion and the same treatment.

Flow immunophenotype is the second confirmatory layer. APL blasts are CD117 bright, CD33 bright, MPO bright, with characteristic absence or dim expression of CD34 and HLA-DR — distinguishing APL from typical CD34-positive, HLA-DR-positive AML. CD13 expression is heterogeneous. Molecular confirmation is by RT-PCR for the PML::RARA fusion transcript or by FISH for t(15;17). Three transcript breakpoints exist (bcr1, bcr2, bcr3); all respond to ATRA, but the breakpoint identity is recorded for later MRD monitoring.

TRAP — "Correct the coagulopathy first, then start ATRA"

A common wrong answer on APL vignettes is the option that prioritises FFP, cryoprecipitate, and platelets before introducing ATRA. The reasoning feels surgical and disciplined, and it is wrong. ATRA addresses the cause of DIC (the procoagulant promyelocyte) and lowers death-from-haemorrhage; product support alone does not. The correct sequence is parallel, not sequential: ATRA is given on morphological suspicion, while the coagulopathy is corrected concurrently with cryoprecipitate (target fibrinogen >150 mg/dL [>1.5 g/L]), FFP, and platelets (target >30–50 × 10^9/L). Do not anticoagulate the DIC. Do not delay ATRA for molecular confirmation. The exam will reward the answer that starts ATRA first.

HIGH-YIELD PEARL — Differentiation syndrome (formerly ATRA syndrome)

In 15–25% of APL patients started on ATRA or arsenic trioxide, the differentiating blasts release inflammatory cytokines and infiltrate tissues, producing a syndrome of fever, weight gain, dyspnea, pulmonary infiltrates, pleural and pericardial effusions, hypotension, and acute kidney injury. The syndrome appears within the first three weeks of therapy and is fatal if untreated. Treatment is intravenous dexamethasone 10 mg twice daily; ATRA is held only if the syndrome is severe. Prophylactic dexamethasone is given when the presenting WBC exceeds 5–10 × 10^9/L. The renamed terminology (differentiation syndrome) reflects that arsenic trioxide produces the same picture by the same mechanism — it is not specific to ATRA.

12.4 ELN 2022 Risk Stratification and Treatment Implications

The European LeukemiaNet 2022 system is the lingua franca of AML prognosis on the wards and the exam. It collapses cytogenetics and molecular genetics into three risk groups that drive whether a patient receives consolidation chemotherapy alone or proceeds to allogeneic stem cell transplantation in first complete remission. The most important conceptual update from ELN 2017 is the simplification of NPM1 with FLT3-ITD: the allelic-ratio distinction is gone. Any FLT3-ITD with NPM1 mutation is now intermediate, regardless of ratio.

ELN 2022 group	Genetic criteria	Approx 5-y OS	Treatment
Favourable	t(8;21)/RUNX1::RUNX1T1; inv(16) or t(16;16)/CBFB::MYH11; NPM1 mutated WITHOUT FLT3-ITD; CEBPA in-frame bZIP mutation (single or biallelic)	>60%	Chemotherapy consolidation; alloSCT generally NOT required in first CR
Intermediate	NPM1 mutated WITH FLT3-ITD (any allelic ratio); NPM1 wild-type with FLT3-ITD; t(9;11)/MLLT3::KMT2A; cytogenetic/molecular findings not assigned to favourable or adverse	30–60%	Consider alloSCT in first CR; MRD-guided decision
Adverse	Monosomy 5, del(5q), monosomy 7, del(17p); complex karyotype (≥3 unrelated abnormalities); monosomal karyotype; t(6;9)/DEK::NUP214; t(v;11q23)/KMT2A-r (other than MLLT3); BCR::ABL1; TP53 mutation at VAF ≥10% (irrespective of mono- or biallelic status); ASXL1, BCOR, EZH2, RUNX1, SF3B1, SRSF2, STAG2, U2AF1, ZRSR2 mutations in absence of favourable	<20%	AlloSCT in first CR; venetoclax-based regimens; clinical trials

Table 12.3. ELN 2022 risk stratification.

STEP 2 BRIDGE — AML induction therapy

Standard induction for fit, non-APL AML is "7+3": cytarabine by continuous infusion for seven days plus an anthracycline (daunorubicin or idarubicin) for three days. FLT3-mutated AML adds midostaurin in newly diagnosed disease; quizartinib is approved with chemotherapy specifically for newly diagnosed FLT3-ITD AML. CD33-positive AML may receive gemtuzumab ozogamicin added to induction in favourable-risk and intermediate-risk disease. Older or unfit patients receive a hypomethylating agent (azacitidine or decitabine) plus venetoclax — a regimen with lower toxicity and durable responses, particularly in NPM1-mutated and IDH-mutated AML. Menin inhibitors — revumenib

(FDA-approved November 2024 for relapsed/refractory KMT2A-rearranged or NPM1-mutated acute leukaemia) and ziftomenib (FDA-approved 2025 for NPM1-mutated AML) — disrupt the menin–KMT2A interaction required for HOX/MEIS1 transcription and are now standard of care in relapsed disease for these subsets. APL is the exception: ATRA plus arsenic trioxide replaces conventional induction in low-to-intermediate-risk APL and produces cure without cytotoxic chemotherapy.

STEP 2 BRIDGE — When does an AML patient need allogeneic stem cell transplantation?

AlloSCT is mandatory in first complete remission for ELN-adverse AML, primary refractory AML, and relapsed AML in second remission. It is generally not required for ELN-favourable AML, where chemotherapy consolidation produces durable cures. Intermediate-risk disease is the decision-making zone; the modern answer is MRD-guided — patients who clear measurable residual disease after consolidation can defer transplant, while MRD-positive patients are referred. The rationale for transplant is the graft-versus-leukaemia (GVL) effect: donor T cells recognise residual leukaemic cells as alloantigenic and eliminate them, an immunological cure unavailable to autologous transplantation. The price is graft-versus-host disease, the central paradox of allo-transplantation. Reduced-intensity conditioning has expanded transplant eligibility into the seventh decade, where most AML actually presents.

STEP 2 BRIDGE — Tumour lysis syndrome — anticipate, do not react

Acute leukaemias with high tumour burden — ALL, particularly T-ALL with hyperleukocytosis or mediastinal mass, and high-WBC AML — collapse on starting cytotoxic therapy. Massive nucleic acid release floods the circulation with potassium, phosphate, and uric acid (a degradation product of purines via xanthine oxidase). Hyperphosphataemia drives hypocalcaemia and tetany; calcium phosphate deposits in renal tubules; uric acid crystals also obstruct tubules — together they cause acute kidney injury, the syndrome's most dangerous endpoint. Prophylaxis is layered: aggressive intravenous hydration to maintain a brisk urine output, allopurinol (a xanthine oxidase inhibitor that prevents new uric acid formation but does not lower existing uric acid), and rasburicase (a recombinant urate oxidase that converts existing uric acid to allantoin, lowering levels within hours). Rasburicase is preferred when baseline uric acid is already high or the tumour burden is large, and it is contraindicated in G6PD deficiency because the hydrogen peroxide byproduct triggers severe haemolysis. The classic exam pattern is the patient three days into induction with hyperkalaemia, hyperphosphataemia, hypocalcaemia, and rising creatinine.

12.5 ALL — Pathogenesis and WHO 2022 Classification

MECHANISM HOOK — Why ALL happens

ALL is the most common malignancy of childhood. It arises from a lymphoid progenitor that has been arrested at an early B-cell or T-cell developmental checkpoint. Two cooperating events drive the disease: a genetic lesion that perturbs lymphoid transcription factors (ETV6::RUNX1, TCF3::PBX1, KMT2A rearrangements, IKZF1 deletions, hyperdiploidy or hypodiploidy) and a second hit affecting the cell cycle, kinase signalling, or DNA repair. The B-cell receptor and T-cell receptor loci are uniquely vulnerable substrates because they undergo physiological RAG-mediated recombination during lymphoid development; aberrant recombination generates many of the recurrent translocations. Childhood B-ALL frequently begins in utero — t(12;21)/ETV6::RUNX1 is detectable on Guthrie cards from healthy newborns who later develop ALL years later, demonstrating that the founder lesion alone is insufficient and that environmental triggers (the "delayed-infection hypothesis") cooperate to produce overt disease. The therapeutic implication is direct: ALL responds to remission-induction chemotherapy that is fundamentally different from AML's 7+3 — vincristine, glucocorticoids, asparaginase, and an anthracycline, with mandatory CNS-directed therapy because the CNS is a sanctuary site.

ALL accounts for approximately 25% of cancers diagnosed in US children under 15 years of age and shows a peak incidence between ages 2 and 5. In adults it is uncommon but more aggressive. Hispanic and white children have higher incidence than Black children in the United States; this demographic distribution matters at the bedside and on the exam. T-ALL accounts for roughly 15% of childhood ALL and 25% of adult ALL.

WHO 2022 entity	Defining feature	Frequency	Prognosis
B-ALL with t(12;21)/ETV6::RUNX1	Cryptic translocation, not visible on conventional karyotype; detected by FISH or RT-PCR	~25% paediatric; ~3% adult	Favourable; >90% long-term survival in children
B-ALL with high hyperdiploidy	>50 chromosomes; trisomies of 4, 10, and 17 most favourable ("triple-trisomy")	~25% paediatric	Favourable; methotrexate accumulates avidly in hyperdiploid blasts
B-ALL with hypodiploidy	<44 chromosomes; near-haploid (<30) is the worst subset; TP53 mutations frequent in low-hypodiploid	~5%	Very poor; near-haploid <20% OS; alloSCT in first CR
B-ALL with t(9;22)/BCR::ABL1 (Ph+)	p190 most common in ALL (vs p210 in CML); TKI-sensitive	~25% adult; 3–5% paediatric	Historically poor; transformed by TKI integration
B-ALL, BCR::ABL1-like (Ph-like)	Gene-expression profile identical to BCR::ABL1+ ALL but no fusion	15% paediatric;	Poor without TKI; precision-medicine

WHO 2022 entity	Defining feature	Frequency	Prognosis
	present; activated kinase signalling from CRLF2-r, JAK2 mutations, ABL-class fusions, PDGFRB, NTRK fusions	25–30% AYA/adult	target
B-ALL with KMT2A rearrangement	t(4;11)/KMT2A::AFF1 most common; many partners; defines infant ALL	~5% overall; ~80% of infant ALL	Very poor; menin inhibitors (revumenib FDA-approved Nov 2024 for relapsed/refractory KMT2A-r acute leukaemia); alloSCT in first CR
B-ALL with t(1;19)/TCF3::PBX1	Classical "pre-B" phenotype with cytoplasmic mu	~5% paediatric	Intermediate; good with intensified therapy
B-ALL with iAMP21	Intrachromosomal amplification of chromosome 21	~2%	Poor without intensified therapy
T-ALL	NOTCH1 mutations in >50%; TAL1, LMO2, TLX1 rearrangements; CDKN2A/B deletion frequent; ETP-ALL (early T-cell precursor) is a distinct very-aggressive subset	15% paediatric; 25% adult	Intermediate; NOTCH1/FBXW7 mutated cases do better; nelarabine in T-cell directed therapy

Table 12.4. WHO 2022 classification of ALL.

12.6 ALL — Clinical Features and Immunophenotyping

The clinical presentation reflects two processes: marrow failure (anaemia, neutropenic fever, bleeding from thrombocytopenia) and lymphoid tissue infiltration. Lymphadenopathy and hepatosplenomegaly are common. Bone pain — particularly at night and in long-bone metaphyses — is a frequent and underappreciated feature in children. T-ALL classically presents with a mediastinal (anterior mediastinum / thymic) mass; the mass may compress the superior vena cava and produce facial swelling, plethora, distended neck veins, and dyspnea — the SVC syndrome. CNS involvement at presentation is detectable in approximately 5% of patients but occult disease is universal, which is why intrathecal methotrexate (with or without cytarabine and hydrocortisone) is given to every ALL patient as CNS prophylaxis. Testicular relapse is a late, sanctuary-site relapse phenomenon unique to B-ALL in boys.

On the smear, lymphoblasts are medium-sized cells with high N:C ratio, fine open chromatin (more open than mature lymphocytes, less open than myeloblasts), inconspicuous nucleoli, and scant agranular cytoplasm. Auer rods are absent — their presence excludes ALL absolutely. Smudge cells (Gumprecht shadows) are common because lymphoblasts are mechanically fragile. The traditional FAB L1/L2/L3 morphological subtyping has been superseded by immunophenotypic and genetic classification, with the historical exception that

L3 morphology (basophilic vacuolated cytoplasm, "starry sky" pattern in nodes) corresponds to mature B-cell neoplasia — Burkitt lymphoma/leukaemia — and is treated as a distinct disease, not as B-ALL.

Immunophenotype and lineage assignment

Marker	B-ALL early pre-B	B-ALL common/pre-B	T-ALL	Significance
TdT	+	+	+	Marker of immaturity; absent in mature B and T neoplasms
CD34	+	+ (most)	± (some)	Progenitor marker; absent in some subtypes (ETV6::RUNX1)
HLA-DR	+	+	NEGATIVE	T-ALL is HLA-DR negative — useful B vs T discriminator
CD19	+	+	–	Pan-B; aberrant on AML with t(8;21) — does NOT make MPAL
cCD79a (cytoplasmic)	+	+	–	Earliest committed B-lineage marker
CD10 (CALLA)	–	+ (common ALL)	±	Defines "common ALL" subtype
CD20	– or dim	Variable	–	Rituximab target; positivity may guide therapy in B-ALL
cCD3 (cytoplasmic)	–	–	+ (lineage-specific)	The ONLY T-lineage-specific marker; surface CD3 is absent in T-ALL
CD7	–	–	+ (most)	T-lineage but not specific; also on some NK and AML
CD5	–	–	+ (most)	Also on CLL and mantle cell — mature B-cell neoplasms
MPO	–	–	–	If positive: reconsider AML or MPAL

Table 12.5. Immunophenotype of ALL.

HIGH-YIELD PEARL — Haematogones are not B-ALL blasts

Haematogones are normal immature B-cell precursors that expand in the marrow during regeneration after chemotherapy, after stem cell transplant, and during recovery from parvovirus B19 — and they are abundant in healthy young children. They can morphologically mimic B-ALL blasts and are the single most common reason a B-ALL relapse is wrongly diagnosed. Flow cytometry is the discriminator. Haematogones show a CONTINUOUS spectrum of B-cell maturation: CD34 high then falling, CD10 high then falling, CD20 progressively rising, surface immunoglobulin appearing at the most mature end. B-ALL blasts are DISCRETE: a single aberrant population in which all cells express the same markers at the same intensity, with no maturation spectrum. Aberrant antigen co-expression (CD33, CD13, or CD7) and uniform CD45-dim staining without progression also flag malignancy. The clinical setting — recovery after induction in a child whose disease was MRD-negative — should raise haematogone suspicion before re-induction is ordered.

Ph-like (BCR::ABL1-like) ALL — the precision-medicine pivot

Ph-like ALL is the most consequential emerging concept in B-ALL. These leukaemias have a gene-expression signature indistinguishable from BCR::ABL1-positive ALL — the same transcriptional fingerprint of activated kinase signalling — but they lack the BCR::ABL1 fusion. The activating lesions are diverse and individually rare: rearrangements of CRLF2 (P2RY8::CRLF2 or IGH::CRLF2; together the most common Ph-like driver, frequently co-mutated with JAK1/2 mutations); ABL-class fusions involving ABL1, ABL2, CSF1R, or PDGFRB (sensitive to ABL-class TKIs such as imatinib and dasatinib); JAK2 fusions (sensitive to ruxolitinib); EPOR rearrangements; and NTRK fusions (sensitive to larotrectinib or entrectinib). Each driver is targetable, but identification requires genomic profiling — typically RNA sequencing — because the lesions are individually too rare for a routine FISH panel to capture them all.

Clinical implications are direct. Ph-like ALL accounts for approximately 15% of paediatric and 25–30% of adolescent/young-adult and adult B-ALL. Outcomes with conventional chemotherapy alone are poor — relapse rates exceed 50%. Outcomes with chemotherapy plus a TKI directed at the specific driver approach those of Ph-positive ALL with imatinib. The exam-level point: in a young adult with B-ALL, aggressive disease, IKZF1 deletion, and BCR::ABL1 negative by FISH, think Ph-like and order RNA sequencing.

IMG-TRAP — Ph-like ALL is invisible to a "Ph chromosome" workup

Trainees who learned haematology in laboratories where the standard ALL workup ends at "send a Ph chromosome by FISH" will systematically misclassify Ph-like ALL. The disease was named for its kinase-activated transcriptional signature, not its cytogenetics; conventional karyotype is normal in many cases, BCR::ABL1 FISH is negative by definition, and a CRLF2 rearrangement requires a CRLF2-specific FISH probe or a transcriptomic assay. On the USMLE, a young adult with B-ALL, normal cytogenetics, BCR::ABL1 negative, IKZF1 deletion, and poor response to standard induction is the Ph-like prompt. The correct answer choice will mention RNA-based screening, kinase-fusion panels, or gene-expression profiling. Do not pick "no further testing required" because the karyotype is normal.

IMG-TRAP — ALL demographics on the USMLE follow US epidemiology

Subtype frequencies in published global series differ substantially from the US distributions used to construct USMLE vignettes. ETV6::RUNX1 is the most common paediatric B-ALL subtype in US and European series and is the implicit "favourable" backdrop for childhood ALL vignettes. Hispanic and white children in the US have higher incidence than Black children, and the peak age is 2 to 5 years. Ph-like ALL is enriched in Hispanic populations and in adolescents and young adults. T-ALL is more common in adolescent boys. Down syndrome confers a 10–20-fold increased ALL risk, and Down syndrome–associated ALL has its own biology (CRLF2 rearrangement is overrepresented and often co-occurs with JAK2 mutation). On the exam, do not import non-US epidemiology into a vignette — the answer key uses US baseline rates. A 4-year-old white boy with bruising, lymphadenopathy, and lymphoblasts is statistically B-ALL with t(12;21), and the favourable-prognosis distractor is correct.

12.7 AML versus ALL — Distinguishing Features

Two questions decide the lineage assignment in any acute leukaemia: are there Auer rods on the smear, and is MPO positive? An Auer rod establishes myeloid lineage on its own and rules out ALL. MPO positivity by cytochemistry or by flow cytometry establishes myeloid lineage in the absence of Auer rods. TdT positivity, in contrast, points toward lymphoid lineage but is not lineage-specific — TdT is also expressed on a minority of AMLs and on the lymphoblastic phase of CML. The single specific T-lineage marker is cytoplasmic CD3 (cCD3). The B-lineage diagnosis requires strong CD19 plus at least one of CD79a, cytoplasmic CD22, or CD10 (or weak CD19 with at least two of these).

Feature	AML	ALL
Peak age	Adults; median ~68 years; M0/M1 in elderly	Children 2–5 years; second smaller adult peak
Auer rods	Present (esp. M2, M3)	ABSENT — pathognomonically excluded
MPO cytochemistry	Positive (≥3% blasts)	Negative
TdT	Negative (rare aberrant +)	Positive in B-ALL and T-ALL
PAS	Diffuse/fine; positive in M6 erythroid	Coarse "block" positive in B-lineage
Flow lineage marker	CD13, CD33, CD117, intracellular MPO	B: CD19 + cCD79a + CD10 or cCD22; T: cCD3
Mediastinal mass	Uncommon (myeloid sarcoma rare)	T-ALL — classic anterior mediastinal mass with SVC syndrome
Gum hypertrophy / skin lesions	Monocytic (M4, M5) and KMT2A-r	Uncommon
CNS sanctuary disease	Most common in M4/M5 and APL	Universal — intrathecal prophylaxis mandatory in all
Tumour lysis risk	Moderate; high in hyperleukocytic AML	HIGH — especially T-ALL with mediastinal mass and hyperleukocytosis
Induction backbone	"7+3" cytarabine + anthracycline; ATRA + ATO for APL; HMA + venetoclax in unfit	Vincristine, glucocorticoid, asparaginase, anthracycline; intrathecal methotrexate; TKI if Ph+
Cure rate	Variable — APL >90%; favourable AML 60–70%; adverse <20% without alloSCT	Paediatric overall ~90%; adult 30–50%; Ph+ improved with TKI

Table 12.6. AML versus ALL — discriminating features.

12.8 Buzzwords and Associations — Vignette Trigger Table

The vignette buzzword is the writer's gift to the reader. Examiners insert specific phrases to trigger specific diagnoses. The table below catalogues the highest-yield associations across acute leukaemias. Memorising it converts dense vignette stems into single-step recognition.

Vignette buzzword / finding	Diagnosis to trigger	One-line "why"
Faggot cells (bundles of Auer rods)	APL — AML with PML::RARA, t(15;17)	Abnormal granule fusion in promyelocytes; pathognomonic
DIC at presentation in acute leukaemia	APL until proven otherwise	Promyelocyte granules release tissue factor and cancer procoagulant
Auer rods + maturing granulocytes + young adult	AML with t(8;21) / RUNX1::RUNX1T1	M2 morphology; CD19 aberrant on blasts; favourable
Marrow eosinophilia with abnormal basophilic granules	AML with inv(16) / CBFB::MYH11	Bilineal differentiation; favourable
Cup-like nuclear invaginations on blasts; CD34 negative; HLA-DR negative	AML with NPM1 mutation	NPM1 mutation aberrant cytoplasmic localisation; FLT3-ITD modulates risk
Gum hypertrophy and skin lesions	Monocytic AML (M4/M5) — often KMT2A rearranged	Monocytic homing to oral mucosa and skin
Myeloid sarcoma (chloroma) at orbit in a child	AML — frequently with t(8;21)	Extramedullary myeloid mass; classify as AML regardless of marrow
Prior breast cancer chemo; new pancytopenia 5–7 years later	Therapy-related AML / AML, myelodysplasia-related	Alkylator latency 5–7 yr; topo-II inhibitor latency 1–3 yr
Down syndrome neonate with circulating blasts that resolve	Transient abnormal myelopoiesis (TAM) — GATA1 mutation	20% progress to ML-DS / acute megakaryoblastic leukaemia by age 4
Adolescent boy with mediastinal mass + lymphocytosis + SVC syndrome	T-ALL	Thymic origin; cCD3+, HLA-DR negative; high TLS risk
Bone pain in a child waking at night; pancytopenia	B-ALL	Marrow infiltration; check smear for blasts
Infant <12 months with hyperleukocytosis and CNS disease	B-ALL with KMT2A rearrangement (t(4;11))	80% of infant ALL is KMT2A-r; very poor prognosis
Adult B-ALL with t(9;22)	Ph+ B-ALL with BCR::ABL1	p190 most common in ALL; add TKI to chemo

Vignette buzzword / finding	Diagnosis to trigger	One-line "why"
Young adult B-ALL, normal karyotype, BCR::ABL1 negative, IKZF1 deletion, poor response	Ph-like ALL	Kinase-activated; needs RNA-seq or kinase-fusion panel
Coarse "block" PAS positivity in lymphoblasts	B-ALL	Glycogen accumulation; classical PAS pattern
Brisk fall in counts after starting induction; rising K, PO_4, urate; falling Ca; AKI	Tumour lysis syndrome	Massive nucleic acid release; rasburicase; aggressive hydration

Table 12.7. Vignette buzzwords and the diagnoses they should trigger.

12.9 USMLE Vignettes

The vignettes below mirror Step 1 and Step 2 CK testing patterns. Stems include the specific lab values and morphological descriptors examiners use as diagnostic anchors. After each correct answer, the rationale walks through the mechanism, and the distractor analysis explains why each wrong answer was placed in the option set.

Vignette 1. A 42-year-old woman with bleeding gums and a coagulopathy

A 42-year-old woman presents to the emergency department with bleeding gums, easy bruising, and fatigue for one week. She has not had fever. Vital signs are temperature 37.2°C, pulse 98/min, blood pressure 118/72 mm Hg. Examination shows mucosal petechiae, bilateral conjunctival haemorrhages, and ecchymoses on both forearms. There is no lymphadenopathy or splenomegaly. Laboratory studies: haemoglobin 8.6 g/dL (86 g/L), platelets 18,000/µL, white blood cells 2,400/µL with 32% blasts. PT is 22 seconds (control 12), aPTT 48 seconds (control 30), fibrinogen 88 mg/dL (0.88 g/L), and D-dimer is markedly elevated. Peripheral smear shows medium-to-large blasts with abundant cytoplasmic azurophilic granules; several blasts contain bundles of needle-shaped reddish cytoplasmic inclusions. A bone marrow biopsy is pending, and FISH for t(15;17) has been sent. Which of the following is the most appropriate next step in management?

- **(A)** Begin all-trans retinoic acid (ATRA) immediately while supporting the coagulopathy with cryoprecipitate, fresh frozen plasma, and platelets.
- **(B)** Withhold all chemotherapy until the FISH result for t(15;17) and the bone marrow morphology are available.
- **(C)** Initiate "7+3" induction with cytarabine and an anthracycline, and treat the coagulopathy with heparin to prevent further fibrin consumption.
- **(D)** Transfuse cryoprecipitate, fresh frozen plasma, and platelets to correct the coagulopathy, and reassess for chemotherapy after fibrinogen exceeds 200 mg/dL.
- **(E)** Perform plasma exchange to remove the procoagulant factors, and start cytotoxic chemotherapy after PT and aPTT normalise.

Best answer: **(A) Begin all-trans retinoic acid (ATRA) immediately while supporting the coagulopathy with cryoprecipitate, fresh frozen plasma, and platelets.**

Rationale. Faggot cells (bundles of Auer rods within a single hypergranular promyelocyte) plus a coagulopathy with hypofibrinogenaemia and elevated D-dimer establish a clinical diagnosis of acute promyelocytic leukaemia (AML with PML::RARA, t(15;17)). The promyelocyte granules release tissue factor and cancer procoagulant, driving disseminated intravascular coagulation that kills patients within hours of presentation if untreated. ATRA binds the PML::RARA fusion protein and forces the malignant promyelocytes to differentiate into mature granulocytes, eliminating the procoagulant source and addressing the cause of the DIC. Product support is given concurrently — cryoprecipitate to maintain fibrinogen above 150 mg/dL, FFP for global coagulation factor replacement, and platelets above 30–50 × 10^9/L. ATRA is started on morphological suspicion alone; molecular confirmation (PML::RARA RT-PCR, t(15;17) FISH) is sent urgently but does not gate therapy.

Distractor analysis. (B) Delaying ATRA for confirmatory testing is a common wrong answer driven by procedural caution; the time cost is paid in fatal haemorrhage. (C) "7+3" is the induction backbone for non-APL AML; APL is treated with ATRA + arsenic trioxide. Heparin in APL DIC is harmful. (D) Correcting the coagulopathy first removes a marker but not the cause — the DIC will recur until the malignant promyelocytes are differentiated or destroyed. (E) Plasma exchange has no role in APL DIC; the fix is mechanistic, not removal.

Vignette 2. A 28-year-old man with fatigue, gingival bleeding, and circulating blasts

A 28-year-old man presents with two months of progressive fatigue, gingival bleeding when brushing his teeth, and a recent painless bruise on his thigh. He has no significant past medical history. Examination shows pallor, mild gingival hypertrophy, and scattered ecchymoses; no lymphadenopathy or organomegaly. Laboratory studies: haemoglobin 7.4 g/dL, platelets 22,000/μL, white blood cells 12,000/μL with 65% blasts. The peripheral smear shows medium-to-large blasts with a high nuclear-to-cytoplasmic ratio, fine open chromatin, prominent nucleoli, pale-blue cytoplasm with occasional azurophilic granules, and a single needle-shaped reddish cytoplasmic inclusion in some cells. A bone marrow biopsy shows 78% blasts. Cytochemistry demonstrates MPO positivity in approximately 40% of the blast population; non-specific esterase is negative. Which of the following is the most likely diagnosis?

- **(A)** Acute lymphoblastic leukaemia (ALL).
- **(B)** Acute myeloid leukaemia (AML).
- **(C)** Mixed-phenotype acute leukaemia (MPAL).
- **(D)** Chronic myeloid leukaemia in blast phase.
- **(E)** Reactive lymphocytosis from acute viral infection.

Best answer: (B) Acute myeloid leukaemia (AML).

Rationale. The needle-shaped reddish cytoplasmic inclusion is an Auer rod, formed by abnormal fusion of azurophilic primary granules. Auer rods are pathognomonic of myeloid lineage and exclude ALL absolutely. MPO positivity by cytochemistry confirms myeloid lineage; the threshold for myeloid assignment by cytochemistry is ≥3% of blasts MPO-positive, which is far exceeded here. Gingival hypertrophy raises the possibility of monocytic differentiation (M4 or M5), but NSE-negative rules out the monocytic component, leaving an MPO-positive AML — most consistent with M2 morphology. The patient should now have flow cytometry, conventional karyotype with FISH, and an NGS panel including FLT3, NPM1, CEBPA, IDH1/2, and TP53 to refine the WHO 2022 entity and ELN 2022 risk group.

Distractor analysis. (A) Auer rods exclude ALL. (C) MPAL requires demonstration of more than one lineage (MPO + cCD3, or strong CD19 with cCD79a/cCD22/CD10) on the same blast population — not yet established here, and the cytochemistry alone supports myeloid only. (D) CML in blast phase requires a preceding chronic phase, splenomegaly, and BCR::ABL1; not described. (E) Reactive lymphocytosis does not produce 78% marrow blasts and does not contain Auer rods.

Vignette 3. A 22-year-old woman with newly diagnosed AML and a favourable cytogenetic abnormality

A 22-year-old woman is found on routine pre-employment evaluation to have haemoglobin 9.2 g/dL, platelets 64,000/μL, and white blood cells 8,000/μL with 22% blasts. She is asymptomatic. Examination is unremarkable. A bone marrow biopsy is performed: 60% myeloid blasts with maturing granulocytes, frequent Auer rods, and dyserythropoiesis. Flow cytometry shows blasts that are CD13+, CD33+, CD117+, MPO+, CD15+, CD34+, and aberrantly CD19-positive. Conventional karyotype shows t(8;21)(q22;q22). Which of the following is the most accurate prognostic assessment for this patient?

- **(A)** Adverse risk; alloSCT in first complete remission is mandatory.
- **(B)** Adverse risk because of the aberrant CD19 expression on myeloid blasts.
- **(C)** Favourable risk; standard induction and consolidation chemotherapy without alloSCT is expected to produce a durable remission.
- **(D)** Intermediate risk; alloSCT decision should be guided by measurable residual disease after consolidation.
- **(E)** Acute promyelocytic leukaemia; treat with ATRA plus arsenic trioxide.

Best answer: (C) Favourable risk; standard induction and consolidation chemotherapy without alloSCT is expected to produce a durable remission.

Rationale. The t(8;21)(q22;q22) translocation produces the RUNX1::RUNX1T1 fusion, which is the defining lesion of one of the core-binding factor AMLs. The companion entity is inv(16) or t(16;16) producing CBFB::MYH11. Both are ELN 2022 favourable-risk AMLs and respond to standard induction (cytarabine + anthracycline) followed by high-dose cytarabine consolidation, with cure rates of 60–70% and complete remission rates above 90%. Allogeneic stem cell transplantation in first CR is not required and is generally reserved for relapse. Aberrant CD19 expression on myeloid blasts is the immunophenotypic hallmark of t(8;21) — it is not a prognostic modifier, simply a marker of the underlying genetic lesion.

Distractor analysis. (A) Confuses RUNX1::RUNX1T1 (favourable) with monosomal/complex karyotype or TP53 (adverse). (B) CD19 here is a fingerprint, not a risk factor. (D) Intermediate risk would be NPM1+FLT3-ITD or KMT2A:MLLT3 — not t(8;21). (E) APL is t(15;17)/PML::RARA, not t(8;21); ATRA + arsenic does not apply here.

Vignette 4. A 64-year-old woman with new pancytopenia six years after breast cancer treatment

A 64-year-old woman with a history of stage II hormone-receptor-positive breast cancer treated with lumpectomy, radiation, and four cycles of doxorubicin plus cyclophosphamide six years ago presents with two months of fatigue and recurrent sinopulmonary infections. She has been in remission from breast cancer. Examination shows pallor and scattered oral petechiae with mild gingival pallor; no lymphadenopathy. Laboratory studies: haemoglobin 8.0 g/dL, platelets 38,000/µL, white blood cells 1,800/µL with 18% blasts. A bone marrow biopsy shows a hypercellular marrow with 32% myeloid blasts, multilineage dysplasia, and ring sideroblasts on iron stain. Karyotype shows del(5q), monosomy 7, and an additional unrelated structural abnormality. NGS demonstrates a TP53 mutation with a variant allele frequency of 38% and an ASXL1 mutation. Which of the following best classifies this leukaemia under WHO 2022?

- **(A)** Acute myeloid leukaemia with PML::RARA.
- **(B)** Acute myeloid leukaemia, myelodysplasia-related (AML-MR).
- **(C)** Acute myeloid leukaemia with NPM1 mutation.
- **(D)** Myelodysplastic syndrome with multilineage dysplasia.
- **(E)** Acute myeloid leukaemia with CEBPA bZIP mutation.

Best answer: (B) Acute myeloid leukaemia, myelodysplasia-related (AML-MR).

Rationale. The blast count (32%) exceeds the 20% threshold required for AML categories that lack a defining genetic fusion. The patient has all three WHO 2022 features that establish AML-MR: prior cytotoxic therapy with an alkylating agent (cyclophosphamide) and an anthracycline (doxorubicin), MDS-related cytogenetics (del(5q), −7, complex karyotype with ≥3 abnormalities), and MDS-related mutations (ASXL1). Under WHO 2022, therapy-related AML is folded into AML-MR when no AML-defining fusion is present. The TP53 mutation at VAF ≥10% is independently sufficient to designate this as ELN 2022 adverse risk and is biologically distinct enough that the ICC 2022 classification recognises AML with mutated TP53 (VAF ≥10%) as a separate adverse-risk entity distinct from AML-MR, whereas WHO HAEM5 retains TP53 as a defining biomarker within AML-MR. Latency of 5–7 years after alkylator exposure is classical (versus 1–3 years for topoisomerase II inhibitors with KMT2A rearrangement). Treatment is generally with hypomethylating agent + venetoclax for unfit patients, and alloSCT is the only intervention with curative potential; outcomes are poor regardless.

Distractor analysis. (A) PML::RARA AML is t(15;17) APL, not described here. (C) NPM1-mutated AML lacks MDS-related cytogenetics or mutations and is favourable when FLT3-ITD is absent. (D) MDS requires <20% blasts; this patient has 32% blasts. (E) CEBPA bZIP AML is favourable risk and not associated with prior chemotherapy or MDS-related cytogenetics.

Vignette 5. A 78-year-old man with a known MDS history and worsening counts

A 78-year-old man has been followed for two years for low-risk myelodysplastic syndrome with a baseline haemoglobin of 9.5 g/dL and platelets of 90,000/µL. He now presents with worsening fatigue. Laboratory studies: haemoglobin 7.2 g/dL, platelets 28,000/µL, white blood cells 1,400/µL with 14% blasts. Bone marrow examination shows a hypercellular marrow with 24% myeloid blasts, trilineage dysplasia, and an absence of Auer rods. Karyotype: 46,XY,del(20q). NGS: SF3B1 mutation (VAF 42%), SRSF2 mutation (VAF 18%). FISH for PML::RARA, RUNX1::RUNX1T1, and CBFB::MYH11 is negative. Which of the following is the most accurate diagnosis under WHO 2022?

- **(A)** Refractory anaemia with excess blasts (RAEB) — terminology is preferred under WHO 2022.
- **(B)** Acute myeloid leukaemia with NPM1 mutation.
- **(C)** Acute myeloid leukaemia, myelodysplasia-related (AML-MR).
- **(D)** Chronic myelomonocytic leukaemia (CMML).
- **(E)** Aplastic anaemia with secondary blast accumulation.

Best answer: (C) Acute myeloid leukaemia, myelodysplasia-related (AML-MR).

Rationale. The 24% blast count exceeds the 20% threshold that separates AML from MDS, and the patient meets multiple AML-MR-defining criteria simultaneously: prior MDS history, multilineage dysplasia, and the WHO 2022–defined MDS-related mutations SF3B1 and SRSF2. (The other defining mutations are ASXL1, BCOR, EZH2, STAG2, U2AF1, and ZRSR2.) The translocation panel is negative, so no AML-defining fusion is present to override the MDS-related qualifier. The diagnosis is AML-MR, and the prognosis is intermediate-to-adverse depending on the cytogenetic complexity and patient fitness. Treatment in this 78-year-old is most likely a hypomethylating agent (azacitidine) with venetoclax; intensive induction is generally not appropriate for this fitness profile.

Distractor analysis. (A) RAEB is the older WHO 2008 terminology; current WHO HAEM5 uses MDS with increased blasts (MDS-IB, 5–19% blasts); ICC 2022 instead creates a separate MDS/AML overlap category for 10–19% blasts, recognising the biological continuum at this interface. (B) NPM1-mutated AML is diagnosed at any blast count but requires NPM1 mutation, which is not present. (D) CMML requires sustained peripheral monocytosis ≥1 × 10^9/L plus monocytic dysplasia; the WBC differential here does not establish that. (E) Aplastic anaemia is a hypocellular marrow without blast accumulation; this marrow is hypercellular with 24% blasts.

Vignette 6. A 4-year-old boy with bruising, lymphadenopathy, and a high WBC

A 4-year-old previously healthy boy is brought in with three weeks of fatigue, intermittent low-grade fevers, and easy bruising. His mother reports that he has been waking at night complaining of pain in his legs. Examination shows pallor, scattered ecchymoses, bilateral non-tender cervical lymphadenopathy, and a palpable spleen tip. Laboratory studies: haemoglobin 7.2 g/dL, platelets 26,000/µL, white blood cells 38,000/µL with 72% blasts. The peripheral smear shows medium-sized blasts with high N:C ratio, fine chromatin, scant agranular cytoplasm, and no Auer rods. Flow cytometry on the blast population: CD45 dim, TdT positive, CD34+, HLA-DR+, CD19+, cCD79a+, CD10 bright, CD20 dim, and MPO negative. FISH demonstrates t(12;21)(p13;q22). Which of the following is the most accurate prognostic statement?

(A) This is the most common subtype of paediatric B-ALL and carries a favourable prognosis with long-term survival above 90%.

(B) This is a Ph-like B-ALL and requires the addition of a tyrosine kinase inhibitor to standard induction.

(C) This is a KMT2A-rearranged B-ALL and requires alloSCT in first complete remission.

(D) This is hypodiploid B-ALL and has a very poor prognosis even with intensified therapy.

(E) This is T-ALL and requires nelarabine in addition to standard ALL induction.

Best answer: (A) This is the most common subtype of paediatric B-ALL and carries a favourable prognosis with long-term survival above 90%.

Rationale. The t(12;21)(p13;q22) translocation produces the ETV6::RUNX1 fusion, the most common genetic abnormality in paediatric B-ALL (~25%) and the prototype favourable-prognosis subtype. The translocation is cryptic — it is not visible on a conventional karyotype and is detected by FISH or by RT-PCR. The classical immunophenotype is TdT+, CD34+, CD19+, cCD79a+, CD10 bright (the "common ALL" phenotype), with CD20 frequently dim or negative. The favourable biology is reflected at the bedside: relapses do occur but are often late and frequently re-respond to chemotherapy, contributing to overall survival rates above 90% in modern multi-agent risk-adapted protocols. Bone pain, especially nocturnal long-bone pain, is a frequent and underappreciated presenting feature of childhood ALL.

Distractor analysis. (B) Ph-like ALL has the same gene-expression signature as Ph+ ALL but lacks BCR::ABL1; ETV6::RUNX1 is a distinct entity. (C) KMT2A-rearranged B-ALL is overwhelmingly an infant disease (<12 months) and is very poor risk; this is a 4-year-old with t(12;21). (D) Hypodiploidy is defined by <44 chromosomes — t(12;21) does not establish hypodiploidy. (E) The cCD3 needed for T-lineage assignment is absent; the CD19/cCD79a/CD10 phenotype is B-lineage.

Vignette 7. A 38-year-old man with newly diagnosed B-ALL and the Philadelphia chromosome

A 38-year-old man presents with two weeks of fatigue and a recent nosebleed. He has no significant past medical history. Examination shows pallor, scattered petechiae, no lymphadenopathy, and no organomegaly. Laboratory studies: haemoglobin 8.4 g/dL, platelets 32,000/µL, white blood cells 84,000/µL with 88% blasts. Bone marrow biopsy: 92% blasts. Flow cytometry: TdT+, CD34+, HLA-DR+, CD19+, cCD79a+, CD10+, MPO negative. Conventional karyotype shows t(9;22)(q34;q11.2), and RT-PCR identifies the

BCR::ABL1 p190 fusion transcript. Which of the following is the most appropriate addition to standard B-ALL induction chemotherapy in this patient?

(A) Imatinib (or another BCR::ABL1 tyrosine kinase inhibitor such as dasatinib).

(B) Rituximab.

(C) Midostaurin.

(D) All-trans retinoic acid (ATRA).

(E) Larotrectinib.

Best answer: (A) Imatinib (or another BCR::ABL1 tyrosine kinase inhibitor such as dasatinib).

Rationale. Adult B-ALL with the Philadelphia chromosome (t(9;22)/BCR::ABL1) is the most common cytogenetic abnormality in adult ALL, accounting for approximately 25% of adult cases (versus only 3–5% of paediatric cases). The BCR::ABL1 fusion in ALL most often produces the smaller p190 protein, distinguishing it from the p210 isoform that predominates in CML. Before the era of targeted therapy, Ph+ B-ALL had a very poor prognosis with chemotherapy alone. The integration of BCR::ABL1 tyrosine kinase inhibitors — imatinib, dasatinib, ponatinib, or, in current paediatric and AYA practice, dasatinib in combination with chemotherapy — has transformed outcomes, raising long-term survival rates several-fold and reducing the role of allogeneic stem cell transplantation in first remission. CNS-penetrant TKIs (dasatinib) are preferred when CNS disease risk is a concern. Allogeneic SCT remains an option for high-risk or MRD-positive patients, but TKIs alone have made chemotherapy-light regimens (TKI + steroid + blinatumomab) viable in many patients.

Distractor analysis. (B) Rituximab targets CD20 and may be added in CD20-positive Ph+ B-ALL but is not the answer to "what addresses the BCR::ABL1 driver." (C) Midostaurin is an FLT3 inhibitor used in FLT3-mutated AML, not in Ph+ ALL. (D) ATRA is for APL (PML::RARA), not Ph+ ALL. (E) Larotrectinib is an NTRK inhibitor for NTRK-fusion–positive cancers (a Ph-like ALL subset, not Ph+ ALL).

Vignette 8. A 16-year-old boy with a mediastinal mass, dyspnea, and lymphocytosis

A 16-year-old boy presents with three weeks of progressive dyspnea on exertion, dry cough, and facial swelling that is worse on waking. Examination shows facial plethora, distended jugular veins, and stridor on lying flat. Vital signs are stable but he prefers to sit upright. A chest radiograph shows a large anterior mediastinal mass with tracheal deviation. Laboratory studies: haemoglobin 11.8 g/dL, platelets 124,000/µL, white blood cells 64,000/µL with 56% lymphoblasts. The peripheral smear shows medium-sized blasts with fine chromatin and scant agranular cytoplasm; no Auer rods. Flow cytometry on the blast population: TdT+, cytoplasmic CD3 positive, surface CD3 negative, CD7+, CD5+, CD2+, CD4+, CD8+ ("double-positive"), CD1a+, CD34 dim, HLA-DR negative, CD19 negative, cCD79a negative, MPO negative. Which of the following diagnoses is most consistent with these findings?

(A) B-cell acute lymphoblastic leukaemia (B-ALL) with t(12;21)/ETV6::RUNX1.

(B) T-cell acute lymphoblastic leukaemia (T-ALL), cortical thymocyte stage.

(C) Acute promyelocytic leukaemia (APL).

(D) Hodgkin lymphoma with leukaemic involvement.

(E) Burkitt lymphoma/leukaemia.

Best answer: (B) T-cell acute lymphoblastic leukaemia (T-ALL), cortical thymocyte stage.

Rationale. The clinical picture is the classical T-ALL presentation: an adolescent male with a thymic-origin anterior mediastinal mass causing superior vena cava syndrome (facial plethora, distended neck veins, orthopnea, stridor) and a high circulating blast count. The immunophenotype is unambiguously T-lineage. Cytoplasmic CD3 (cCD3) is the only T-lineage-specific marker — surface CD3 is characteristically absent in T-ALL. HLA-DR negativity in an acute leukaemia points strongly toward T-lineage. The CD4+/CD8+ "double-positive" pattern with CD1a expression localises this T-ALL to the cortical thymocyte stage of T-cell development, the most frequent T-ALL subset and a prognostically favourable position within T-ALL. The patient is at high risk for tumour lysis syndrome on initiating cytoreduction; aggressive hydration and rasburicase prophylaxis are indicated. Steroid pre-treatment over 5–7 days before full induction is sometimes used to debulk hyperleukocytic T-ALL and reduce TLS risk.

Distractor analysis. (A) B-ALL would express CD19 and cCD79a and would not be cCD3-positive. (C) APL does not produce a mediastinal mass; the morphology and HLA-DR/CD34 pattern are not those of APL. (D) Hodgkin lymphoma can produce a mediastinal mass but does not present with circulating lymphoblasts at this volume. (E) Burkitt lymphoma/leukaemia has a mature B-cell phenotype (sIg+, CD20+, CD10+, MYC translocated, TdT negative); cCD3 is absent.

Vignette 9. A 19-year-old with T-ALL three days into induction

A 19-year-old man with newly diagnosed T-ALL and a mediastinal mass began induction chemotherapy three days ago. He has been receiving intravenous fluids at twice maintenance and is on allopurinol 300 mg daily. He now develops generalised muscle cramps, perioral tingling, and a single brief tonic-clonic seizure. Vital signs are temperature 37.4°C, pulse 118/min, blood pressure 138/86 mm Hg. Laboratory studies: potassium 6.8 mEq/L, phosphate 8.4 mg/dL (2.7 mmol/L), corrected calcium 6.8 mg/dL (1.7 mmol/L), uric acid 14.2 mg/dL (845 µmol/L), creatinine 2.4 mg/dL (212 µmol/L) (baseline 0.9 mg/dL), and lactate dehydrogenase 1,420 U/L. Urinalysis shows uric acid crystals. Which of the following is the most appropriate next step?

- **(A)** Add rasburicase intravenously, intensify intravenous hydration, and treat the hyperkalaemia and hypocalcaemia urgently.
- **(B)** Hold all chemotherapy until renal function recovers, and continue allopurinol at the same dose.
- **(C)** Initiate haemodialysis as the first intervention without administering rasburicase.
- **(D)** Increase allopurinol to 600 mg daily and add urinary alkalinisation with intravenous sodium bicarbonate.
- **(E)** Replace calcium aggressively to a normal range; this will resolve the rest of the metabolic abnormalities.

Best answer: (A) Add rasburicase intravenously, intensify intravenous hydration, and treat the hyperkalaemia and hypocalcaemia urgently.

Rationale. This is established tumour lysis syndrome — laboratory and clinical TLS by Cairo–Bishop criteria — driven by the massive nucleic acid release from a large T-ALL tumour burden lysing in response to induction. The mechanistic chain: nucleic acids degrade to hypoxanthine → xanthine → uric acid via xanthine oxidase, releasing potassium and phosphate from cells. Hyperphosphataemia drives reciprocal hypocalcaemia (calcium phosphate precipitation) and contributes to acute kidney injury through intratubular calcium phosphate deposition. Allopurinol blocks xanthine oxidase and prevents new uric acid formation, but it does not lower already-formed uric acid — once uric acid is high, allopurinol is too slow. Rasburicase is a recombinant urate oxidase that converts existing uric acid to allantoin, lowering urate within hours. Aggressive hydration sustains tubular flow. Urinary alkalinisation, once standard, is now generally avoided when rasburicase is used because alkaline urine promotes calcium phosphate precipitation. Hyperkalaemia and symptomatic hypocalcaemia (the seizure) require urgent correction in parallel. Rasburicase is contraindicated in G6PD deficiency because the hydrogen peroxide byproduct triggers severe oxidative haemolysis — screen if uncertain.

Distractor analysis. (B) Stopping chemotherapy with persistent tumour burden does not address the cause. (C) Haemodialysis is reserved for refractory hyperkalaemia, oligo-anuric AKI, or persistent severe metabolic derangement after medical therapy fails. (D) Allopurinol cannot reverse existing hyperuricaemia, and bicarbonate alkalinisation now causes more harm than good. (E) Calcium replacement alone treats the symptom, not the cause; aggressive calcium repletion in the setting of hyperphosphataemia worsens metastatic calcification.

Vignette 10. A 20-year-old woman with a viral illness and "atypical" lymphocytes — the elimination test

A 20-year-old previously healthy college student presents with one week of fatigue, sore throat, and low-grade fever. Examination shows tonsillar enlargement with greyish-white exudates, bilateral cervical lymphadenopathy, mild hepatosplenomegaly, and a faint truncal maculopapular rash that began two days after she was started on amoxicillin elsewhere. Laboratory studies: haemoglobin 13.4 g/dL, platelets 168,000/µL, white blood cells 16,000/µL with 18% large mononuclear cells described by the laboratory as "atypical lymphocytes" — large cells with abundant deeply basophilic cytoplasm with scalloped borders abutting adjacent red cells, eccentric nuclei, and condensed chromatin. There are no blasts. A heterophile antibody test is positive. Which of the following best explains the laboratory picture and is the most appropriate next step?

- **(A)** Reactive lymphocytosis from infectious mononucleosis (Epstein–Barr virus); the cells are activated cytotoxic T lymphocytes responding to EBV-infected B cells, and supportive care is indicated.
- **(B)** Acute lymphoblastic leukaemia presenting subtly; immediately perform a bone marrow biopsy and start induction chemotherapy.
- **(C)** Acute myeloid leukaemia; perform a peripheral blood flow cytometry panel for myeloid markers and arrange for induction.
- **(D)** Hairy cell leukaemia; arrange for tartrate-resistant acid phosphatase staining and pursue cladribine therapy.
- **(E)** Burkitt lymphoma in leukaemic phase; arrange for an LDH, urgent bone marrow biopsy, and tumour lysis prophylaxis.

Best answer: (A) Reactive lymphocytosis from infectious mononucleosis (Epstein–Barr virus); the cells are activated cytotoxic T lymphocytes responding to EBV-infected B cells, and supportive care is indicated.

Rationale. The clinical syndrome — sore throat with exudative tonsillitis, posterior and anterior cervical lymphadenopathy, splenomegaly, fatigue, and a maculopapular rash precipitated by amoxicillin (a classical reaction in 80–90% of EBV-mononucleosis patients exposed to ampicillin or amoxicillin) — combined with a positive heterophile (Monospot) antibody test, establishes EBV-infectious mononucleosis. The "atypical lymphocytes" (Downey cells) are not blasts: they are activated CD8-positive cytotoxic T lymphocytes mounting an immune response against EBV-infected B cells. Morphologically they have abundant deeply basophilic cytoplasm with characteristic scalloped borders that mould around adjacent red cells, eccentric nuclei, and condensed (mature) chromatin — the chromatin pattern is the key discriminator from a true blast, which has fine, open, "blast" chromatin with prominent nucleoli. Reactive lymphocytes are TdT-negative and CD3-positive (mature T-cell phenotype). Treatment is supportive; the splenomegaly justifies avoidance of contact sports for several weeks because of splenic rupture risk. Avoid corticosteroids unless airway compromise develops.

Distractor analysis. (B) ALL produces blasts with fine open chromatin and prominent nucleoli, not the dense chromatin of activated lymphocytes; the platelet count and haemoglobin would also typically be lower at this WBC. The amoxicillin rash and heterophile positivity make IM the right answer. (C) AML lineage requires Auer rods or MPO positivity; nothing here suggests AML. (D) Hairy cell leukaemia presents in middle-aged men with pancytopenia and splenomegaly — not this clinical picture. (E) Burkitt presents with rapidly enlarging masses and very high LDH; the heterophile positivity and amoxicillin rash here belong to a different disease.

12.10 Discriminators — Pearls and Traps

The remaining boxes target the wrong-answer patterns examiners reuse. Each pearl is a discriminator that converts a vignette into a single-step diagnosis; each trap is a wrong answer that looks correct because it follows from training reflexes that are appropriate elsewhere but not on this question.

HIGH-YIELD PEARL — What an Auer rod actually is

An Auer rod is not a generic "leukaemic" inclusion. It is an abnormal crystalline aggregate of fused azurophilic primary granules, found only in cells of myeloid lineage with primary granule production. Auer rods stain positively with myeloperoxidase, Sudan Black B, and PAS. They are most prominent in AML M2 (RUNX1::RUNX1T1), AML M3 (PML::RARA — the bundled "faggot cell" form), and high-grade myelodysplastic neoplasms with excess blasts. They are absent in lymphoid lineage, and an Auer rod on an "atypical lymphocyte" is not an Auer rod — re-examine the morphology. The exam corollary: Auer rod present → myeloid lineage → exclude ALL.

HIGH-YIELD PEARL — MRD is the dominant prognostic variable in ALL

Measurable residual disease (MRD) is arguably the single most important prognostic tool in ALL. It guides both intensification (MRD-positive after induction = high risk; escalate to alloSCT, blinatumomab, or CAR-T) and de-escalation (MRD-negative throughout = low risk; reduce consolidation toxicity). Two methods are clinically validated: multiparameter flow cytometry detecting the leukaemia-associated immunophenotype (sensitivity 10^{-4}) and allele-specific PCR or next-generation sequencing of the clonal IGH or T-cell receptor gene rearrangement (sensitivity 10^{-5} to 10^{-6}). MRD negativity at the end of induction (typically day 29 in paediatric protocols) is associated with event-free survival above 90%. MRD positivity at the end of consolidation is the strongest single predictor of relapse and the principal indication for alloSCT in first complete remission. The exam-level statement: "MRD-positive at end of consolidation" is a prompt for transplant, not for "continuing the same regimen and re-checking later."

HIGH-YIELD PEARL — Acute leukaemias in Down syndrome

Children with Down syndrome have an approximately 10–20-fold increased risk of acute leukaemia, but the spectrum is age-stratified and biologically distinct. In the neonatal period, ~10% of Down syndrome infants develop transient abnormal myelopoiesis (TAM) with circulating megakaryoblasts that resolve spontaneously over weeks to months — driven by somatic GATA1 mutations on a background of trisomy 21. Approximately 20% of TAM patients later develop myeloid leukaemia of Down syndrome (ML-DS, formerly AMKL), peaking before age 4 and curable with reduced-intensity chemotherapy. After age 4, the leukaemia spectrum shifts toward B-ALL, with CRLF2 rearrangements (a Ph-like driver) overrepresented. Down syndrome ALL has historically shown higher induction mortality and inferior outcomes; modern protocols compensate with risk-adapted dose modification.

TRAP — "TdT positive, therefore ALL"

TdT is a marker of immaturity, not of lineage. It is expressed in B-ALL, T-ALL, and approximately 20% of AMLs as an aberrant marker — particularly in AML M0 (minimal differentiation) and AML M1. The blast in lymphoblastic transformation of CML is also TdT-positive. Lineage assignment never rests on TdT alone. Confirm myeloid lineage with MPO (cytochemistry, IHC, or flow cytometry) or with monocytic markers (≥2 of NSE, CD11c, CD14, CD64, lysozyme); confirm B-lineage with strong CD19 plus one of cCD79a, cCD22, or CD10 (or weak CD19 with two of the three); confirm T-lineage with cytoplasmic CD3. The wrong-answer pattern: a vignette mentions "TdT-positive blasts" and the test-taker reflexively picks ALL despite an Auer rod or MPO positivity in the same stem.

TRAP — Hyperleukocytosis with leukostasis is not the same as APL DIC

Two distinct emergencies in acute leukaemia look superficially similar in the first hour and require opposite responses. Hyperleukocytosis with leukostasis (typically AML with WBC >100,000/µL, especially monocytic AML) presents with respiratory distress, neurological symptoms (headache, confusion, focal deficits), and visual disturbance from microvascular obstruction by adherent blasts; treatment is leukapheresis or hydroxyurea cytoreduction with prompt induction, and platelet transfusions are kept conservative because they paradoxically worsen blood viscosity. APL DIC presents with bleeding, hypofibrinogenaemia, and elevated D-dimer; the WBC may be low or normal in classical APL or high in the microgranular variant; treatment is ATRA on morphological suspicion plus aggressive product support to maintain fibrinogen and platelet thresholds. The wrong-answer pattern: applying leukostasis-style restraint on transfusion to an APL patient with bleeding, or applying APL-style ATRA to a hyperleukocytic non-APL AML.

IMG-TRAP — The "investigate first, treat later" reflex meets APL

Trainees educated in laboratory-led diagnostic systems often internalise an admirable rule: do not treat without a confirmed diagnosis. The rule fails in APL. The mortality from waiting for a PML::RARA RT-PCR result, or even for a t(15;17) FISH report, is the dominant determinant of early death — patients die from intracranial haemorrhage in the first 24 hours, not from misclassification of a non-APL AML as APL. ATRA itself is well-tolerated; if the suspected APL turns out to be a non-APL AML on confirmation, ATRA is simply discontinued. If the suspected APL is APL, those hours of ATRA exposure are the hours that prevented the fatal haemorrhage. On the USMLE, the answer that starts ATRA on morphology — bundled Auer rods, hypergranular promyelocytes, DIC — without waiting for molecular confirmation is the correct answer. The "send the molecular test and decide when it returns" option is a trap.

12.11 Quick Recall — One-Page Chapter Compression

QUICK RECALL — Acute Leukaemias

Definition. AML = ≥20% myeloid blasts (or any blast count for most defining genetic abnormalities under WHO 2022). ALL = lymphoblast accumulation in marrow/blood; TdT+, MPO−, no Auer rods.

Auer rod. Myeloid lineage. Pathognomonic. Faggot cell (bundle in one promyelocyte) =

APL.

APL. t(15;17)/PML::RARA. HLA-DR negative, CD34 typically negative. DIC at presentation. Start ATRA on morphology — do not wait for molecular confirmation. Add arsenic trioxide. Differentiation syndrome in 15–25%: dexamethasone.

AML core-binding factor. t(8;21)/RUNX1::RUNX1T1 (M2 morphology, aberrant CD19, dyserythropoiesis); inv(16)/CBFB::MYH11 (marrow eosinophilia). ELN favourable. No alloSCT in CR1.

AML with NPM1 mutation. CD34 negative, HLA-DR negative, cup-like nuclei. Favourable IF FLT3-ITD absent. NPM1 + FLT3-ITD = intermediate.

AML adverse cytogenetics. Complex karyotype, monosomy 5 or 7, del(17p), TP53 mutation, BCR::ABL1, t(6;9), KMT2A-r (other than MLLT3). AlloSCT in CR1.

AML-MR. Prior MDS, MDS-related cytogenetics, or MDS-related mutations (ASXL1, BCOR, EZH2, SF3B1, SRSF2, STAG2, U2AF1, ZRSR2). Absorbs most therapy-related AML without a defining fusion.

B-ALL favourable. t(12;21)/ETV6::RUNX1 (cryptic, FISH-detected) and high hyperdiploidy (especially trisomies 4, 10, 17). Paediatric. Long-term survival >90%.

B-ALL adverse. Hypodiploidy <44 chromosomes (especially near-haploid <30). KMT2A rearrangement (infant ALL). Ph+ (BCR::ABL1) without TKI. iAMP21 without intensification.

Ph-like ALL. No BCR::ABL1 but kinase-activated. CRLF2-r (most common; +JAK2 mutation), ABL-class fusions, JAK2 fusions, NTRK fusions. Detection requires RNA-seq or kinase-fusion panel. TKI matched to driver.

T-ALL. Adolescent boys; mediastinal mass with SVC syndrome; cCD3+, surface CD3−, HLA-DR negative, CD7+, CD5+. NOTCH1 mutated in >50%. ETP-ALL is a distinct very-aggressive subset.

TLS. Hyperuricaemia, hyperkalaemia, hyperphosphataemia, hypocalcaemia, AKI. Allopurinol prevents new urate; rasburicase clears existing urate (contraindicated in G6PD deficiency). Aggressive hydration.

AlloSCT in AML. CR1 for ELN-adverse, primary refractory, relapsed in CR2. MRD-guided in intermediate. GVL effect drives cure. APL almost never needs alloSCT.

Ph+ ALL therapy. Add TKI (imatinib or dasatinib) to chemotherapy. Has transformed outcomes; dasatinib preferred when CNS-penetration matters.

Haematogones vs B-ALL. Haematogones = continuous maturation spectrum on flow. B-ALL = discrete monotypic aberrant population. Setting: post-chemo or post-transplant marrow regeneration favours haematogones.

— End of Chapter 12 —

CHAPTER 13

Chapter 13 — Chronic Leukaemias and Myeloproliferative Neoplasms

BIG PICTURE

Chronic leukaemias and myeloproliferative neoplasms are clonal expansions of mature or near-mature blood cells that proliferate without the differentiation block that defines acute leukaemia. The four classical Philadelphia-negative MPNs (PV, ET, PMF, and the MPN-unclassifiable group) are unified by JAK-STAT pathway activation through JAK2, CALR, or MPL mutations. CML is the Philadelphia-positive prototype and the founding example of targeted oncology therapy. CLL is a mature B-cell lymphoid neoplasm grouped here by clinical chronicity rather than by lineage. Mastery of this chapter rests on three pivots: which kinase is activated, which morphological pattern is in the marrow, and which clinical complication kills the patient first.

MECHANISM HOOK — Why Philadelphia-negative MPNs happen

A single biology unifies polycythaemia vera, essential thrombocythaemia, and primary myelofibrosis: constitutive activation of JAK-STAT signalling in a haematopoietic stem cell. JAK2 V617F, present in >95% of PV and approximately half of ET and PMF, is a gain-of-function mutation in the pseudokinase domain of JAK2 that locks the kinase in an active conformation. The mutant JAK2 transduces signalling through cytokine receptors that normally require ligand engagement — EPO-R drives autonomous erythropoiesis (PV), MPL drives autonomous megakaryopoiesis (ET, PMF), and G-CSFR drives granulopoiesis. CALR mutations (frame-shift insertions or deletions in exon 9) generate a mutant calreticulin that binds and constitutively activates MPL, producing the same downstream signal in the absence of JAK2 mutation. MPL mutations (W515L, W515K) directly activate the thrombopoietin receptor. The three-driver framework — JAK2, CALR, MPL — explains why MPNs share clinical features (thrombosis, splenomegaly, marrow hypercellularity) and why a single kinase inhibitor (ruxolitinib, a JAK1/2 inhibitor) is active across the spectrum. CML is the kinase-driven outlier: BCR::ABL1 from t(9;22) drives a constitutively active ABL1 tyrosine kinase that phosphorylates a different downstream signalling network (RAS-MAPK, PI3K-AKT, JAK-STAT collaterally), producing the panmyeloid expansion of CML.

13.1 Chronic Myeloid Leukaemia — The Targeted Therapy Paradigm

Chronic myeloid leukaemia is a clonal myeloproliferative neoplasm defined by the BCR::ABL1 fusion oncogene arising from the Philadelphia chromosome, t(9;22)(q34;q11.2). The translocation fuses the BCR gene on chromosome 22 to the ABL1 tyrosine kinase gene on chromosome 9; the fusion protein is a constitutively active tyrosine kinase that phosphorylates substrates across RAS-MAPK, PI3K-AKT, and JAK-STAT pathways, producing uncontrolled myeloid proliferation, impaired apoptosis, and reduced stromal adhesion (allowing circulating progenitors). The introduction of imatinib in 2001 transformed CML from a disease with a median survival of three to five years into a condition in which most patients diagnosed in early chronic phase have a life expectancy approaching that of the general population. CML accounts for approximately 15% of adult leukaemias in the US, with a median age at diagnosis near 65.

In CML, the BCR breakpoint is most commonly in the major breakpoint cluster region (M-bcr) producing the p210 fusion protein. This contrasts with Ph+ B-ALL, where the minor breakpoint (m-bcr) producing the smaller p190 protein predominates. The distinction matters: a p210 transcript in a patient with leukocytosis points to CML; a p190 transcript in a patient with lymphoblasts points to Ph+ B-ALL. Both are sensitive to BCR::ABL1 TKIs, but the disease frameworks and treatment regimens differ.

Three phases of CML

Over 90% of patients are diagnosed in chronic phase, often incidentally on a routine CBC showing leukocytosis. Symptoms when present are fatigue, early satiety from massive splenomegaly, left upper quadrant discomfort, weight loss, and night sweats. The peripheral blood shows the diagnostic myeloid spectrum: marked leukocytosis (typically 50–300 × 10^9/L), the full left shift from myeloblasts through promyelocytes, myelocytes, metamyelocytes, bands, and mature neutrophils, and the two pathognomonic findings — basophilia and eosinophilia. Absolute basophilia is the single most reliable morphological clue distinguishing CML from a leukemoid reaction. The leukocyte alkaline phosphatase (LAP) score is low or zero in CML, distinguishing it from reactive leukocytosis (high LAP).

Accelerated phase is defined by rising blast counts (10–19% of marrow or peripheral blood blasts under WHO 2022), persistent basophilia ≥20%, cytogenetic clonal evolution beyond the Philadelphia chromosome (additional Ph, trisomy 8, isochromosome 17q, trisomy 19), unexplained thrombocytopenia <100 × 10^9/L or thrombocytosis >1,000 × 10^9/L unresponsive to therapy, and resistance to TKI therapy. Blast phase (blast crisis) is defined by ≥20% blasts in marrow or blood or by extramedullary blast proliferation (a chloroma). Approximately two-thirds of blast crises are myeloid and one-third are lymphoid (almost always B-lineage). The lymphoid blast crisis is treated with ALL-style induction plus a TKI, and the myeloid blast crisis is treated with AML-style induction plus a TKI; both ultimately require allogeneic stem cell transplantation if remission is achieved.

Feature	Chronic phase	Accelerated phase	Blast phase
Marrow / blood blasts	<10%	10–19% (WHO 2022)	≥20% or extramedullary blast proliferation
Basophils	Elevated; <20%	≥20%	Variable; often very high
Platelets	Normal or elevated	<100 × 10^9/L (not therapy-induced) OR >1,000 × 10^9/L unresponsive	Often thrombocytopenic
Cytogenetics	Ph chromosome only	Clonal evolution: +Ph, +8, i(17q), +19	Markedly abnormal karyotype; additional mutations
TKI response	Excellent; major molecular response	Reduced; switch TKI; consider alloSCT	Poor; treat as AML or ALL plus TKI; alloSCT

Feature	Chronic phase	Accelerated phase	Blast phase
	achievable		if remission

Table 13.1. WHO 2022 phase criteria for CML.

HIGH-YIELD PEARL — Distinguishing CML from a leukemoid reaction
A leukemoid reaction is a neutrophilic leukocytosis (typically 30–50 × 10^9/L) with a left shift driven by infection, severe inflammation, glucocorticoids, or G-CSF therapy. It can be morphologically confusing because the smear shows myelocytes and metamyelocytes alongside mature neutrophils. Three discriminators settle the diagnosis. First, basophilia: leukemoid reactions do not show basophilia, while basophilia is nearly universal in CML. Second, leukocyte alkaline phosphatase (LAP) score: high in leukemoid reaction (the neutrophils are functional and reactive), low or zero in CML (the clonal neutrophils have reduced LAP activity). Third, BCR::ABL1: present in CML, absent in leukemoid reaction. Toxic granulation, Döhle bodies, and a clear infectious source point to a reactive process. The vignette signal: leukocytosis with basophilia → CML; leukocytosis with toxic granulation, an obvious infection, and a high LAP score → leukemoid reaction.

13.2 Treatment of CML and Tyrosine Kinase Inhibitor Resistance

First-line therapy for chronic-phase CML is a BCR::ABL1 tyrosine kinase inhibitor. Five agents are now FDA-approved for newly diagnosed disease: imatinib (first-in-class, longest safety record), the second-generation ATP-pocket inhibitors dasatinib, nilotinib, and bosutinib (deeper, faster molecular responses), and the first-in-class STAMP-pocket allosteric inhibitor asciminib (FDA-approved first-line October 2024 based on the ASC4FIRST trial showing superior 48-week MMR versus investigator-selected TKIs; NCCN Category 1 preferred). Asciminib binds the ABL myristoyl pocket allosterically rather than the ATP-binding pocket, giving it a distinct toxicity profile and retained activity against most ATP-pocket resistance mutations. Ponatinib is a third-generation TKI with activity against the T315I "gatekeeper" mutation, which causes resistance to all earlier-generation ATP-pocket TKIs. Risk stratification at diagnosis uses the ELTS (EUTOS Long-Term Survival) score — now preferred over Sokal because it is age-stratified and predicts CML-related death rather than overall survival; Sokal and EUTOS scores remain in use.

Treatment response is monitored by quantitative RT-PCR for the BCR::ABL1 transcript reported on the International Scale (IS). Major molecular response (MMR) is defined as BCR::ABL1 IS ≤0.1%. Deep molecular response (MR4.0 or MR4.5) corresponds to ≤0.01% and ≤0.0032%, respectively. Patients with sustained deep molecular response for at least two years can be considered for treatment-free remission with TKI discontinuation under close monitoring. Failure to achieve BCR::ABL1 IS ≤10% at three months or ≤1% at twelve months prompts mutational analysis and consideration of TKI switch. The T315I mutation, which substitutes isoleucine for threonine at the gatekeeper position of the ATP-binding pocket, blocks imatinib, dasatinib, nilotinib, and bosutinib; ponatinib and asciminib retain activity. Allogeneic stem cell transplantation is reserved for accelerated and blast phase, multi-TKI resistance, or T315I in patients without ponatinib access.

STEP 2 BRIDGE — Choosing a TKI for CML

Comorbidity profile drives TKI selection more than efficacy in many cases. Imatinib has the longest safety record but slower deep responses; common toxicities are oedema, muscle cramps, and rash. Dasatinib is associated with pleural effusion and pulmonary arterial hypertension — avoid in patients with pulmonary disease — and with platelet dysfunction beyond its thrombocytopenia (gastrointestinal bleeding risk). Nilotinib carries a QT-prolongation risk and a class-specific risk of arterial occlusive events (myocardial infarction, peripheral arterial disease, cerebrovascular events) — avoid in patients with established cardiovascular disease. Bosutinib produces self-limited diarrhoea and transaminitis. Ponatinib has the highest cardiovascular risk and is reserved for T315I or multi-TKI failure. The "exam" pattern: T315I mutation → ponatinib (or asciminib); cardiovascular history → imatinib or bosutinib over nilotinib and ponatinib; pulmonary disease → avoid dasatinib.

TRAP — "BCR::ABL1 positive — therefore CML"

A BCR::ABL1 positive result on RT-PCR is not by itself diagnostic of CML; it is also positive in Ph+ B-ALL and a subset of AML. The transcript identity matters. p210 (M-bcr breakpoint) predominates in CML; p190 (m-bcr breakpoint) predominates in Ph+ B-ALL; p230 (µ-bcr) is the rare neutrophilic CML variant. The clinical and morphological context disambiguates: lymphoblasts → Ph+ B-ALL; chronic myeloid spectrum with basophilia → CML; new-onset acute leukaemia in an adult with t(9;22) and lineage on flow cytometry decides AML with BCR::ABL1 versus Ph+ ALL versus CML in blast crisis. Do not equate the molecular finding with a single disease — examiners use this trap to reward integration over reflex.

13.3 Polycythaemia Vera

Polycythaemia vera is the prototype Philadelphia-negative MPN driven by JAK2 V617F (>95% of cases) or, in 3–5%, by JAK2 exon 12 mutations. The disease produces autonomous panmyelosis with a dominant erythroid phenotype: elevated haemoglobin and haematocrit, leukocytosis with mature granulocytes, and thrombocytosis. Median age at presentation is approximately 60. Symptoms reflect hyperviscosity (headache, dizziness, blurred vision, plethora, erythromelalgia — burning pain in the extremities relieved by cold), pruritus after warm showers (aquagenic pruritus, attributed to mast-cell activation), and gout (from urate overproduction by the expanded myeloid mass). Hepatosplenomegaly is common.

The most consequential complication is thrombosis — both arterial (myocardial infarction, stroke) and venous, including the unusual splanchnic locations: hepatic vein (Budd-Chiari syndrome), portal vein, and mesenteric vein thromboses. Hyperviscosity, qualitative platelet abnormalities, and a pro-thrombotic milieu drive these events. Haemorrhage from acquired von Willebrand disease (very high platelet counts adsorb high-molecular-weight VWF multimers) coexists in some patients, producing a paradoxical bleeding-and-clotting phenotype. Long-term, PV can transform to post-PV myelofibrosis (15–20% over 20 years) or to AML (3–10%, accelerated by alkylator exposure).

WHO 2022 diagnostic criteria for PV

Criterion	WHO 2022 definition
Major 1	Haemoglobin >16.5 g/dL (men) or >16.0 g/dL (women); OR haematocrit >49% (men) or >48% (women); OR red cell mass >25% above mean predicted
Major 2	Bone marrow hypercellularity for age with trilineage proliferation (panmyelosis): erythroid, granulocytic, and megakaryocytic, with pleomorphic mature megakaryocytes of varying size
Major 3	JAK2 V617F or JAK2 exon 12 mutation
Minor	Subnormal serum erythropoietin level
Diagnosis	All three major criteria; OR major 1 and 2 plus the minor criterion

Table 13.2. WHO 2022 PV criteria.

Treatment is risk-adapted. All PV patients receive low-dose aspirin (unless contraindicated) and therapeutic phlebotomy to maintain haematocrit below 45%. High-risk patients — age >60, prior thrombosis, or both — receive cytoreductive therapy: hydroxyurea is the first-line agent; ropeginterferon alfa-2b is preferred in younger patients and in pregnancy; ruxolitinib is approved for hydroxyurea-resistant or hydroxyurea-intolerant disease and produces durable spleen and symptom control. Aquagenic pruritus often responds to selective serotonin reuptake inhibitors or to ruxolitinib in refractory cases.

HIGH-YIELD PEARL — JAK2 V617F is not specific to PV

JAK2 V617F is the dominant driver mutation in PV (>95%) but it is also present in approximately 50–60% of essential thrombocythaemia and 50–60% of primary myelofibrosis. The mutation alone does not establish a diagnosis — the clinical phenotype (which lineage is over-represented), the marrow morphology, and the EPO level are required. The corollary is more useful: a JAK2 V617F–negative patient with absolute erythrocytosis still requires evaluation for a JAK2 exon 12 mutation before PV is excluded, because exon 12 mutations account for 3–5% of PV and are associated with a more pure erythroid phenotype.

13.4 Essential Thrombocythaemia

Essential thrombocythaemia is an MPN of the megakaryocyte lineage producing sustained thrombocytosis (platelet count ≥450 × 10^9/L by WHO 2022) without erythrocytosis or significant marrow fibrosis. Driver mutations are JAK2 V617F (50–60%), CALR (20–25%), and MPL (3–5%); approximately 10–15% are "triple-negative" with no detectable driver mutation but a clonal disease. Median age at diagnosis is approximately 60, with a smaller second peak in young women in the third or fourth decade. Clinical features cluster around vasomotor symptoms (headache, dizziness, paresthesias, erythromelalgia), thrombosis (more often arterial than venous), and bleeding from acquired von Willebrand disease at very high platelet counts.

The diagnostic challenge is distinguishing ET from reactive thrombocytosis (iron deficiency, infection, inflammation, post-splenectomy, malignancy) and from the early "prefibrotic" stage of primary myelofibrosis. Marrow biopsy is decisive: ET shows enlarged, hyperlobated mature megakaryocytes in loose clusters without the dense, tight clustering, the cytologic atypia, or the reticulin fibrosis of prefibrotic PMF. Mutation status further refines diagnosis — a CALR mutation in a thrombocytotic patient is essentially diagnostic of an MPN.

Treatment is risk-adapted. Low-risk patients (age ≤60, no thrombosis, JAK2 wild-type) receive observation or low-dose aspirin alone. High-risk patients (age >60, prior thrombosis, or extreme thrombocytosis with bleeding risk) receive cytoreduction with hydroxyurea (first-line), anagrelide (selective megakaryocyte inhibitor), or interferon alfa. Anagrelide is associated with palpitations, headache, and fluid retention and is reserved for hydroxyurea intolerance or resistance.

IMG-TRAP — CALR-mutated MPN has a different prognosis than JAK2-mutated MPN

A common training reflex is to treat all MPN driver mutations as equivalent surrogates for "MPN" without further clinical implication. This collapses important prognostic distinctions used on USMLE CK questions. In essential thrombocythaemia, CALR-mutated disease has a lower thrombosis rate than JAK2 V617F–mutated disease and a generally more indolent course, while triple-negative disease has variable outcomes. In primary myelofibrosis, CALR type 1 mutations carry a more favourable prognosis than JAK2 V617F or CALR type 2, and the MIPSS70 and MIPSS70+ v2.0 prognostic scores integrate driver mutation type with high-risk somatic mutations (ASXL1, EZH2, IDH1/2, SRSF2, U2AF1 Q157) to risk-stratify patients. The exam-level pattern: a young woman with thrombocytosis and a CALR mutation has a different long-term forecast than a 70-year-old with JAK2 V617F PMF and an ASXL1 mutation, and the answer choice that recognises the CALR-favorability or the high-molecular-risk-mutation panel will reward you.

13.5 Primary Myelofibrosis

Primary myelofibrosis is the most aggressive of the Philadelphia-negative MPNs. Driver mutations are JAK2 V617F (50–60%), CALR (20–35%), and MPL (5–10%); approximately 10% are triple-negative. PMF has two recognised stages — prefibrotic and overt fibrotic. The prefibrotic stage shows hypercellular marrow with megakaryocytic atypia (dense clustering, cloud-like nuclei, abnormal nucleoplasmic ratios) without significant reticulin fibrosis; it is the stage that is most often misdiagnosed as ET. The fibrotic stage shows marrow reticulin and collagen fibrosis (MF grade 2 or 3), an osteosclerotic component in advanced disease, and a leukoerythroblastic peripheral blood picture: nucleated red cells, immature granulocytes, and dacrocytes (teardrop cells) reflecting marrow architectural disruption.

Clinical features include progressive anaemia, hypercatabolic symptoms (fatigue, weight loss, night sweats, low-grade fever), and massive splenomegaly from extramedullary haematopoiesis. Hepatomegaly is also common, and extramedullary haematopoiesis can occur in unusual sites including pleura and dura. Risk stratification uses MIPSS70 or MIPSS70+ v2.0, which integrate driver mutation type, high-molecular-risk mutations (ASXL1, EZH2, IDH1/2, SRSF2, U2AF1 Q157), karyotype, blast count, haemoglobin, platelet count, and constitutional symptoms.

Treatment is symptom-directed and risk-adapted. Low-risk asymptomatic patients are observed. Symptomatic patients receive ruxolitinib (a JAK1/2 inhibitor that produces durable spleen-volume reduction and improves constitutional symptoms regardless of mutation status), fedratinib (alternative JAK2 inhibitor for ruxolitinib-intolerant patients), or pacritinib (preferred when platelet count is below $50 \times 10^9/L$ because it lacks myelosuppression at lower platelet counts). Allogeneic stem cell transplantation is the only curative option and is offered to fit patients with intermediate-2 or high-risk disease. Approximately 10–20% of patients transform to AML over 10 years, and this transformation is largely refractory to conventional induction.

HIGH-YIELD PEARL — The leukoerythroblastic blood picture

A leukoerythroblastic blood picture is defined by the simultaneous presence of immature granulocytes (myelocytes, metamyelocytes), nucleated red blood cells, and dacrocytes (teardrop-shaped red cells) on the peripheral smear. The pattern reflects displacement of marrow architecture and forced extramedullary haematopoiesis. The differential is short and high-yield: primary myelofibrosis, marrow infiltration by metastatic carcinoma (particularly breast and prostate), advanced lymphoma involvement of marrow, severe sepsis or haemolysis, and miliary tuberculosis or disseminated fungal infection. The vignette signal: a patient with massive splenomegaly, weight loss, and a leukoerythroblastic smear is PMF until proven otherwise; a patient with known breast or prostate cancer and a leukoerythroblastic smear has marrow metastases until proven otherwise. The discriminator is the marrow biopsy with reticulin staining.

13.6 MDS/MPN Overlap — Chronic Myelomonocytic Leukaemia

CMML is the most common MDS/MPN overlap entity, defined by sustained peripheral blood monocytosis (≥0.5 × 10^9/L absolute count and ≥10% of the white cell differential), one or more dysplastic features, and exclusion of CML, atypical CML, and chronic eosinophilic leukaemia. Two clinical subtypes are recognised: a myeloproliferative form with leukocytosis and splenomegaly, and a myelodysplastic form with cytopenias. Recurrent mutations include TET2 (60%), SRSF2 (50%), ASXL1 (40%), and CBL (15%). The disease is age-skewed (median 70+) and progresses to AML in 15–30% over 3–5 years. Treatment is hypomethylating-agent based (azacitidine, decitabine) for higher-risk disease; alloSCT is the only curative option and is offered to fit younger patients. Atypical CML (BCR::ABL1-negative) and juvenile myelomonocytic leukaemia (RAS-pathway driven, in children) are the related MDS/MPN entities; both are exam-relevant primarily as Ph-negative discriminators in a vignette describing CML-like leukocytosis.

TRAP — "Persistent monocytosis means CMML"
Sustained monocytosis is necessary but not sufficient for CMML. Reactive monocytosis from chronic inflammation (tuberculosis, inflammatory bowel disease, autoimmune disease), recovery from infection, splenectomy, and certain drugs (G-CSF) all produce sustained monocyte elevations. The CMML diagnosis additionally requires dysplasia (≥10% of cells in at least one lineage), exclusion of other MPNs, and ideally a clonal marker (TET2, SRSF2, ASXL1 mutations or a clonal cytogenetic abnormality). Reactive monocytosis lacks dysplasia and clonal mutations. Apply the TET2/SRSF2/ASXL1 panel before committing.

13.7 Chronic Lymphocytic Leukaemia / Small Lymphocytic Lymphoma

MECHANISM HOOK — Why CLL happens
CLL is a clonal expansion of mature CD5-positive B lymphocytes that fail to undergo apoptosis. Two collaborating biological forces produce the disease. The first is constitutive B-cell receptor (BCR) signalling — chronic, often antigen-independent BCR engagement drives downstream activation of LYN, SYK, BTK (Bruton tyrosine kinase), PI3Kδ, and BCL2-mediated survival. The second is dysregulated apoptosis: BCL2 protein is over-expressed in essentially all CLL cells, blocking the intrinsic apoptotic pathway. The therapeutic implication is direct and elegant — both pathways can be pharmacologically inhibited. Ibrutinib, acalabrutinib, and zanubrutinib (BTK inhibitors) cut the BCR signal at the kinase. Venetoclax (a BCL2 inhibitor) restores the apoptotic threshold. Together they have replaced cytotoxic chemotherapy as first-line therapy for most CLL patients. The IGHV mutational status of the malignant clone is the dominant biological prognostic variable: IGHV-mutated CLL (>2% deviation from germline) arises from post-germinal-centre B cells and is associated with indolent disease; IGHV-unmutated CLL arises from pre-germinal-centre B cells and is associated with aggressive disease and the need for earlier therapy.

CLL is the most common adult leukaemia in Western populations, with a median age at diagnosis near 70 and a male predominance. Most patients are diagnosed asymptomatically on a routine CBC showing absolute lymphocytosis. When symptomatic, patients present with painless lymphadenopathy, splenomegaly, fatigue, or autoimmune complications. Cytopenias may reflect either marrow infiltration (Rai stage III/IV: anaemia or thrombocytopenia from bone-marrow effacement) or autoimmune destruction (autoimmune haemolytic anaemia in 5–10%, immune thrombocytopenia in 2–5%). The peripheral smear is unmistakable when interpreted in context: small mature-appearing lymphocytes with clumped "block" chromatin, scant cytoplasm, and abundant smudge cells (Gumprecht shadows) reflecting the mechanical fragility of the malignant clone.

Diagnosis and immunophenotype

The diagnostic criterion is an absolute lymphocyte count of ≥5 × 10^9/L of clonal B lymphocytes sustained for ≥3 months, with the characteristic immunophenotype on flow cytometry: CD19+, CD5+, CD23+, CD20 dim, CD79b dim, surface immunoglobulin (sIg) dim with κ or λ light-chain restriction. The CD5 positivity overlaps with mantle cell lymphoma, but mantle cell is CD23-negative, has bright CD20, and carries t(11;14)/CCND1::IGH (cyclin D1 over-expression on IHC). The Matutes score (also called the CLL score or CLLflow score) integrates CD5, CD23, CD79b, FMC7, and surface Ig intensity to distinguish CLL from other small B-cell lymphomas. SLL is the same disease presenting with predominant tissue (lymph node) involvement and a peripheral lymphocyte count below 5 × 10^9/L; treatment principles are identical.

Marker	CLL	MCL	FL	MZL	HCL
CD5	+	+	–	–	–
CD23	+	NEGATIVE	–	–	–
CD20	Dim	Bright	Bright	Bright	Bright
CD10	–	–	+	–	–
CD103/ CD25/CD11c	–	–	–	±	TRIPLE +
Cyclin D1	–	+ (IHC)	–	–	+ (weak)
Genetics	del(13q), trisomy 12, del(11q)/ATM , del(17p)/TP53	t(11;14)/ CCND1	t(14;18)/BCL2	Variable	BRAF V600E

Table 13.3. CD5+ small B-cell neoplasms and key discriminators (MCL = mantle cell lymphoma, FL = follicular lymphoma, MZL = marginal zone lymphoma, HCL = hairy cell leukaemia).

HIGH-YIELD PEARL — Smudge cells point to CLL

Smudge cells (Gumprecht shadows) are nuclear remnants of mechanically fragile lymphocytes that have ruptured during smear preparation. They are abundant in CLL and uncommon in reactive lymphocytosis or in other small B-cell neoplasms. Adding a drop of albumin to the blood prior to smear preparation reduces smudge cell formation when an accurate differential is required. A high smudge-cell count has been associated with a more indolent CLL course in some series. The exam vignette signal: an older patient with absolute lymphocytosis of small mature-appearing lymphocytes with abundant smudge cells is CLL — flow cytometry confirms.

CLL prognosis, staging, and treatment

Staging uses the Rai (US) and Binet (European) systems. Rai stage 0 (lymphocytosis only) and stage I (lymphocytosis with lymphadenopathy) are low-risk; stage II (with hepatomegaly or splenomegaly) is intermediate; stages III (anaemia from marrow infiltration) and IV (thrombocytopenia from marrow infiltration) are high-risk. Beyond stage, the prognostically dominant variables are IGHV mutational status, FISH cytogenetic abnormalities (del(17p) and del(11q) are adverse; del(13q) alone is favourable; trisomy 12 is intermediate), and TP53 mutational status.

First-line therapy for treatment-naive CLL is now a targeted-agent regimen: a BTK inhibitor (acalabrutinib or zanubrutinib preferred over ibrutinib for cardiovascular safety) given continuously, or venetoclax plus obinutuzumab given as a fixed-duration regimen (12 months). FCR (fludarabine, cyclophosphamide, rituximab) retains a role only in young, fit IGHV-mutated patients without del(17p) or TP53 mutation, where it can produce long-term plateau survival. Patients with del(17p) or TP53 mutation should never receive purine-analogue chemotherapy (chemotherapy-resistant by virtue of TP53 loss) and require BTK or BCL2 inhibitor therapy. For relapsed disease — particularly after covalent BTK inhibitor failure with C481-mutated resistance — pirtobrutinib (a non-covalent reversible BTK inhibitor, FDA-approved 2023) restores BTK inhibition and is now standard for that setting. Richter transformation — emergence of a high-grade large B-cell lymphoma in a patient with CLL — occurs in 5–10% of CLL patients and is treated with aggressive lymphoma-directed therapy (R-EPOCH or stem-cell transplant); the prognosis remains poor.

STEP 2 BRIDGE — del(17p)/TP53 in CLL changes everything

The 17p deletion encompasses the TP53 locus, and CLL with del(17p) — or with TP53 mutation in the absence of deletion — is fundamentally chemorefractory. Cytotoxic chemotherapy depends on intact TP53 to drive apoptosis after DNA damage; loss of TP53 abrogates this response. Patients with del(17p) who receive FCR have a markedly inferior progression-free survival compared with del(17p) patients receiving BTK inhibitors. The clinical rule: FISH for del(17p) and sequencing for TP53 mutations are mandatory before any treatment decision in CLL, and a positive result mandates a targeted-agent regimen — never chemotherapy.

13.9 Hairy Cell Leukaemia

Hairy cell leukaemia is a rare indolent mature B-cell neoplasm with a distinctive morphology and a near-universal driver mutation. Patients are typically middle-aged men presenting with pancytopenia, monocytopenia (a striking and often diagnostic finding), and massive splenomegaly without lymphadenopathy. The bone marrow aspirate is frequently a "dry tap" because of accompanying reticulin fibrosis; the trephine biopsy shows a diffuse infiltrate of medium-sized lymphoid cells with eccentric reniform nuclei and abundant pale cytoplasm with fine cytoplasmic projections — the "fried egg" appearance on H&E. The hairy cells are TRAP (tartrate-resistant acid phosphatase) positive. Flow cytometry shows the diagnostic CD20-bright, CD25+, CD11c+, CD103+ phenotype with characteristic surface immunoglobulin restriction.

The driver mutation is BRAF V600E, present in essentially all classical hairy cell leukaemia cases. The "variant" form (HCL-v) lacks BRAF V600E, has a more aggressive course, and does not respond to standard cladribine therapy. Treatment of classical HCL is a single course of cladribine (2-CdA) or pentostatin, both purine-analogue drugs, producing long-term remissions in approximately 80% of patients. Vemurafenib (a BRAF V600E inhibitor) is active in relapsed disease and in the rare patient who cannot tolerate purine analogues. Moxetumomab pasudotox (anti-CD22 immunotoxin) is approved for relapsed disease.

HIGH-YIELD PEARL — Recognising hairy cell leukaemia

Three findings together are essentially diagnostic of hairy cell leukaemia and are the discriminators examiners use: absolute monocytopenia (a profoundly low monocyte count is unusual in any other condition), massive splenomegaly without significant lymphadenopathy, and a marrow trephine showing the "fried egg" cells with TRAP positivity and the CD25+, CD103+, CD11c+ phenotype on flow. The single-step molecular confirmation is BRAF V600E mutation testing. The vignette signal: a middle-aged man with pancytopenia, monocytopenia, and splenomegaly is hairy cell leukaemia until proven otherwise; the answer set will include a "fried egg" or TRAP-positive descriptor.

13.10 Buzzwords and Associations — Vignette Trigger Table

Vignette buzzword / finding	Diagnosis to trigger	One-line "why"
Leukocytosis with basophilia and eosinophilia; full myeloid spectrum	Chronic myeloid leukaemia (BCR::ABL1, p210)	Constitutive ABL1 kinase; basophilia is the discriminator from leukemoid reaction
Low LAP score (leukocyte alkaline phosphatase)	CML	Clonal granulocytes have reduced LAP activity
TKI failure with T315I gatekeeper mutation	Switch to ponatinib (or asciminib)	T315I blocks all earlier-generation BCR::ABL1 TKIs
Hct >55%, plethora, pruritus after warm shower, low EPO	Polycythaemia vera (JAK2 V617F)	Autonomous EPO-independent erythropoiesis suppresses endogenous EPO
Erythromelalgia (burning pain in hands/feet relieved by cold)	PV or ET	Microvascular platelet aggregation; aspirin-responsive
Hepatic vein thrombosis (Budd-Chiari) in a young patient	PV (or other MPN)	Splanchnic thrombosis is the MPN-defining complication
Persistent thrombocytosis $>450 \times 10^9$/L without iron deficiency	Essential thrombocythaemia	JAK2 (50–60%), CALR (20–25%), or MPL (3–5%); marrow biopsy decides
Leukoerythroblastic blood with teardrop cells (dacrocytes), massive splenomegaly, weight loss	Primary myelofibrosis	Marrow architectural disruption; extramedullary haematopoiesis
Older patient, absolute lymphocytosis, smudge cells, CD5+ CD23+ CD20-dim B cells	Chronic lymphocytic leukaemia	CD23 distinguishes CLL from mantle cell lymphoma
CLL with rapidly enlarging single node, B symptoms, high LDH	Richter transformation (DLBCL)	Aggressive transformation; biopsy the dominant node
Middle-aged man with pancytopenia, monocytopenia, massive splenomegaly, dry tap	Hairy cell leukaemia (BRAF V600E)	Marrow fibrosis from hairy cells produces the dry tap
"Fried egg" cells on marrow biopsy; TRAP positive; CD25/CD103/CD11c triple positive	Hairy cell leukaemia	Classic morphology and triple-positive immunophenotype
Sustained monocytosis $\geq 1 \times 10^9$/L with dysplasia	Chronic myelomonocytic leukaemia	TET2, SRSF2, ASXL1 mutations support clonality

Vignette buzzword / finding	Diagnosis to trigger	One-line "why"
Toxic granulation, Döhle bodies, high LAP, identifiable infection	Leukemoid reaction (NOT CML)	Reactive process — no basophilia, high LAP, no BCR::ABL1

Table 13.4. Vignette buzzwords for chronic leukaemias and MPNs.

13.11 USMLE Vignettes

Ten vignettes follow, weighted toward the most heavily tested entities: CML pathogenesis and TKI selection, the JAK2-driven MPN spectrum, and CLL prognosis-driven therapy. Each vignette includes lab values examiners use as anchors and rationales that walk through the mechanism rather than merely the answer.

Vignette 1. A 58-year-old man with leukocytosis on a routine CBC

A 58-year-old man is referred to haematology after a routine pre-operative CBC for elective hernia repair shows a leukocytosis. He reports several months of mild fatigue and early satiety. Examination shows a palpable spleen 6 cm below the costal margin; no lymphadenopathy. Laboratory studies: haemoglobin 11.2 g/dL, platelets 540,000/µL, white blood cells 142,000/µL with 2% blasts, 4% promyelocytes, 12% myelocytes, 18% metamyelocytes, 14% bands, 38% segmented neutrophils, 7% basophils, 3% eosinophils, 2% lymphocytes. The leukocyte alkaline phosphatase score is 8 (low). FISH detects the t(9;22)(q34;q11.2) translocation and RT-PCR identifies the BCR::ABL1 p210 fusion transcript. Which of the following is the most appropriate first-line therapy?

- **(A)** A BCR::ABL1 tyrosine kinase inhibitor — imatinib, dasatinib, nilotinib, bosutinib, or asciminib.
- **(B)** Allogeneic stem cell transplantation in first chronic phase.
- **(C)** Hydroxyurea monotherapy without molecular monitoring.
- **(D)** Splenectomy followed by interferon alfa.
- **(E)** Induction chemotherapy with "7+3" cytarabine and an anthracycline.

Best answer: (A) A BCR::ABL1 tyrosine kinase inhibitor — imatinib, dasatinib, nilotinib, bosutinib, or asciminib.

Rationale. The clinical picture is classical chronic-phase CML: a middle-aged man with marked leukocytosis, the full myeloid spectrum (blasts, promyelocytes, myelocytes, metamyelocytes, bands, segmented neutrophils), basophilia, mild thrombocytosis, splenomegaly, a low LAP score, and confirmed BCR::ABL1 by FISH and RT-PCR. The blast count is below 10%, basophils are below 20%, and there are no accelerated-phase features — chronic phase. First-line therapy is a BCR::ABL1 TKI. Five agents are now FDA-approved first-line: imatinib (longest safety record), dasatinib, nilotinib, bosutinib, and asciminib (FDA-approved first-line October 2024 based on superior 48-week MMR in ASC4FIRST; NCCN Category 1 preferred). Asciminib is a STAMP-pocket allosteric inhibitor mechanistically distinct from the ATP-pocket TKIs. Second-generation ATP-pocket TKIs (dasatinib, nilotinib) produce faster, deeper molecular responses and may be preferred in younger patients, in higher-risk ELTS or Sokal scores, or when treatment-free remission is the long-term goal. Treatment response is monitored by quantitative RT-PCR on the International Scale; the goal at 12 months is BCR::ABL1 IS ≤1%, and major molecular response (≤0.1%) is the durable target.

Distractor analysis. (B) AlloSCT is reserved for accelerated/blast phase, multi-TKI failure, or T315I without ponatinib access. (C) Hydroxyurea controls the WBC but does not produce cytogenetic or molecular response and is not standard of care. (D) Splenectomy is not a CML therapy; interferon has been displaced by TKIs. (E) "7+3" induction is for AML, not chronic-phase CML.

Vignette 2. A 62-year-old woman in CML chronic phase three years into imatinib who develops resistance

A 62-year-old woman has been on imatinib 400 mg daily for chronic-phase CML for three years. She achieved a complete cytogenetic response at 12 months and major molecular response at 18 months. At her routine 36-month follow-up, BCR::ABL1 IS has risen from 0.05% (12 months ago) to 1.8% (6 months ago) to 12% today. She has been compliant with imatinib (verified pill counts and trough drug levels in range). A repeat bone marrow biopsy shows chronic-phase morphology with 4% blasts. BCR::ABL1 kinase domain sequencing is performed and identifies a T315I mutation. Which of the following is the most appropriate next step?

- **(A)** Switch to nilotinib at maximum tolerated dose.
- **(B)** Switch to ponatinib (or asciminib).
- **(C)** Increase imatinib to 800 mg daily.
- **(D)** Add hydroxyurea to imatinib for cytoreduction.
- **(E)** Proceed directly to allogeneic stem cell transplantation without further TKI therapy.

Best answer: (B) Switch to ponatinib (or asciminib).

Rationale. Rising BCR::ABL1 transcript levels in a compliant CML patient indicate either disease progression or acquired TKI resistance via a kinase-domain mutation. Sequencing identifies T315I — a substitution of isoleucine for threonine at the gatekeeper position of the ABL1 ATP-binding pocket. T315I confers resistance to imatinib, dasatinib, nilotinib, and bosutinib because the bulky isoleucine side chain prevents these TKIs from binding the kinase pocket. Ponatinib (a third-generation TKI designed to accommodate the T315I mutation) and asciminib (a STAMP-class inhibitor that binds the myristoyl pocket allosterically and is unaffected by ATP-pocket mutations) retain activity. Ponatinib carries significant cardiovascular risk; the dose has been refined (15–30 mg) to balance efficacy and toxicity. AlloSCT remains an option in patients without ponatinib or asciminib access or in those who progress despite these agents.

Distractor analysis. (A) Nilotinib does not overcome T315I. (C) Imatinib dose escalation does not overcome T315I and risks toxicity without benefit. (D) Hydroxyurea is a cytoreductive agent that does not address the kinase resistance. (E) AlloSCT is appropriate only after exhausting effective TKI options.

Vignette 3. A 62-year-old man with plethora, pruritus after showers, and elevated haematocrit

A 62-year-old man presents with three months of headache, dizziness, blurred vision, and intense pruritus after warm showers. He has noted facial plethora and a recent episode of severe burning pain in his fingers and toes that resolved with aspirin. Examination shows a ruddy complexion, non-tender splenomegaly 4 cm below the costal margin, and no lymphadenopathy. Laboratory studies: haemoglobin 19.4 g/dL, haematocrit 58%, platelets 612,000/µL, white blood cells 14,000/µL with normal differential. Serum erythropoietin is 2.4 mIU/mL (low; reference 4–24). JAK2 V617F mutation is detected. Bone marrow biopsy shows hypercellularity for age with trilineage proliferation and pleomorphic megakaryocytes. Which of the following best describes the appropriate management strategy?

- **(A)** Therapeutic phlebotomy to maintain haematocrit below 45%, low-dose aspirin, and cytoreduction with hydroxyurea given the patient's age >60 years (high-risk PV by

NCCN/ELN criteria).

(B) Therapeutic phlebotomy alone to maintain haematocrit below 45%, with no other intervention required.

(C) Anticoagulation with warfarin and observation without phlebotomy.

(D) Splenectomy and erythropoiesis-stimulating agent administration.

(E) Allogeneic stem cell transplantation.

Best answer: (A) Therapeutic phlebotomy to maintain haematocrit below 45%, low-dose aspirin, and cytoreduction with hydroxyurea given the patient's age >60 years (high-risk PV by NCCN/ELN criteria).

Rationale. The patient meets all WHO 2022 PV diagnostic criteria: haemoglobin >16.5 g/dL (major 1), trilineage marrow hypercellularity with pleomorphic megakaryocytes (major 2), JAK2 V617F (major 3), and subnormal EPO (minor). Erythromelalgia (burning pain in extremities relieved by cold or aspirin), aquagenic pruritus, and plethora are classical. Risk stratification places age >60 or prior thrombosis into high-risk; at 62 this patient meets the age criterion. Standard PV therapy for high-risk patients is the triad of phlebotomy (target Hct <45% — the CYTO-PV trial demonstrated reduced cardiovascular events at this threshold), low-dose aspirin (reduces thrombosis), and cytoreduction (hydroxyurea is first-line; ropeginterferon alfa-2b is preferred in younger patients and pregnancy; ruxolitinib for hydroxyurea intolerance/resistance). Aquagenic pruritus often responds to SSRIs or to ruxolitinib in refractory cases.

Distractor analysis. (B) Phlebotomy alone is appropriate only for the lowest-risk PV — younger patients without thrombosis history and without extreme thrombocytosis or hyperviscosity. (C) Anticoagulation without addressing the underlying erythrocytosis fails to address the cause. (D) Splenectomy is not standard PV management; ESAs are contraindicated. (E) AlloSCT is reserved for transformation to post-PV myelofibrosis or AML.

Vignette 4. A 28-year-old woman with persistent thrombocytosis and a CALR mutation

A 28-year-old woman is found to have a platelet count of 920,000/µL on a routine CBC. She is asymptomatic. Iron studies show ferritin 78 ng/mL and normal iron saturation. C-reactive protein is normal. There is no recent infection, surgery, or splenectomy. Repeat platelet count six weeks later is 870,000/µL. Bone marrow biopsy shows enlarged hyperlobated mature megakaryocytes in loose clusters without significant reticulin fibrosis and no blast excess. JAK2 V617F is negative. CALR exon 9 sequencing identifies a 52-base-pair deletion (type 1 CALR mutation). Which of the following statements about her diagnosis and management is most accurate?

(A) She has essential thrombocythaemia; observation alone is reasonable, with low-dose aspirin if vasomotor symptoms develop, given her low-risk profile.

(B) She has essential thrombocythaemia; high-risk features mandate immediate hydroxyurea and aspirin.

(C) She has primary myelofibrosis; ruxolitinib is indicated.

(D) She has reactive thrombocytosis; iron supplementation is the appropriate next step.

(E) She has chronic myeloid leukaemia; a BCR::ABL1 TKI should be initiated.

Best answer: (A) She has essential thrombocythaemia; observation alone is reasonable, with low-dose aspirin if vasomotor symptoms develop, given her low-

risk profile.

Rationale. Sustained thrombocytosis ≥450 × 10^9/L with the characteristic megakaryocytic morphology of ET (enlarged hyperlobated mature megakaryocytes in loose clusters, no significant fibrosis), a normal-iron status, and a clonal driver mutation (CALR type 1) establishes the WHO 2022 diagnosis of essential thrombocythaemia. The CALR type 1 mutation in ET is associated with a more indolent course than JAK2 V617F. Risk stratification (IPSET-thrombosis) places age ≤60, no prior thrombosis, and absence of cardiovascular risk factors into the very-low-risk category. JAK2-wild-type ET further reduces the thrombosis risk. Low-risk ET can be observed; low-dose aspirin is added when vasomotor symptoms develop or in the presence of cardiovascular risk factors. Cytoreduction is reserved for high-risk patients (age >60, prior thrombosis, or extreme thrombocytosis with bleeding from acquired von Willebrand disease).

Distractor analysis. (B) High-risk features (age >60, prior thrombosis) are absent; reflexive cytoreduction is overtreatment. (C) PMF requires marrow fibrosis and a different megakaryocyte morphology. (D) Reactive thrombocytosis would not have a clonal CALR mutation and the iron studies are normal. (E) CML is BCR::ABL1 positive and morphologically distinct.

Vignette 5. A 68-year-old woman with progressive splenomegaly and a leukoerythroblastic blood picture

A 68-year-old woman presents with one year of progressive fatigue, ten-pound weight loss, drenching night sweats, and increasing abdominal fullness. Examination shows pallor, massive splenomegaly extending to the iliac crest, and hepatomegaly. Laboratory studies: haemoglobin 8.2 g/dL, platelets 84,000/µL, white blood cells 18,000/µL with 4% blasts, 8% myelocytes, 6% metamyelocytes, 8% nucleated red blood cells, and prominent teardrop-shaped red cells (dacrocytes). LDH is 1,180 U/L. Bone marrow aspiration is unsuccessful (dry tap); the trephine biopsy shows marked reticulin and collagen fibrosis (MF-3) with atypical megakaryocyte clusters and increased cellularity. JAK2 V617F is detected. ASXL1 mutation is also present. Which of the following is the best initial therapy for symptom control in this patient?

- **(A)** Ruxolitinib.
- **(B)** Imatinib.
- **(C)** Hydroxyurea monotherapy.
- **(D)** Therapeutic phlebotomy.
- **(E)** Splenectomy as the first intervention before any pharmacologic therapy.

Best answer: (A) Ruxolitinib.

Rationale. The clinical picture is classical primary myelofibrosis: progressive constitutional symptoms (weight loss, night sweats, fatigue), massive splenomegaly from extramedullary haematopoiesis, anaemia, and a leukoerythroblastic peripheral blood smear with dacrocytes. The marrow trephine confirms MF-3 fibrosis with atypical megakaryocytes. JAK2 V617F is the most common driver mutation in PMF; ASXL1 is a high-molecular-risk mutation that worsens prognosis. Ruxolitinib (a JAK1/2 inhibitor) is first-line for symptomatic PMF and produces durable spleen volume reduction and improvement in constitutional symptoms regardless of driver mutation status. Pacritinib is preferred when the platelet count is below 50 × 10^9/L. Allogeneic stem cell transplantation is the only curative option and should be offered to fit patients with high-risk MIPSS70 or MIPSS70+ v2.0 scores; this patient at 68 with multiple high-molecular-risk mutations (JAK2 plus ASXL1) qualifies for transplant evaluation in parallel.

Distractor analysis. (B) Imatinib targets BCR::ABL1, which is not present. (C) Hydroxyurea controls counts and may help splenomegaly modestly but does not match ruxolitinib for symptom and spleen response. (D) Phlebotomy is for PV, not for PMF (where anaemia, not erythrocytosis, dominates). (E) Splenectomy in PMF carries high perioperative morbidity and mortality and is reserved for refractory transfusion-dependent splenomegaly after pharmacologic options fail.

Vignette 6. A 72-year-old man with absolute lymphocytosis and smudge cells

A 72-year-old man is found on routine evaluation to have an absolute lymphocyte count of 28,000/µL. He is asymptomatic. Examination shows mild non-tender bilateral cervical lymphadenopathy and a palpable spleen tip; no hepatomegaly. Laboratory studies: haemoglobin 13.1 g/dL, platelets 168,000/µL, white blood cells 32,000/µL with 88% lymphocytes. The peripheral smear shows small mature-appearing lymphocytes with clumped "block" chromatin and abundant smudge cells. Flow cytometry on peripheral blood: CD19+, CD5+, CD23+, CD20 dim, CD79b dim, surface immunoglobulin dim with κ light-chain restriction. FISH shows del(13q) as the sole abnormality. IGHV is mutated (4.5% deviation from germline). TP53 is wild-type. Which of the following is the most appropriate management strategy?

- **(A)** Observation with serial CBC and clinical assessment ("watchful waiting"); no therapy is indicated until clinical progression occurs.
- **(B)** Immediate initiation of acalabrutinib regardless of stage.
- **(C)** FCR (fludarabine, cyclophosphamide, rituximab) chemoimmunotherapy.
- **(D)** Allogeneic stem cell transplantation as consolidation.
- **(E)** Splenectomy followed by venetoclax monotherapy.

Best answer: (A) Observation with serial CBC and clinical assessment ("watchful waiting"); no therapy is indicated until clinical progression occurs.

Rationale. The diagnosis is CLL: absolute B-lymphocyte count ≥5 × 10^9/L (this patient has 28 × 10^9/L) with the characteristic CD19+, CD5+, CD23+, CD20-dim, CD79b-dim, surface-Ig-dim phenotype. Smudge cells on the smear are consistent. The patient has Rai stage I (lymphocytosis with lymphadenopathy; haemoglobin and platelets are preserved), favourable cytogenetics (del(13q) alone is the most favourable single FISH abnormality), IGHV mutated (favourable), and TP53 wild-type. CLL with these features is biologically indolent. Multiple prospective trials have shown that early treatment of asymptomatic CLL does not improve overall survival regardless of stage, and the standard of care for asymptomatic Rai stage 0–II CLL without high-risk features remains observation. Indications to initiate therapy (per iwCLL criteria) are progressive marrow failure (anaemia or thrombocytopenia from infiltration), massive or progressive splenomegaly, massive or progressive lymphadenopathy, progressive lymphocytosis with rapid doubling time (<6 months) or significant constitutional symptoms, autoimmune cytopenias unresponsive to corticosteroids, or symptomatic extranodal involvement.

Distractor analysis. (B) Initiating BTK inhibitor in asymptomatic indolent CLL exposes the patient to chronic toxicity without survival benefit. (C) FCR is now reserved for fit younger patients with IGHV-mutated, TP53-wild-type CLL who require treatment, not for observation candidates. (D) AlloSCT is reserved for high-risk relapsed/refractory disease. (E) Splenectomy is not first-line CLL management.

Vignette 7. A 65-year-old woman with CLL and a deletion 17p

A 65-year-old woman with previously low-risk CLL has been followed for two years. She now presents with progressive fatigue, painless cervical and axillary lymphadenopathy, and a haemoglobin that has fallen from 12.4 to 8.9 g/dL over six months. Platelets are 95,000/µL. Bone marrow biopsy shows >70% replacement by CLL cells. Flow cytometry confirms her CLL phenotype unchanged. Repeat FISH now shows del(17p) in 65% of cells. TP53 sequencing identifies a missense mutation. IGHV remains unmutated. She is otherwise functionally well and has no significant comorbidities. Which of the following is the most appropriate first-line therapy?

(A) A BTK inhibitor (acalabrutinib or zanubrutinib) as continuous therapy, OR venetoclax plus obinutuzumab as fixed-duration therapy.

(B) FCR (fludarabine, cyclophosphamide, rituximab) chemoimmunotherapy.

(C) Bendamustine plus rituximab.

(D) Chlorambucil monotherapy.

(E) High-dose methylprednisolone alone.

Best answer: (A) A BTK inhibitor (acalabrutinib or zanubrutinib) as continuous therapy, OR venetoclax plus obinutuzumab as fixed-duration therapy.

Rationale. CLL with del(17p) or TP53 mutation is fundamentally chemorefractory: the cytotoxic drugs depend on intact TP53 to drive apoptosis after DNA damage, and TP53 loss abrogates this response. Patients with del(17p) treated with FCR have markedly inferior progression-free survival compared with del(17p) patients receiving targeted agents. The current standard of care for treatment-naive del(17p)/TP53-mutated CLL is either continuous BTK inhibitor (acalabrutinib and zanubrutinib are preferred over ibrutinib for cardiovascular safety) or fixed-duration venetoclax plus obinutuzumab. Both produce substantially better outcomes than any chemoimmunotherapy regimen. The clinical rule: any CLL patient requires FISH for del(17p) and TP53 sequencing before treatment; a positive result mandates targeted therapy and excludes chemoimmunotherapy.

Distractor analysis. (B) FCR is contraindicated in del(17p)/TP53-mutated disease. (C) Bendamustine-rituximab is also chemoimmunotherapy and shares the chemorefractory issue with del(17p). (D) Chlorambucil monotherapy is reserved for very frail patients without targeted-agent options and is suboptimal regardless of TP53 status today. (E) High-dose corticosteroids are used short-term for autoimmune cytopenias in CLL but are not disease-directed therapy.

Vignette 8. A 54-year-old man with pancytopenia, monocytopenia, and splenomegaly

A 54-year-old man presents with fatigue and recurrent sinopulmonary infections over six months. Examination shows pallor, no lymphadenopathy, and a spleen palpable 8 cm below the costal margin. Laboratory studies: haemoglobin 9.4 g/dL, platelets 88,000/µL, white blood cells 2,200/µL with 14% neutrophils, 80% lymphocytes, 1% monocytes (absolute monocyte count 22/µL), and 5% atypical lymphocytes. The peripheral smear shows medium-sized mononuclear cells with eccentric nuclei and abundant pale cytoplasm with fine projections. A bone marrow aspirate yields no spicules ("dry tap"). The trephine biopsy shows a diffuse infiltrate of medium-sized lymphoid cells with reniform nuclei surrounded by abundant pale cytoplasm — described as a "fried egg" appearance — and increased reticulin. Flow cytometry on the marrow shows the lymphoid cells are CD19+, CD20 bright, CD25+, CD11c+, CD103+, with κ light-chain restriction. Which of the following molecular findings would be most expected, and what is the appropriate first-line therapy?

(A) BRAF V600E mutation; cladribine (or pentostatin) as a single course.

(B) JAK2 V617F mutation; ruxolitinib.

(C) BCR::ABL1 p210 fusion; imatinib.

(D) MYD88 L265P mutation; ibrutinib plus rituximab.

(E) CALR type 1 mutation; aspirin and observation.

Best answer: (A) BRAF V600E mutation; cladribine (or pentostatin) as a single course.

Rationale. The diagnosis is hairy cell leukaemia. The triad of pancytopenia with absolute monocytopenia, massive splenomegaly without lymphadenopathy, and the dry tap with "fried egg" cells on trephine is essentially diagnostic. The CD20-bright, CD25+, CD11c+, CD103+ phenotype is the classic immunophenotypic signature. Classical HCL is driven by BRAF V600E in essentially all cases (the variant form, HCL-v, is BRAF-wild-type, more aggressive, and does not respond to standard cladribine therapy). First-line treatment is a single course of cladribine (2-CdA) or pentostatin, both purine-analogue drugs that produce long-term remissions in approximately 80% of patients. Vemurafenib (a BRAF V600E inhibitor) and moxetumomab pasudotox (anti-CD22 immunotoxin) are second-line options for relapsed disease.

Distractor analysis. (B) JAK2 V617F drives PV/ET/PMF and ruxolitinib treats myelofibrosis — neither matches the fried-egg morphology and dry tap. (C) BCR::ABL1 is CML or Ph+ ALL. (D) MYD88 L265P drives Waldenström macroglobulinaemia (lymphoplasmacytic lymphoma with IgM monoclonal gammopathy and hyperviscosity), not HCL. (E) CALR type 1 is an MPN driver in ET/PMF, not HCL.

Vignette 9. A 68-year-old man with CLL who develops a rapidly enlarging single node with B symptoms

A 68-year-old man with a five-year history of Rai stage II CLL on observation presents with two months of weight loss, drenching night sweats, and a single rapidly enlarging right cervical lymph node measuring 6 × 5 cm. He has no other new adenopathy. Laboratory studies show his stable CLL parameters but a markedly elevated lactate dehydrogenase at 1,640 U/L (reference upper limit 250). Excisional biopsy of the cervical node shows a diffuse infiltrate of large cells with vesicular nuclei, prominent nucleoli, and frequent mitotic figures, replacing nodal architecture. Immunohistochemistry: CD20+, CD79a+, CD5+ (consistent with CLL origin), with a Ki-67 proliferation index of 85%. EBV in situ hybridisation is negative. Which of the following best explains the clinical picture and indicates the appropriate next step?

- **(A)** Richter transformation of the underlying CLL to diffuse large B-cell lymphoma; treat with R-EPOCH or equivalent aggressive lymphoma-directed therapy and consider stem cell transplantation.
- **(B)** CLL progression alone; intensify ibrutinib dose and continue observation of the node.
- **(C)** Reactive lymphadenopathy from concurrent infection; perform infectious workup before any treatment.
- **(D)** Hodgkin lymphoma–type Richter transformation; treat with ABVD chemotherapy.
- **(E)** Tuberculous lymphadenitis; start RIPE anti-tuberculous therapy.

Best answer: (A) Richter transformation of the underlying CLL to diffuse large B-cell lymphoma; treat with R-EPOCH or equivalent aggressive lymphoma-directed therapy and consider stem cell transplantation.

Rationale. Richter transformation is the emergence of an aggressive lymphoma, most commonly DLBCL, in a patient with underlying CLL. It occurs in 5–10% of CLL patients over the disease course and presents with a triad of rapid focal lymph node growth, B symptoms (fever, weight loss, night sweats), and very high LDH. The transformed clone is most often clonally related to the CLL (sharing the same IGHV rearrangement) and retains CLL-derived markers (CD5, CD20). The Ki-67 proliferation index in DLBCL is high (typically 60–95%), confirming the aggressive biology. Treatment requires lymphoma-directed therapy: R-EPOCH (rituximab, etoposide, prednisone, vincristine, cyclophosphamide, doxorubicin) is the most commonly used regimen; allogeneic SCT is considered in fit patients who achieve response. Outcomes remain poor (median survival under one year for clonally related Richter), and Richter transformation is the dominant cause of disease-related death in modern CLL. The minority subset of clonally unrelated Richter has a substantially better prognosis and is treated like de novo DLBCL. EBV-positive Richter is uncommon and pathobiologically distinct.

Distractor analysis. (B) CLL progression produces gradual generalised lymphadenopathy, not a single rapidly enlarging node with very high LDH. (C) Reactive lymphadenitis produces pain, tenderness, and lower LDH; the biopsy here shows large-cell lymphoma. (D) Hodgkin-type Richter is a recognised but minority form; the histology described (CD20+, CD79a+, large vesicular cells) is DLBCL, not Hodgkin. (E) Tuberculous lymphadenitis produces granulomatous inflammation, not large-cell lymphoma.

Vignette 10. A 24-year-old man with leukocytosis, fever, and a known infection — the elimination test

A 24-year-old previously healthy man presents to the emergency department with three days of high fever, productive cough, and right-sided pleuritic chest pain. Examination shows temperature 39.4°C, pulse 118/min, blood pressure 112/68 mm Hg, respiratory rate 24/min, and a focal area of bronchial breath sounds and crackles over the right middle lobe. Chest radiograph shows a right middle lobe consolidation. Laboratory studies: haemoglobin 13.8 g/dL, platelets 380,000/µL, white blood cells 64,000/µL with 18% bands, 4% myelocytes, 2% metamyelocytes, 70% segmented neutrophils with prominent toxic granulation, Döhle bodies, and cytoplasmic vacuolation, 4% lymphocytes, 2% monocytes, no basophilia, and no eosinophilia. The leukocyte alkaline phosphatase score is 280 (high). Blood cultures are sent. Which of the following best explains the laboratory findings and is the most appropriate next step?

- **(A)** Leukemoid reaction from community-acquired pneumonia; admit, start empiric antibiotics for community-acquired pneumonia, and reassess the WBC after antimicrobial therapy.
- **(B)** Chronic myeloid leukaemia with concurrent pneumonia; send BCR::ABL1 RT-PCR, start hydroxyurea, and treat the pneumonia.
- **(C)** AML in blast crisis from undiagnosed CML; arrange urgent bone marrow biopsy and start induction chemotherapy.
- **(D)** Polycythaemia vera with infection-related leukocytosis; phlebotomise and start aspirin.
- **(E)** Chronic neutrophilic leukaemia (CSF3R-driven); send CSF3R T618I sequencing and start ruxolitinib.

Best answer: (A) Leukemoid reaction from community-acquired pneumonia; admit, start empiric antibiotics for community-acquired pneumonia, and reassess the WBC after antimicrobial therapy.

Rationale. Three findings together exclude CML and establish a leukemoid reaction. First, the absence of basophilia: basophilia is nearly universal in chronic-phase CML and absent in reactive leukocytosis. Second, the high LAP score (280): clonal granulocytes in CML have low or zero LAP activity, while reactive granulocytes have high LAP activity.

Third, the morphological signs of activation — toxic granulation, Döhle bodies, cytoplasmic vacuolation — are features of reactive (cytokine-stimulated) neutrophils responding to an obvious infectious stimulus, not features of clonal CML. The clinical setting (febrile young adult with focal lobar pneumonia) is consistent with severe bacterial sepsis driving cytokine-mediated bone-marrow output. The appropriate next step is empiric antibiotic therapy for community-acquired pneumonia (a beta-lactam plus a macrolide, or a respiratory fluoroquinolone), with reassessment of the WBC after 48–72 hours of effective antimicrobial therapy. Resolution of the leukocytosis with treatment of the infection confirms the reactive process. Persistence of leukocytosis beyond infection control prompts BCR::ABL1 testing.

Distractor analysis. (B) Reflexive BCR::ABL1 testing in this clinical context is reasonable as confirmation but is not the immediate next step; the high LAP and absent basophilia argue strongly against CML. (C) "Blast crisis" requires ≥20% blasts; this WBC differential does not show that. (D) PV is defined by erythrocytosis, not by neutrophilic leukocytosis. (E) Chronic neutrophilic leukaemia is rare, requires CSF3R T618I or T615A mutation, and typically lacks the toxic granulation and identifiable infection seen here.

13.12 Closing Discriminators

HIGH-YIELD PEARL — Splanchnic vein thrombosis as a presentation of MPN

Hepatic vein (Budd-Chiari syndrome), portal vein, and mesenteric vein thrombosis are over-represented as presenting features of myeloproliferative neoplasms, particularly polycythaemia vera and essential thrombocythaemia. The vignette pattern is a young to middle-aged patient with new abdominal pain, ascites, and hepatomegaly (Budd-Chiari) or with portal hypertension and a normal-appearing liver imaging without cirrhosis. JAK2 V617F testing should be performed in any patient with unexplained splanchnic thrombosis even when blood counts are normal — masked PV (with iron deficiency from chronic GI losses or with plasma volume expansion in cirrhosis) can normalise the haematocrit and hide the underlying disease. The "exam" pattern: a young woman with Budd-Chiari and a normal CBC who is JAK2 V617F positive has occult PV, not idiopathic Budd-Chiari, and requires phlebotomy and aspirin once the splanchnic thrombosis is anticoagulated.

HIGH-YIELD PEARL — Autoimmune cytopenias in CLL

Autoimmune complications occur in 5–15% of CLL patients and are diagnostically distinct from marrow infiltration. Autoimmune haemolytic anaemia (AIHA) is most common, typically warm-antibody (IgG, panreactive); the direct antiglobulin test is positive, haemolytic markers (LDH, indirect bilirubin, reticulocyte count) are elevated, and haptoglobin is low. Immune thrombocytopenia (ITP) and pure red cell aplasia (PRCA) are less common. Crucially, autoimmune cytopenias in CLL do NOT upstage the patient to Rai III/IV — those stages require marrow-infiltration-derived cytopenias. AIHA in CLL is treated initially with corticosteroids (prednisone 1 mg/kg) followed by rituximab if refractory; CLL-directed therapy is intensified only if the cytopenia is refractory or recurrent or if the CLL itself otherwise meets treatment criteria. The exam vignette: a CLL patient with new anaemia, positive DAT, elevated LDH and bilirubin, and reticulocytosis is AIHA — start prednisone, do not yet escalate CLL therapy.

TRAP — Not all polycythaemia is PV

Erythrocytosis (elevated haematocrit) has many causes; PV is one of them. The first step in any erythrocytosis workup is the EPO level. Low EPO points to PV (autonomous erythropoiesis suppresses endogenous EPO); normal-to-high EPO points to secondary erythrocytosis. Causes of high-EPO erythrocytosis include hypoxia-driven (chronic hypoxic lung disease, sleep apnea, high altitude, cyanotic congenital heart disease, heavy smoking with elevated COHb) and inappropriate-EPO-production (renal cell carcinoma, hepatocellular carcinoma, cerebellar haemangioblastoma, polycystic kidney disease, post-renal-transplant erythrocytosis). Apparent (relative) polycythaemia from plasma volume contraction (severe dehydration, diuretics, Gaisbock syndrome in obese hypertensive males) shows normal red cell mass on isotope dilution. The wrong-answer pattern: assuming PV in any patient with elevated haematocrit and prescribing phlebotomy and aspirin without checking EPO. The discriminator answer is "check serum EPO first."

IMG-TRAP — "If the count is high, treat" reflex applied to CLL is wrong

Trainees educated where every leukaemia diagnosis prompts immediate cytoreduction tend to mistreat CLL on USMLE vignettes. Asymptomatic Rai stage 0 to II CLL — even with a lymphocyte count of 100 × 10^9/L — does not require therapy. Multiple prospective trials (CLL1, the German CLL Study Group experience) have demonstrated that early treatment of asymptomatic CLL does not improve overall survival. The treatment thresholds (iwCLL criteria) are clinical, not numerical: progressive marrow failure (Rai III/IV anaemia or thrombocytopenia from infiltration), bulky or progressive lymphadenopathy or splenomegaly, lymphocyte doubling time <6 months at counts >30 × 10^9/L, autoimmune cytopenias unresponsive to corticosteroids, or significant constitutional symptoms (the iwCLL B-symptom equivalents). The exam-correct answer for an asymptomatic Rai stage 0–II patient — even with a striking absolute lymphocyte count — is observation. Treatment intensity is determined by indication, not by count alone.

13.13 Quick Recall

QUICK RECALL — Chronic Leukaemias and MPNs

CML. t(9;22)/BCR::ABL1 (p210). Leukocytosis with full myeloid spectrum, basophilia, eosinophilia, low LAP. Three phases: chronic (<10% blasts), accelerated (10–19%, ≥20% basophils), blast (≥20% blasts). First-line: BCR::ABL1 TKI (imatinib, dasatinib, nilotinib, bosutinib, or asciminib — first-line FDA-approved Oct 2024). T315I → ponatinib or asciminib. Risk score: ELTS preferred over Sokal.

TKI selection. Cardiovascular disease: avoid nilotinib, ponatinib. Pulmonary disease: avoid dasatinib (pleural effusions, PAH). T315I: ponatinib or asciminib.

PV. JAK2 V617F (>95%) or JAK2 exon 12 (3–5%). WHO 2022: 3 majors (Hb threshold + panmyelosis + JAK2) or majors 1+2 plus low EPO. Plethora, aquagenic pruritus, erythromelalgia, gout, splanchnic thrombosis. Treatment: phlebotomy to Hct <45%, aspirin, hydroxyurea (high-risk), ruxolitinib (refractory).

ET. JAK2 (50–60%), CALR (20–25%), MPL (3–5%). Sustained platelets ≥450 × 10^9/L without erythrocytosis or significant fibrosis. Loose mature megakaryocyte clusters. Low-risk: observation ± aspirin. High-risk: cytoreduction.

PMF. JAK2/CALR/MPL drivers. Prefibrotic and fibrotic stages. Leukoerythroblastic blood with dacrocytes. Massive splenomegaly, weight loss, night sweats. MIPSS70/MIPSS70+ v2.0 risk. Ruxolitinib for symptoms; alloSCT for cure.

CMML. Sustained monocytosis ≥1 × 10^9/L (or ≥0.5 × 10^9/L plus ≥10% of WBC) plus dysplasia. TET2/SRSF2/ASXL1/CBL mutations. Two clinical subtypes (myeloproliferative, myelodysplastic). HMA for higher-risk; alloSCT only cure.

CLL phenotype. CD19+, CD5+, CD23+, CD20 dim, CD79b dim, sIg dim with light-chain restriction. Smudge cells. Distinguish from MCL (CD23 negative, cyclin D1+, t(11;14)).

CLL prognosis drivers. IGHV mutated (favourable) vs unmutated (adverse). FISH: del(13q) favourable; trisomy 12 intermediate; del(11q)/ATM, del(17p)/TP53 adverse. TP53 mutation = chemorefractory.

CLL treatment thresholds. iwCLL criteria. Asymptomatic Rai 0–II = observation regardless of count. del(17p)/TP53 = NEVER chemoimmunotherapy; use BTK inhibitor (acalabrutinib/zanubrutinib) or venetoclax + obinutuzumab.

Richter transformation. Rapidly enlarging single node with B symptoms and very high LDH in a CLL patient. Biopsy. R-EPOCH; alloSCT for fit responders. Median survival <1 year for clonally related Richter.

Hairy cell leukaemia. BRAF V600E. Pancytopenia + monocytopenia + massive splenomegaly without lymphadenopathy. Dry tap. "Fried egg" cells. TRAP+. CD20 bright, CD25+, CD11c+, CD103+. Cladribine (single course) or pentostatin → 80% long-term remission. HCL-v: BRAF wild-type, more aggressive.

Leukemoid reaction discriminators. High LAP, no basophilia, identifiable infection/inflammation, BCR::ABL1 negative. Toxic granulation and Döhle bodies. Resolves with treatment of the underlying cause.

Erythrocytosis workup. Step 1: serum EPO. Low → PV (JAK2 V617F → exon 12 if negative). Normal-high → secondary (hypoxia-driven or autonomous EPO production: RCC, HCC, cerebellar haemangioblastoma, PCKD, post-renal-transplant).

Splanchnic vein thrombosis. Budd-Chiari, portal vein, mesenteric vein thrombosis can be MPN presentations. Test JAK2 V617F even with normal CBC (masked PV).

Autoimmune cytopenias in CLL. Warm AIHA most common; positive DAT, haemolytic markers. Treat with prednisone → rituximab if refractory. Does NOT upstage CLL.

— End of Chapter 13 —

CHAPTER 14

Chapter 14 — Lymphomas: Hodgkin and Non-Hodgkin

BIG PICTURE

Lymphomas are clonal neoplasms of mature lymphocytes — predominantly B cells, with a smaller T-cell and rare NK-cell subset. The classical division between Hodgkin lymphoma and non-Hodgkin lymphoma is morphological and historical: Hodgkin lymphoma is a single B-cell malignancy with a distinctive minority population of malignant cells (Reed-Sternberg cells) embedded in a non-malignant inflammatory infiltrate, while non-Hodgkin lymphoma encompasses a broad family of B-cell, T-cell, and NK-cell malignancies. Two organising principles unlock the classification on the USMLE: stage of B-cell development at which the malignancy arose (pre-germinal centre, germinal centre, post-germinal centre), and the dominant cytogenetic translocation. Each combination predicts the clinical phenotype, the buzzword, and the answer.

MECHANISM HOOK — Why most B-cell lymphomas trace to the germinal centre

The germinal centre (GC) is a transient anatomical structure within secondary lymphoid follicles where activated B cells undergo somatic hypermutation (SHM) and class-switch recombination (CSR) to produce high-affinity antibodies. Both processes are driven by activation-induced cytidine deaminase (AID), an enzyme that intentionally introduces DNA breaks. The GC is therefore an environment of programmed genomic instability, and B cells that survive this process and exit as memory B cells or plasma cells have completed a high-risk maturation step. When SHM or CSR misfires, AID-induced double-strand breaks at immunoglobulin loci can be aberrantly joined to oncogenes — the molecular origin of t(14;18) joining BCL2 to IGH (follicular lymphoma), t(11;14) joining CCND1 to IGH (mantle cell, derived from naive pre-GC B cells), t(8;14) joining MYC to IGH (Burkitt lymphoma, post-GC origin), and the BCL6 rearrangements (3q27) in DLBCL — partnering with IGH or with various non-Ig genes. The cell-of-origin framework explains the clinical phenotype: pre-GC malignancies (mantle cell) tend to be CD5+ and aggressive; GC-derived malignancies (follicular, Burkitt, GCB-DLBCL) carry the apoptosis-blocking translocations; post-GC malignancies (ABC-DLBCL, plasma cell neoplasms, marginal zone lymphomas) reflect the next maturation step. WHO 2022 reorganises lymphoma classification along this developmental axis.

14.1 Hodgkin Lymphoma

Hodgkin lymphoma is divided in WHO 2022 into two biologically distinct entities: classical Hodgkin lymphoma (cHL, ~95%) and nodular lymphocyte-predominant B-cell lymphoma (NLPBL, formerly nodular lymphocyte-predominant Hodgkin lymphoma). Classical HL is further divided morphologically into four subtypes: nodular sclerosis (NSHL, ~70%), mixed cellularity (MCHL), lymphocyte-rich (LRHL), and lymphocyte-depleted (LDHL). The pathological hallmark of cHL is the Reed-Sternberg cell — a large binucleate or multinucleate cell with prominent eosinophilic "owl-eye" nucleoli, derived from a germinal centre B cell that has paradoxically extinguished most of its B-cell gene expression program. The malignant cells constitute only 1–5% of the tumour mass; the bulk of the lesion is a non-malignant inflammatory infiltrate of small lymphocytes, eosinophils, plasma cells, neutrophils, and histiocytes recruited by cytokines secreted by the Hodgkin and Reed-Sternberg (HRS) cells.

The HRS immunophenotype is decisive and counterintuitive. HRS cells are CD30 strongly positive (the defining marker, and the target of brentuximab vedotin), CD15 positive (membrane and Golgi pattern), CD20 negative or dim (aberrant loss of B-cell program), CD79a negative, PAX5 dim positive (the surviving residual B-cell transcription factor), CD45 negative, and OCT2/BOB1 negative (which explains the absence of immunoglobulin expression). EBV-LMP1 is positive in 30–80% of cases depending on subtype — highest in mixed cellularity and lymphocyte-depleted subtypes. The CD30+/CD15+/CD45− pattern distinguishes HRS cells from anaplastic large cell lymphoma, which is also CD30 positive but CD45 positive and (in the systemic ALK+ form) ALK positive.

Hodgkin lymphoma subtypes

Subtype	Morphology	Background	Demographics / clinical
Nodular sclerosis (NSHL)	Lacunar variant RS cells (retraction artefact); collagen bands dividing the node into nodules	Mixed eosinophils, neutrophils, plasma cells, lymphocytes; sclerosis prominent	Young adults (15–35); female preponderance; mediastinal mass classic
Mixed cellularity (MCHL)	Classical RS cells abundant	Eosinophils, plasma cells, histiocytes prominent; no sclerosis	Bimodal — children and elderly; EBV in ~70%; immunosuppression-associated
Lymphocyte-rich (LRHL)	RS cells sparse, in nodular or diffuse small-lymphocyte background	Predominantly small lymphocytes; few eosinophils; can mimic NLPBL	Older males; excellent prognosis
Lymphocyte-depleted (LDHL)	RS cells numerous, may form sheets	Few lymphocytes; fibrosis or necrosis	HIV-associated; elderly; retroperitoneal disease; worst-prognosis cHL
NLPBL (was NLPHL)	Lymphocyte-predominant ("popcorn") cells with multilobated folded nuclei	Abundant small lymphocytes and histiocytes in nodular pattern; no eosinophils or plasma cells	Young males; peripheral lymphadenopathy; indolent but late relapse; treated like indolent NHL

Table 14.1. Hodgkin lymphoma subtypes (WHO 2022).

Classical HL versus NLPBL — immunophenotypic discriminators

Marker	Classical HL (RS cells)	NLPBL (LP / popcorn cells)
CD30	STRONGLY POSITIVE (defining)	Negative

Marker	Classical HL (RS cells)	NLPBL (LP / popcorn cells)
CD15	Positive (membrane + Golgi)	Negative
CD20	Negative or dim	STRONGLY POSITIVE (retained B-cell)
CD45 (LCA)	Negative	POSITIVE — key discriminator
PAX5	Dim positive	Strong positive
OCT2 / BOB1	Negative (lost; explains absent Ig)	Positive
EBV-LMP1	Positive in 30–80%	Negative
Treatment	ABVD ± radiation; brentuximab + AVD in advanced; PD-1 blockade in relapse	Indolent NHL approach: rituximab ± radiation; observation in select stage IA

Table 14.2. Classical HL versus NLPBL — immunophenotype.

HIGH-YIELD PEARL — Reed-Sternberg-like cells are not specific to Hodgkin lymphoma

Cells morphologically resembling Reed-Sternberg cells appear in several non-Hodgkin contexts: anaplastic large cell lymphoma (CD30+, CD45+, ALK+ in systemic ALK+ form), T-cell/histiocyte-rich large B-cell lymphoma (CD20+, CD45+), EBV-driven post-transplant lymphoproliferative disorder, and even in florid infectious mononucleosis (rare HRS-like cells in inflamed lymph nodes). The diagnosis of cHL rests on the immunophenotypic triad CD30+ / CD15+ / CD45− in cells with the appropriate morphology and the appropriate inflammatory background. Morphology alone — even with classic RS appearance — is insufficient on the USMLE; confirm with IHC.

STEP 2 BRIDGE — Treating classical Hodgkin lymphoma

Stage drives intensity. Early-stage favourable cHL (stage I–II without bulky disease, B symptoms, or high ESR) is treated with abbreviated chemotherapy (ABVD × 2–4 cycles) plus involved-site radiation, achieving cure rates above 90%. Early-stage unfavorable disease receives more cycles of chemotherapy plus radiation. Advanced-stage cHL (stage III–IV) — current US first-line is nivolumab + AVD (N-AVD) per SWOG S1826 (NEJM 2024), which showed superior 2-year PFS (92% vs 83%) and better tolerability than brentuximab + AVD (BV-AVD); BV-AVD and full-course ABVD × 6 cycles remain acceptable alternatives. The shift away from bleomycin (pulmonary toxicity) and from BV (peripheral neuropathy, infections in older patients) reflects the cumulative late-effects burden in a curable disease. Relapsed/refractory cHL is treated with PD-1 blockade (nivolumab or pembrolizumab) — cHL has the highest response rate to PD-1 blockade of any malignancy, driven by 9p24.1 amplification and consequent PD-L1 over-expression. Brentuximab vedotin (anti-CD30 antibody-drug conjugate) and stem cell transplantation are also effective options in relapsed disease. Late effects of HL therapy — secondary breast cancer (radiotherapy-associated), cardiac toxicity (anthracycline plus radiation), and infertility — are major considerations in younger patients and shape de-escalation strategies.

14.2 Mature B-Cell Non-Hodgkin Lymphomas

Diffuse large B-cell lymphoma (DLBCL)

DLBCL is the most common non-Hodgkin lymphoma worldwide and accounts for approximately 30% of adult NHL in the United States. It is morphologically a diffuse proliferation of large B cells with vesicular nuclei, prominent nucleoli, and a high mitotic rate, replacing nodal architecture. WHO 2022 classifies DLBCL principally by cell of origin (COO): germinal-centre B-cell type (GCB) and activated B-cell type (ABC), distinguished by the Hans IHC algorithm (CD10, BCL6, IRF4/MUM1) or by gene-expression profiling. GCB-DLBCL has a substantially better prognosis with R-CHOP than ABC-DLBCL, which is driven by chronic active B-cell receptor signalling and dependence on NF-κB.

Two molecularly defined high-risk subgroups are essential to recognise. Double-hit lymphoma (DHL; WHO 2022 calls these "large B-cell lymphoma with MYC and BCL2 rearrangements") shows MYC rearrangement plus BCL2 rearrangement (with or without BCL6) by FISH break-apart probes. DHL accounts for ~5% of DLBCL, is overwhelmingly GCB-COO, and has very poor outcomes with R-CHOP — intensified regimens such as DA-EPOCH-R or R-CODOX-M/IVAC are preferred. Double-expressor lymphoma (DEL) shows MYC protein over-expression (≥40% by IHC) plus BCL2 protein over-expression (≥50% by IHC) without gene rearrangement; DEL is more common (~30% of DLBCL), has intermediate prognosis, and is treated with R-CHOP or with intensified regimens depending on risk. The exam point: DHL is defined by FISH (gene rearrangement); DEL is defined by IHC (protein); they are not interchangeable.

HIGH-YIELD PEARL — Double-hit and double-expressor lymphoma

Double-hit lymphoma (DHL) is now formally classified by WHO 2022 as "large B-cell lymphoma with MYC and BCL2 rearrangements." It requires confirmation of both MYC rearrangement AND BCL2 rearrangement on FISH break-apart probes — IHC is insufficient. Double-expressor lymphoma (DEL) requires MYC protein ≥40% and BCL2 protein ≥50% by IHC, with NO gene rearrangement on FISH. Vignettes describing "MYC and BCL2 over-expression" are ambiguous unless they specify whether the finding is by IHC (DEL) or by FISH (DHL). The treatment implication is direct: DHL is too aggressive for R-CHOP and needs intensified therapy; DEL receives R-CHOP with awareness of inferior outcomes. Note that under WHO 2022 the previous "MYC + BCL6" rearrangement (without BCL2) is no longer a "hit" lymphoma and is reported as DLBCL or HGBL NOS.

Burkitt lymphoma

Burkitt lymphoma is one of the fastest-growing human tumours, with a doubling time of approximately 24–48 hours and a Ki-67 proliferation index of essentially 100%. It is defined by a MYC rearrangement, most commonly t(8;14)/MYC::IGH (~80%), with light-chain partners t(2;8)/IGK::MYC and t(8;22)/MYC::IGL accounting for the remainder. Morphologically, Burkitt shows medium-sized cells with multiple basophilic nucleoli, basophilic cytoplasm with prominent lipid vacuoles, and a "starry sky" pattern at low power produced by tingible-body macrophages ingesting the abundant apoptotic tumour cells. The immunophenotype is CD20+, CD10+, BCL6+, BCL2 NEGATIVE (a critical discriminator from DHL, which expresses BCL2), Ki-67 ~100%, and TdT NEGATIVE (which discriminates from B-ALL with mature B-cell phenotype, formerly called L3-ALL).

Three clinical variants are recognised. The endemic form occurs in equatorial Africa, presents with a jaw or facial bone mass in children, and is EBV-positive in over 95% of cases — the prototype of EBV-driven malignancy. The sporadic form occurs in the United States and Europe, presents with abdominal disease (ileocecal mass, mesenteric or retroperitoneal nodes), and is EBV-positive in approximately 30%. The immunodeficiency-associated form (HIV) is EBV-positive in approximately 40%. All three variants are treated with intensified short-duration chemotherapy regimens (DA-EPOCH-R for adults; paediatric protocols based on COG or LMB89). Tumour lysis syndrome at induction is essentially universal and demands rasburicase prophylaxis.

IMG-TRAP — "Starry sky pattern means Burkitt"

The starry-sky pattern is high-yield but not specific. It appears in any high-grade B-cell lymphoma with a high apoptotic rate — Burkitt lymphoma classically, but also in double-hit lymphoma and in some high-grade B-cell lymphomas not otherwise specified. The discriminator is BCL2 status: Burkitt is BCL2 NEGATIVE; DHL is BCL2 positive (by IHC) and BCL2 rearranged (by FISH). Vignettes that describe "starry sky with BCL2 positivity by IHC" are NOT Burkitt — they are pointing toward DHL or HGBL. The exam-correct discriminator is the BCL2 result, not the starry-sky pattern alone. CD10 and BCL6 positivity overlap; Ki-67 close to 100% favours Burkitt but is not pathognomonic. FISH for MYC, BCL2, and BCL6 rearrangements is the definitive workup.

Follicular lymphoma

Follicular lymphoma is the most common indolent B-cell lymphoma in the United States. The cytogenetic hallmark is t(14;18)(q32;q21)/IGH::BCL2, present in approximately 90% of cases, juxtaposing BCL2 under IGH enhancer control and producing constitutive BCL2 over-expression that prevents apoptosis of germinal-centre B cells. Morphologically, follicular lymphoma shows a nodular/follicular growth pattern of centrocytes (small cleaved cells) and centroblasts (large transformed cells with nucleoli). The immunophenotype is CD20+, CD10+, BCL6+, BCL2 POSITIVE — and BCL2 expression in a follicular pattern is the specific discriminator from reactive germinal centres (where germinal-centre B cells are BCL2 negative).

WHO 2022 has abolished the 1, 2, 3A grading of classic FL because grades 1 through 3A behave similarly; classic FL is now reported without grade. The former grade 3B is reclassified as a separate aggressive entity, follicular large B-cell lymphoma (FLBL), and is treated as DLBCL. Treatment of classical follicular lymphoma is risk-adapted: asymptomatic low-tumour-burden disease can be observed (the GELF criteria define indications for treatment); symptomatic or high-tumour-burden disease is treated with rituximab plus chemotherapy (R-CHOP, R-bendamustine, or R-CVP). Maintenance rituximab prolongs progression-free survival. Transformation to DLBCL occurs in approximately 2–3% per year and is treated with DLBCL-directed therapy.

Mantle cell lymphoma

Mantle cell lymphoma arises from naive pre-germinal-centre B cells of the mantle zone. The defining cytogenetic abnormality is t(11;14)(q13;q32)/CCND1::IGH, juxtaposing cyclin D1 under IGH enhancer control and producing constitutive cyclin D1 over-expression and forced cell-cycle entry. Cyclin D1 nuclear positivity by IHC is the diagnostic marker. The immunophenotype is CD5+, CD20 BRIGHT (compared with CLL's dim CD20), CD23 NEGATIVE (the key discriminator from CLL), FMC7 positive, cyclin D1 positive (nuclear IHC), and SOX11 positive in most cases. SOX11-negative MCL has a more indolent IGHV-mutated non-nodal phenotype and is sometimes managed with observation. Blastoid and pleomorphic variants are aggressive; TP53 mutation confers very poor prognosis regardless of variant.

Clinically, mantle cell lymphoma typically presents in older men with widespread disease — generalised lymphadenopathy, splenomegaly, marrow involvement, and a striking pattern of GI tract involvement (lymphomatous polyposis affecting the entire bowel) that should prompt MCL consideration in any patient with multiple GI lymphoid polyps. Treatment is intensive in younger fit patients (cytarabine-based induction such as R-DHAP or hyperCVAD followed by autologous stem cell transplant in first remission), while older patients receive less-intensive R-bendamustine or R-CHOP with maintenance rituximab. BTK inhibitors (acalabrutinib and zanubrutinib for relapsed disease; pirtobrutinib for BTK-resistant relapse — ibrutinib's MCL indication was withdrawn from the US market in December 2023) and CD19-directed CAR-T therapy (brexucabtagene autoleucel) are effective in relapsed disease.

Marginal zone lymphomas and lymphoplasmacytic lymphoma

Marginal zone lymphomas (MZLs) are indolent B-cell neoplasms arising from post-germinal-centre marginal-zone B cells. Three subtypes are recognised: extranodal MZL of mucosa-associated lymphoid tissue (MALT lymphoma), splenic MZL, and nodal MZL. MALT lymphomas of the stomach are causally linked to chronic Helicobacter pylori infection in approximately 70% — antigen-driven proliferation of mucosal B cells produces a clonal expansion that is dependent on the antigen in early disease and may regress completely with H. pylori eradication, particularly in lymphomas without t(11;18)/API2::MALT1. The t(11;18) translocation predicts antibiotic resistance and the need for additional therapy. Other MALT-associated organisms include Borrelia burgdorferi (cutaneous MALT in Europe), Chlamydia psittaci (ocular adnexal MALT), and Campylobacter jejuni (immunoproliferative small intestinal disease, IPSID). Splenic MZL is associated with hepatitis C virus and may regress with antiviral therapy.

Lymphoplasmacytic lymphoma (LPL), when associated with an IgM monoclonal gammopathy, is termed Waldenström macroglobulinaemia. The driver mutation is MYD88 L265P, present in over 90% of cases and a near-specific diagnostic marker. CXCR4 mutations occur in ~30% and predict reduced response to ibrutinib. Clinical features reflect the IgM paraprotein: hyperviscosity (headache, blurred vision, retinal haemorrhages, mucosal bleeding), peripheral neuropathy from anti-MAG antibodies, type I or type II cryoglobulinaemia, and cold agglutinin disease. Treatment uses BTK inhibitors (ibrutinib, zanubrutinib) or rituximab-based chemoimmunotherapy. Plasmapheresis is the immediate intervention for symptomatic hyperviscosity.

HIGH-YIELD PEARL — H. pylori-associated gastric MALT

A patient with biopsy-proven gastric MALT lymphoma should always have H. pylori testing. If H. pylori is positive, the first-line treatment is triple-therapy eradication (a proton pump inhibitor plus clarithromycin plus amoxicillin or metronidazole) — not chemotherapy or radiation. Approximately 70–80% of H. pylori-positive gastric MALT lymphomas regress completely after successful eradication, with durable remissions. The exception is t(11;18)/API2::MALT1-positive lymphoma, which is generally antibiotic-resistant and requires additional therapy (rituximab ± chemotherapy or involved-site radiation). H. pylori-negative gastric MALT lymphoma also responds poorly to antibiotics. The exam vignette: gastric MALT + positive H. pylori + no t(11;18) → triple therapy alone is the correct first-line answer.

14.3 Translocations and Diagnostic Markers — One-Glance Reference

Lymphoma	Translocation	Gene fusion	Diagnostic marker / pearl
Follicular lymphoma	t(14;18)(q32;q21)	IGH::BCL2	CD10+, BCL6+, BCL2+ in follicular pattern (vs reactive GC: BCL2 negative)
Mantle cell lymphoma	t(11;14)(q13;q32)	CCND1::IGH	Cyclin D1+ nuclear; CD5+, CD23−, CD20 bright; SOX11+
Burkitt lymphoma	t(8;14) — most; t(2;8); t(8;22)	MYC::IGH (or MYC + IGK/IGL)	CD10+, BCL6+, BCL2 NEGATIVE, Ki-67 ~100%, TdT−; "starry sky"
DLBCL — double-hit	MYC + BCL2 rearrangements (FISH)	Various	GCB-COO; very poor with R-CHOP; intensified regimens
MALT lymphoma	t(11;18)(q21;q21)	API2::MALT1	Antibiotic-resistant gastric MALT; consider H. pylori eradication only if negative
Anaplastic large cell lymphoma (ALK+)	t(2;5)(p23;q35) — most	NPM1::ALK	CD30+, CD45+, ALK+, T-cell origin; favourable prognosis vs ALK−
Anaplastic large cell lymphoma (ALK−)	DUSP22-IRF4 r; TP63 r	Various	CD30+, ALK−; DUSP22-rearranged: better prognosis; TP63-rearranged: very poor
Lymphoplasmacytic lymphoma / Waldenström	No defining translocation	MYD88 L265P (>90%); CXCR4 (~30%)	IgM monoclonal gammopathy; hyperviscosity; CXCR4 mut → reduced ibrutinib response
Adult T-cell leukaemia/lymphom a	No characteristic translocation	HTLV-1 integration	Endemic Japan, Caribbean; "flower cells"; hypercalcaemia; CD4+, CD25+
Mycosis fungoides / Sézary syndrome	No characteristic translocation	Variable epigenetic lesions	CD3+, CD4+, CD7−; cerebriform "Sézary" cells; Pautrier microabscesses (epidermotropism)
Extranodal NK/T-cell lymphoma, nasal type	No characteristic translocation	EBV-driven	Midfacial necrosis ("lethal midline granuloma"); CD56+, EBER+; cytotoxic NK or T phenotype

Table 14.3. High-yield translocations and markers across mature lymphoid neoplasms.

MECHANISM HOOK — Why mature T-cell lymphomas are different

Mature T-cell lymphomas account for only 10–15% of NHL but disproportionately occupy USMLE space because each entity has a near-pathognomonic clinical or histological signature. Three biological themes organise them. First, T-cell receptor specialisation — anaplastic large cell lymphoma derives from cytotoxic T cells expressing CD30; angioimmunoblastic T-cell lymphoma (AITL) derives from follicular helper T cells (TFH) and recapitulates the TFH phenotype (CD4+, CXCL13+, PD-1+, BCL6+, ICOS+); cutaneous T-cell lymphomas (mycosis fungoides, Sézary syndrome) derive from skin-resident memory CD4+ T cells. Second, virally driven oncogenesis — adult T-cell leukaemia/lymphoma (ATLL) is HTLV-1 driven and endemic in southwestern Japan, the Caribbean basin, and parts of west Africa; extranodal NK/T-cell lymphoma nasal type is EBV driven. Third, epigenetic and TCR-pathway lesions — RHOA G17V mutations, TET2, IDH2, and DNMT3A loss-of-function mutations recur across the peripheral T-cell lymphoma spectrum and define AITL biology in particular. The treatment implication is sobering: most mature T-cell lymphomas have inferior outcomes to their B-cell counterparts and lack effective targeted agents (with the exception of brentuximab vedotin for CD30+ entities and HDAC inhibitors and anti-CCR4 antibody for ATLL). Allogeneic transplant remains the only curative modality for many.

14.4 Mature T-Cell and NK-Cell Lymphomas

Peripheral T-cell lymphoma, NOS and angioimmunoblastic T-cell lymphoma

Peripheral T-cell lymphoma not otherwise specified (PTCL-NOS) is the largest and most heterogeneous subgroup of mature T-cell lymphoma — a diagnosis of exclusion when no specific PTCL entity fits. Patients are typically older adults presenting with generalised lymphadenopathy, B symptoms, and frequent extranodal involvement. Outcomes with CHOP or CHOEP are inferior to B-cell DLBCL outcomes; intensified regimens with autologous stem cell transplantation in first remission are standard for fit younger patients.

Angioimmunoblastic T-cell lymphoma (AITL) is a distinctive PTCL derived from follicular helper T cells. Under WHO 5th edition (HAEM5/2022), AITL is now formally classified as "nodal T-follicular helper (TFH) cell lymphoma, angioimmunoblastic-type" (nTFHL-AI), grouped with two related entities (nTFHL-follicular and nTFHL-NOS) sharing TFH origin; "AITL" remains in widespread clinical use. Patients present with generalised lymphadenopathy, hepatosplenomegaly, drenching night sweats, polyclonal hypergammaglobulinaemia (often confused initially with autoimmune disease), and a constellation of immune-mediated phenomena including rash, autoimmune cytopenias, and Coombs-positive haemolytic anaemia. The lymph node histology is characteristic: a polymorphous infiltrate with prominent high endothelial venules in a "tree-bark" pattern, expanded follicular dendritic cell meshworks (CD21 positive), scattered EBV-positive large B-cells, and clonal CD4+ TFH cells expressing PD-1, CXCL13, BCL6, and ICOS. The recurrent somatic mutations are RHOA G17V (~70%), TET2 (~80%), DNMT3A, and IDH2 — the same epigenetic-pathway mutations seen in clonal haematopoiesis and CMML, suggesting a shared myeloid-T-lymphoid clonal evolution. Treatment is CHOEP-based chemotherapy with autologous transplant in first remission, or alloSCT in younger fit patients; outcomes remain poor (5-year overall survival approximately 30–40%).

Anaplastic large cell lymphoma

Anaplastic large cell lymphoma (ALCL) is a CD30+ T-cell or null-cell lymphoma defined by large pleomorphic cells with horseshoe-shaped or "hallmark" nuclei and abundant cytoplasm. Three subtypes are clinically and prognostically distinct. Systemic ALK-positive ALCL is most common in children and young adults, carries the t(2;5)(p23;q35)/NPM1::ALK translocation in approximately 80% of cases, expresses ALK protein by IHC (cytoplasmic and nuclear), and has the most favourable prognosis. Systemic ALK-negative ALCL occurs in older adults, has historically been considered intermediate-prognosis, and is now subdivided molecularly: DUSP22-IRF4 rearrangement (~30%) confers a favourable prognosis approaching ALK-positive ALCL, while TP63 rearrangement (~10%) confers a very poor prognosis. Primary cutaneous ALCL is a localised skin disease with an indolent course and is treated with local therapy. Breast implant–associated ALCL is a separate entity characterised by ALK-negative disease arising in the capsule of textured breast implants; capsulectomy is curative in most cases. Brentuximab vedotin (anti-CD30 antibody-drug conjugate) is highly effective in CD30+ ALCL and is incorporated into first-line therapy.

IMG-TRAP — ALK status changes ALCL prognosis dramatically

A common reflex is to treat all ALCL as a single entity. The reality is that prognosis is stratified by molecular subgroup: ALK-positive ALCL has 5-year overall survival of approximately 70–90%; ALK-negative ALCL with DUSP22-IRF4 rearrangement approaches ALK-positive outcomes (~90%); ALK-negative ALCL without DUSP22 has 5-year survival of approximately 40–50%; ALK-negative ALCL with TP63 rearrangement has 5-year survival under 20%. The clinical rule: any patient with ALCL requires ALK testing AND, if ALK-negative, additional FISH for DUSP22 and TP63 rearrangements before treatment intensity is decided. The exam-correct answer for an ALK-positive ALCL patient is brentuximab + CHP (CHP-BV) with curative intent and excellent outcomes; for a TP63-rearranged ALK-negative case, the answer is intensified therapy with alloSCT consolidation in fit patients.

Mycosis fungoides and Sézary syndrome

Mycosis fungoides (MF) is the most common cutaneous T-cell lymphoma. The clinical course progresses through patch, plaque, and tumour stages over years to decades. Patches resemble eczema or psoriasis and respond unpredictably to topical steroids; plaques are well-demarcated, infiltrated, often pruritic; tumours are nodular and may ulcerate. Histology shows an epidermotropic infiltrate of small atypical CD4+ T cells in the upper dermis with collections within the epidermis termed Pautrier microabscesses — the diagnostic histological hallmark. The immunophenotype is CD3+, CD4+, CD7 NEGATIVE (loss of CD7 distinguishes neoplastic from reactive T cells), with TCR clonality on molecular studies. Sézary syndrome is the leukaemic phase of cutaneous T-cell lymphoma, defined by erythroderma (>80% body surface area), generalised lymphadenopathy, and ≥1,000/µL circulating Sézary cells (atypical CD4+ T cells with cerebriform nuclei). Treatment is stage-driven: early-stage MF with topical agents and phototherapy (PUVA, narrowband UVB); advanced disease with systemic agents (bexarotene, brentuximab vedotin for CD30+ disease, mogamulizumab anti-CCR4, romidepsin); alloSCT for selected aggressive disease.

Adult T-cell leukaemia/lymphoma

Adult T-cell leukaemia/lymphoma (ATLL) is caused by HTLV-1 infection and is endemic in southwestern Japan, the Caribbean basin, parts of central and west Africa, and Iran. The lifetime risk of ATLL among HTLV-1 carriers is approximately 5%, with a latency of decades from infection to malignancy. Four clinical variants are recognised: acute (the most common; rapid course with leukocytosis, lymphadenopathy, hepatosplenomegaly, hypercalcaemia, and rash), lymphomatous (lymph node–predominant with no peripheral blood involvement), chronic (more indolent), and smoldering (least aggressive). The peripheral blood shows characteristic "flower cells" — atypical lymphocytes with multilobated convoluted nuclei resembling petals. Hypercalcaemia is a near-defining feature of acute ATLL, mediated by parathyroid hormone–related protein (PTHrP) and RANKL secretion. The immunophenotype is CD3+, CD4+, CD25+ (constitutively over-expressed), CD7 negative. First-line treatment of aggressive ATLL is interferon-α plus zidovudine for chronic and smoldering forms; multi-agent chemotherapy with mogamulizumab (anti-CCR4) for acute and lymphomatous forms. Outcomes remain poor; alloSCT is the only curative option.

Extranodal NK/T-cell lymphoma, nasal type

Extranodal NK/T-cell lymphoma, nasal type is an EBV-driven aggressive lymphoma most common in East Asia and Latin America. The classic presentation is destructive midfacial necrosis — historically called "lethal midline granuloma" — involving the nasal cavity, palate, and orbit, with rapid local progression. The neoplastic cells are typically of NK origin (CD2+, surface CD3 negative, cytoplasmic CD3-epsilon positive, CD56+, EBER positive by in situ hybridisation, with cytotoxic granules: granzyme B, perforin, TIA-1). Aggressive non-anthracycline-based regimens with concurrent or sandwich radiation (SMILE: dexamethasone, methotrexate, ifosfamide, L-asparaginase, etoposide; or modern variants like AspaMetDex) produce response rates around 80% in localised disease. Disseminated disease has dismal outcomes despite intensified therapy.

Langerhans cell histiocytosis — a brief note

Langerhans cell histiocytosis (LCH) is grouped here for completeness as a histiocytic neoplasm with overlapping clinical contexts. LCH cells are bone-marrow-derived myeloid cells that aberrantly express the Langerhans cell phenotype: CD1a positive, S100 positive, CD207 (Langerin) positive, with characteristic Birbeck granules on electron microscopy ("tennis racket" appearance). The driver mutation is BRAF V600E in approximately half of cases, with other MAPK-pathway mutations (MAP2K1, ARAF, RAF1) accounting for most of the remainder. Clinical presentations span an enormous range: solitary bony lesions ("eosinophilic granuloma") in older children, multifocal bone disease, multisystem disease in young children with risk-organ involvement (liver, spleen, haematopoietic system), and the historical eponymous syndromes — Hand-Schüller-Christian disease (lytic skull lesions, exophthalmos, diabetes insipidus) and Letterer-Siwe disease (multisystem disease in infants). Treatment is risk-adapted: single-system disease with curettage or local therapy; multisystem disease with vinblastine plus prednisone, with BRAF or MEK inhibition for refractory or progressive disease.

14.5 Buzzwords and Associations — Vignette Trigger Table

Vignette buzzword / finding	Diagnosis to trigger	One-line "why"
Young adult, mediastinal mass, "owl-eye" binucleate cells, CD30+ CD15+ CD45−	Classical Hodgkin lymphoma (nodular sclerosis)	RS cells; lacunar variant; female predominance
"Popcorn cells" with multilobated nuclei; CD20+, CD45+, CD30−	NLPBL (was NLPHL)	B-cell lymphoma; treated like indolent NHL
Diffuse large cells with vesicular nuclei; CD20+; replaces nodal architecture	DLBCL	Most common NHL; subtype by Hans algorithm or GEP
Starry sky pattern, Ki-67 ~100%, BCL2 NEGATIVE, t(8;14)/MYC::IGH	Burkitt lymphoma	BCL2 negativity discriminates from DHL
Endemic Burkitt — child, jaw mass, equatorial Africa, EBV+	Endemic Burkitt lymphoma	EBV+ in >95%; jaw is anatomical hallmark
Indolent nodal lymphoma, t(14;18)/IGH::BCL2, BCL2+ in follicular pattern	Follicular lymphoma	BCL2 in follicular pattern distinguishes neoplastic from reactive GC
Older man, GI lymphomatous polyposis, CD5+ CD23 NEGATIVE, cyclin D1+	Mantle cell lymphoma	t(11;14)/CCND1::IGH; CD23 negative distinguishes from CLL
Gastric MALT lymphoma + H. pylori positive + no t(11;18)	First-line: H. pylori eradication therapy	70–80% regress with antibiotics; t(11;18) predicts antibiotic resistance
IgM monoclonal gammopathy + hyperviscosity + MYD88 L265P	Waldenström macroglobulinaemia (LPL)	Plasmapheresis for symptomatic hyperviscosity
Erythroderma + circulating CD4+ T cells with cerebriform nuclei	Sézary syndrome	Leukaemic phase of cutaneous T-cell lymphoma
Pautrier microabscesses on skin biopsy; CD3+, CD4+, CD7−	Mycosis fungoides	Epidermotropism; CD7 loss is the neoplastic signal
Caribbean origin + lymphoma + hypercalcaemia + "flower cells" + CD25+	Adult T-cell leukaemia/lymphoma (HTLV-1)	PTHrP/RANKL-driven hypercalcaemia; mogamulizumab + chemotherapy
Midfacial necrosis ("lethal midline granuloma") + CD56+ + EBER+	Extranodal NK/T-cell lymphoma, nasal type	EBV-driven; SMILE-based therapy + radiation

Vignette buzzword / finding	Diagnosis to trigger	One-line "why"
Generalised lymphadenopathy + polyclonal hypergammaglobulinaemia + Coombs+ AIHA + EBV+ B cells	Angioimmunoblastic T-cell lymphoma	TFH origin; RHOA G17V, TET2, IDH2, DNMT3A mutations
CD30+ pleomorphic cells with horseshoe nuclei; ALK+; t(2;5)	Anaplastic large cell lymphoma, ALK+	Most common in children/young adults; favourable prognosis
Birbeck granules ("tennis rackets") on EM; CD1a+, CD207+	Langerhans cell histiocytosis	BRAF V600E in ~50%; risk-adapted treatment

Table 14.4. High-yield vignette buzzwords for lymphomas.

14.6 USMLE Vignettes

Ten vignettes follow, weighted toward the most heavily tested entities: Hodgkin lymphoma, DLBCL, Burkitt, follicular and mantle cell lymphoma, and the high-frequency T-cell entities (mycosis fungoides, ALCL, ATLL). Stems include the lab values and morphological descriptors examiners use as anchors.

Vignette 1. A 24-year-old woman with a mediastinal mass and night sweats

A 24-year-old woman presents with three months of progressive fatigue, drenching night sweats, a 12-pound unintentional weight loss, and a non-productive cough. She denies fever or recent travel. Examination shows a palpable left supraclavicular lymph node 2.5 cm in diameter, no other adenopathy, and clear lung fields. Chest CT shows a 9 × 7 cm anterior mediastinal mass with mediastinal and right hilar lymphadenopathy. Excisional biopsy of the supraclavicular node shows a nodular pattern with bands of collagen sclerosis dividing the node into cellular nodules; within the nodules are large cells with retraction artefact ("lacunar cells") and rare classical binucleate cells with prominent eosinophilic nucleoli, in a mixed background of small lymphocytes, eosinophils, and plasma cells. Immunohistochemistry shows the large cells are CD30+, CD15+, PAX5 dim positive, CD20 negative, CD45 negative, and EBV-LMP1 negative. Which of the following is the most appropriate diagnosis and treatment?

- **(A)** Classical Hodgkin lymphoma, nodular sclerosis subtype; nivolumab + AVD (N-AVD) per SWOG S1826 — preferred first-line for advanced or bulky disease with B symptoms; BV-AVD and ABVD remain acceptable.
- **(B)** Anaplastic large cell lymphoma, ALK-positive; CHP plus brentuximab vedotin (CHP-BV).
- **(C)** Diffuse large B-cell lymphoma, primary mediastinal subtype; R-CHOP or DA-EPOCH-R.
- **(D)** Nodular lymphocyte-predominant B-cell lymphoma; rituximab with or without involved-site radiation.
- **(E)** Reactive lymphadenitis from infectious mononucleosis; supportive care only.

Best answer: (A) Classical Hodgkin lymphoma, nodular sclerosis subtype; nivolumab + AVD (N-AVD) per SWOG S1826 — preferred first-line for advanced or bulky disease with B symptoms; BV-AVD and ABVD remain acceptable.

Rationale. The clinical picture is classic for nodular-sclerosis classical Hodgkin lymphoma in a young woman: anterior mediastinal mass, B symptoms (night sweats and weight loss), and a peripheral nodal biopsy. The histology is diagnostic — collagen sclerosis dividing the node into cellular nodules, lacunar cells, and classical Reed-Sternberg cells in a mixed inflammatory background. The CD30+/CD15+/CD45− immunophenotype with dim PAX5 confirms HRS cells. This patient's disease is bulky (9 × 7 cm) with B symptoms — treated as advanced. Current US first-line for advanced or bulky cHL is nivolumab + AVD (N-AVD) based on SWOG S1826 (NEJM 2024), which demonstrated superior 2-year PFS (92% vs 83%) and better tolerability versus brentuximab + AVD (BV-AVD); BV-AVD and ABVD remain acceptable alternatives. For early-stage favourable cHL (stage I–II without bulk, B symptoms, or other risk factors), abbreviated ABVD (2–4 cycles) plus involved-site radiation remains standard. Cure rates exceed 80% across stages. PD-1 blockade (nivolumab, pembrolizumab) and brentuximab vedotin are the dominant relapse therapies.

Distractor analysis. (B) ALCL is also CD30+ but is CD45 POSITIVE and ALK+ in the systemic ALK+ form. (C) Primary mediastinal large B-cell lymphoma is also a young-woman, mediastinal-mass entity but is CD20 POSITIVE — the IHC distinguishes. (D) NLPBL has popcorn cells, CD20+, CD45+, and lacks the collagen sclerosis. (E) Infectious mononucleosis can produce reactive lymphadenitis and even occasional HRS-like cells but does not produce the architectural pattern of nodular sclerosis HL.

Vignette 2. A 28-year-old man with cervical lymphadenopathy and "popcorn" cells

A 28-year-old man notes a slowly enlarging right cervical lymph node over six months. He has no fever, weight loss, or night sweats. Examination shows a single 3 cm non-tender right cervical node with no other adenopathy, no hepatosplenomegaly, and an otherwise normal physical examination. CBC and LDH are normal. Excisional biopsy shows a vaguely nodular pattern with abundant small reactive lymphocytes and histiocytes, with scattered large cells whose nuclei are multilobated and folded ("popcorn" cells). Immunohistochemistry on the large cells shows CD20 strongly positive, CD45 positive, OCT2 positive, BOB1 positive, CD30 negative, CD15 negative, and EBV-LMP1 negative. Which of the following is the most likely diagnosis?

- **(A)** Nodular lymphocyte-predominant B-cell lymphoma (NLPBL).
- **(B)** Classical Hodgkin lymphoma, lymphocyte-rich subtype.
- **(C)** T-cell/histiocyte-rich large B-cell lymphoma.
- **(D)** Reactive follicular hyperplasia.
- **(E)** Angioimmunoblastic T-cell lymphoma.

Best answer: (A) Nodular lymphocyte-predominant B-cell lymphoma (NLPBL).

Rationale. The defining cell of NLPBL is the lymphocyte-predominant (LP) cell, also called the "popcorn cell" for its multilobated folded nuclei. NLPBL is a B-cell lymphoma reclassified by WHO 2022 (formerly NLPHL) and is biologically distinct from classical Hodgkin lymphoma. The immunophenotype confirms the diagnosis: CD20 strongly positive (retained B-cell program), CD45 positive (the key discriminator from classical HL, which is CD45 negative), OCT2 and BOB1 positive (intact transcription program for immunoglobulin expression), and CD30 and CD15 negative (the hallmark cHL markers). Clinically, NLPBL presents in young to middle-aged men with peripheral lymphadenopathy without B symptoms; the course is indolent, with late relapses but high overall survival. Treatment is risk-adapted: stage IA disease can be observed or treated with involved-site radiation alone; symptomatic or higher-stage disease is treated with rituximab (often with chemotherapy or radiation). Transformation to T-cell/histiocyte-rich large B-cell lymphoma occurs in approximately 5–10% over time.

Distractor analysis. (B) Lymphocyte-rich classical HL has classical RS cells in a lymphocyte-rich background and is CD30+/CD15+/CD45−; the popcorn morphology and CD20+/CD45+ phenotype excludes cHL. (C) T-cell/histiocyte-rich large B-cell lymphoma has scattered large neoplastic B cells in a background of T cells and histiocytes; it is more aggressive and lacks the nodular pattern. (D) Reactive hyperplasia would lack large neoplastic cells with clonal rearrangement. (E) AITL is a T-cell lymphoma with TFH-derived neoplastic cells, not B-cell.

Vignette 3. A 64-year-old man with diffuse large B-cell lymphoma and the COO

question

A 64-year-old man presents with three months of bilateral axillary lymphadenopathy, night sweats, and a 10-pound weight loss. CT shows multiple enlarged nodes above and below the diaphragm and a 6 cm para-aortic mass; bone marrow biopsy is uninvolved. Excisional biopsy of an axillary node shows diffuse effacement of nodal architecture by sheets of large B cells with vesicular nuclei, prominent nucleoli, and brisk mitotic activity. Immunohistochemistry by the Hans algorithm: CD10 positive, BCL6 positive, IRF4/MUM1 negative — consistent with germinal-centre B-cell (GCB) cell-of-origin. FISH break-apart probes: MYC negative, BCL2 negative, BCL6 negative. IPI score is intermediate-high. Which of the following is the most appropriate first-line therapy?

(A) R-CHOP × 6 cycles (rituximab plus cyclophosphamide, doxorubicin, vincristine, prednisone).

(B) DA-EPOCH-R for double-hit lymphoma.

(C) R-CODOX-M/IVAC for Burkitt lymphoma.

(D) ABVD for Hodgkin lymphoma.

(E) BTK inhibitor monotherapy with ibrutinib.

Best answer: (A) R-CHOP × 6 cycles (rituximab plus cyclophosphamide, doxorubicin, vincristine, prednisone).

Rationale. The diagnosis is DLBCL, GCB cell-of-origin, without high-risk molecular features (no MYC, BCL2, or BCL6 rearrangement on FISH; no double-hit; not specified as double-expressor). Standard first-line therapy is R-CHOP for six cycles, with response assessment by interim PET and end-of-treatment PET. The Hans algorithm assigns COO using three IHC markers: CD10, BCL6, and IRF4/MUM1. CD10 positive OR (CD10 negative + BCL6 positive + MUM1 negative) defines GCB; the alternative pattern defines non-GCB (ABC-type). GCB-DLBCL has substantially better outcomes with R-CHOP than ABC-DLBCL. Polatuzumab vedotin (anti-CD79b ADC) added to R-CHP has shown improved progression-free survival in the POLARIX trial in IPI ≥2 disease. CAR-T therapy (axicabtagene ciloleucel, lisocabtagene maraleucel, tisagenlecleucel) is approved for relapsed/refractory disease and is replacing autologous transplant in the second-line setting in many cases.

Distractor analysis. (B) DA-EPOCH-R is reserved for double-hit lymphoma (MYC + BCL2 rearrangements) — this case has neither rearrangement. (C) R-CODOX-M/IVAC is for Burkitt lymphoma — Ki-67 close to 100% and MYC rearrangement are required. (D) ABVD is for Hodgkin lymphoma. (E) BTK inhibitor monotherapy is not standard first-line DLBCL therapy.

Vignette 4. A 38-year-old man with a rapidly enlarging abdominal mass and tumour lysis risk

A 38-year-old man presents with three weeks of rapidly progressive abdominal distension, early satiety, and an 8-pound weight loss. Examination shows a large palpable right abdominal mass and prominent ileocecal fullness. CT shows a 12 × 10 cm ileocecal mass with mesenteric and retroperitoneal lymphadenopathy. Laboratory studies: LDH 2,640 U/L, uric acid 8.9 mg/dL, creatinine 1.1 mg/dL. Core biopsy of the mass shows medium-sized cells with multiple basophilic nucleoli, abundant basophilic cytoplasm with lipid vacuoles, and a "starry sky" pattern produced by tingible-body macrophages. Immunohistochemistry: CD20 positive, CD10 positive, BCL6 positive, BCL2 NEGATIVE, Ki-67 approximately 100%, TdT negative. FISH: MYC rearranged (t(8;14)/MYC::IGH); BCL2 not rearranged. EBV in situ hybridisation negative. HIV testing is negative. Which of the following is the most appropriate management plan?

- **(A)** Initiate dose-adjusted EPOCH-R or R-CODOX-M/IVAC with intensive tumour lysis prophylaxis (rasburicase, aggressive hydration, allopurinol; close electrolyte monitoring) and CNS prophylaxis with intrathecal methotrexate.
- **(B)** R-CHOP × 6 cycles without specific tumour lysis prophylaxis.
- **(C)** ABVD chemotherapy with involved-site radiation.
- **(D)** Surgical resection of the mass followed by observation.
- **(E)** Single-agent rituximab with watchful waiting.

Best answer: (A) Initiate dose-adjusted EPOCH-R or R-CODOX-M/IVAC with intensive tumour lysis prophylaxis (rasburicase, aggressive hydration, allopurinol; close electrolyte monitoring) and CNS prophylaxis with intrathecal methotrexate.

Rationale. The case is sporadic Burkitt lymphoma in an HIV-negative adult: ileocecal mass, very high LDH, MYC rearrangement (t(8;14)/MYC::IGH), BCL2 NEGATIVE (a critical discriminator from double-hit lymphoma — DHL is BCL2 positive), Ki-67 essentially 100%, and TdT negative (excluding mature-B-phenotype B-ALL). Burkitt has the highest tumour doubling time of any human cancer and one of the highest tumour lysis risks. First-line treatment uses intensified short-duration regimens (DA-EPOCH-R with prophylactic intrathecal methotrexate, R-CODOX-M/IVAC, or hyperCVAD-MA in some centres). All Burkitt patients require aggressive tumour lysis prophylaxis from the moment of diagnosis: rasburicase (strongly preferred to allopurinol when uric acid is elevated and the burden is high), aggressive intravenous hydration, frequent electrolyte monitoring (potassium, phosphorus, calcium, uric acid), and ICU readiness. CNS prophylaxis with intrathecal methotrexate is mandatory because CNS relapse is a recognised pattern in Burkitt.

Distractor analysis. (B) R-CHOP is inadequate for Burkitt — outcomes with R-CHOP are markedly inferior to intensified regimens. (C) ABVD treats Hodgkin lymphoma. (D) Surgery is not curative for Burkitt; Burkitt is a chemosensitive disease. (E) Watchful waiting in this aggressive disease would be fatal within weeks.

Vignette 5. A 58-year-old man with indolent lymphadenopathy and t(14;18)

A 58-year-old man notes painless bilateral cervical and inguinal lymphadenopathy that has been stable for six months. He is asymptomatic — no fever, night sweats, weight loss, or fatigue. Examination shows multiple non-tender cervical, axillary, and inguinal nodes, none larger than 3 cm; spleen tip palpable. CBC, LDH, and renal function are normal. Excisional biopsy of an inguinal node shows effacement of nodal architecture by closely packed neoplastic follicles with attenuated mantle zones; the follicles contain a mixture of small cleaved cells (centrocytes) and larger transformed cells (centroblasts). Immunohistochemistry: CD20 positive, CD10 positive, BCL6 positive, BCL2 POSITIVE within the follicles. FISH: t(14;18)(q32;q21)/IGH::BCL2. Which of the following best describes the diagnosis and the appropriate next step?

- **(A)** Follicular lymphoma; observation ("watch and wait") is appropriate given the absence of GELF criteria for treatment.
- **(B)** Follicular lymphoma; immediate R-CHOP × 6 cycles.
- **(C)** Reactive follicular hyperplasia; reassurance and routine follow-up.

(D) Diffuse large B-cell lymphoma transformed from follicular; DA-EPOCH-R.

(E) Mantle cell lymphoma; cytarabine-based induction with autologous transplant.

Best answer: (A) Follicular lymphoma; observation ("watch and wait") is appropriate given the absence of GELF criteria for treatment.

Rationale. The diagnosis is follicular lymphoma: the architecture (closely packed neoplastic follicles), morphology (centrocytes and centroblasts), immunophenotype (CD20+, CD10+, BCL6+, and crucially BCL2+ in a follicular pattern — the discriminator from reactive germinal centres, which are BCL2 negative), and cytogenetics (t(14;18)/IGH::BCL2 in approximately 90% of FL). Asymptomatic FL without high tumour burden is observed. The GELF criteria define indications to initiate treatment: nodal or extranodal mass >7 cm, three or more nodal sites each >3 cm, B symptoms, splenomegaly extending below the umbilicus, ascites or pleural effusion, leukaemic phase $>5 \times 10^9/L$ circulating lymphoma cells, cytopenias from marrow infiltration, or compression of vital organs. This patient meets none of these criteria. Multiple prospective trials have shown that early treatment of asymptomatic low-tumour-burden FL does not improve overall survival. Observation with serial imaging and clinical assessment is the standard of care. Note: WHO 2022 has abolished the 1, 2, 3A grading of classic FL because grades 1–3A behave similarly; classic FL is now reported without grade.

Distractor analysis. (B) Immediate R-CHOP in asymptomatic low-tumour-burden FL is overtreatment without survival benefit. (C) Reactive follicular hyperplasia would be BCL2 negative within germinal centres and would lack t(14;18). (D) Transformation to DLBCL would show diffuse large-cell morphology, not preserved follicular architecture. (E) Mantle cell lymphoma is CD5+, CD23−, cyclin D1+, with t(11;14), not t(14;18).

Vignette 6. A 67-year-old man with widespread GI lymphomatous polyposis

A 67-year-old man presents with three months of fatigue, mild diarrhoea, and a 6-pound weight loss. CBC shows haemoglobin 11.4 g/dL, platelets 195,000/µL, and absolute lymphocyte count 4,600/µL. CT shows generalised lymphadenopathy, splenomegaly, and multiple polypoid lesions throughout the small bowel and colon. Colonoscopy reveals dozens of polyps from the rectum to the caecum. Biopsy of a representative polyp shows a diffuse infiltrate of monomorphic small to medium lymphoid cells with irregular nuclear contours. Immunohistochemistry: CD20 BRIGHT, CD5 positive, CD23 NEGATIVE, FMC7 positive, cyclin D1 positive (nuclear), SOX11 positive. FISH confirms t(11;14)(q13;q32)/CCND1::IGH. TP53 sequencing is wild-type. Which of the following is the most likely diagnosis?

- **(A)** Mantle cell lymphoma with multiple lymphomatous polyposis.
- **(B)** Chronic lymphocytic leukaemia / small lymphocytic lymphoma.
- **(C)** Marginal zone lymphoma involving the bowel.
- **(D)** Burkitt lymphoma.
- **(E)** Follicular lymphoma in unusual extranodal distribution.

Best answer: (A) Mantle cell lymphoma with multiple lymphomatous polyposis.

Rationale. The morphology (small to medium monomorphic cells with irregular nuclei), immunophenotype (CD20 bright, CD5+, CD23 NEGATIVE — the key discriminator from CLL, which is CD23 positive — FMC7+, cyclin D1+, SOX11+), and cytogenetics (t(11;14)/CCND1::IGH) are pathognomonic for mantle cell lymphoma. Lymphomatous polyposis — multiple lymphomatous polyps throughout the GI tract — is a characteristic and often striking pattern of MCL involvement and should prompt MCL consideration in any patient with multiple GI lymphoid polyps. Treatment in fit younger patients combines cytarabine-based induction (R-DHAP, hyperCVAD/MA, or Nordic regimen) with autologous stem cell transplant in first remission. Older or less fit patients receive R-bendamustine or R-CHOP with maintenance rituximab. BTK inhibitors (acalabrutinib and zanubrutinib; pirtobrutinib for BTK-resistant relapse — ibrutinib's MCL indication was withdrawn from the US market in December 2023) and CD19-directed CAR-T therapy (brexucabtagene autoleucel) are highly effective in relapsed disease. TP53 mutation confers very poor prognosis regardless of variant or treatment.

Distractor analysis. (B) CLL/SLL is CD23 POSITIVE and CD20 dim — the inverse of MCL's phenotype. (C) Marginal zone lymphoma is CD5 negative and lacks t(11;14). (D) Burkitt is CD20+, CD10+, BCL2 negative, Ki-67 ~100%, with MYC rearrangement, not t(11;14). (E) Follicular lymphoma is CD10+ with t(14;18), and lymphomatous polyposis is not a typical FL pattern.

Vignette 7. A 55-year-old woman with gastric MALT lymphoma and H. pylori

A 55-year-old woman presents with three months of upper abdominal discomfort, postprandial bloating, and minimal weight loss. Upper endoscopy shows gastric mucosal nodularity in the antrum and body without ulceration or mass. Biopsy shows a dense lymphoid infiltrate of small to medium centrocyte-like cells in the lamina propria, with characteristic lymphoepithelial lesions (lymphoid cells infiltrating gastric glands). Immunohistochemistry: CD20 positive, CD5 negative, CD10 negative, CD23 negative, BCL2 positive, cyclin D1 negative. Helicobacter pylori is positive on rapid urease test and confirmed on histology. FISH for t(11;18)(q21;q21)/API2::MALT1 is NEGATIVE. Endoscopic ultrasound shows disease confined to mucosa and submucosa (T1). Bone marrow biopsy is uninvolved. Which of the following is the most appropriate first-line therapy?

(A) Triple-therapy H. pylori eradication (proton pump inhibitor + clarithromycin + amoxicillin) with endoscopic surveillance to confirm regression.

(B) Rituximab plus bendamustine chemoimmunotherapy.

(C) Involved-site radiation therapy as initial treatment.

(D) Total gastrectomy with adjuvant chemotherapy.

(E) Single-agent rituximab as the only intervention.

Best answer: (A) Triple-therapy H. pylori eradication (proton pump inhibitor + clarithromycin + amoxicillin) with endoscopic surveillance to confirm regression.

Rationale. Gastric MALT lymphoma in an H. pylori–positive patient without t(11;18) is the textbook indication for first-line antibiotic eradication therapy. Approximately 70–80% of H. pylori–positive gastric MALT lymphomas regress completely with successful eradication; remissions are durable in most patients. The first-line eradication regimen is a 14-day course of a proton pump inhibitor plus clarithromycin plus amoxicillin (or metronidazole if penicillin-allergic); local antibiotic resistance patterns may favour bismuth quadruple therapy in some regions. Endoscopic surveillance with biopsies is performed at 3 months to confirm H. pylori eradication and at 6 and 12 months to confirm lymphoma regression. Persistent lymphoma at 12 months despite eradication, or t(11;18)-positive disease (predicting antibiotic resistance), or H. pylori–negative MALT requires additional therapy: rituximab ± chemotherapy, or involved-site radiation.

Distractor analysis. (B) Chemoimmunotherapy is reserved for antibiotic-refractory disease, t(11;18)-positive disease, or advanced-stage disease. (C) Radiation is effective for localised gastric MALT but is not first-line when antibiotic eradication has a 70–80% chance of cure. (D) Total gastrectomy was historical management before recognition of the H. pylori link and is no longer indicated. (E) Rituximab monotherapy is not first-line for H. pylori–positive disease without prior eradication attempt.

Vignette 8. A 60-year-old man with progressive erythroderma and circulating atypical T cells

A 60-year-old man has a 12-year history of patchy pruritic skin lesions previously diagnosed as eczema and treated intermittently with topical steroids. Over the past 18 months the patches have coalesced into infiltrated plaques and now generalised erythroderma covering >90% of body surface area, with intractable pruritus, fissuring, and chronic pain. He has lost 15 pounds. Examination shows generalised erythroderma, scaling, ectropion, palmar and plantar hyperkeratosis, and bilateral cervical and axillary lymphadenopathy. Laboratory studies: haemoglobin 11.0 g/dL, platelets 145,000/µL, white blood cells 18,000/µL with 60% atypical lymphocytes — medium-sized cells with deeply convoluted "cerebriform" nuclei. Flow cytometry on peripheral blood: clonal CD3+, CD4+, CD7 NEGATIVE T cells; absolute "Sézary cell" count is 4,200/µL. Skin biopsy shows an epidermotropic infiltrate of atypical CD4+ T cells with collections within the epidermis (Pautrier microabscesses). Which of the following is the most likely diagnosis?

(A) Sézary syndrome (the leukaemic phase of cutaneous T-cell lymphoma).

(B) Mycosis fungoides, plaque stage, without leukaemic involvement.

(C) Adult T-cell leukaemia/lymphoma (ATLL) — HTLV-1 driven.

(D) Atopic dermatitis with secondary bacterial colonisation.

(E) Drug reaction with eosinophilia and systemic symptoms (DRESS).

Best answer: (A) Sézary syndrome (the leukaemic phase of cutaneous T-cell lymphoma).

Rationale. Sézary syndrome is the leukaemic variant of cutaneous T-cell lymphoma, defined by the triad of erythroderma covering >80% body surface area, generalised lymphadenopathy, and a circulating clonal CD4+ T-cell population (≥1,000/µL Sézary cells with cerebriform nuclei) demonstrating CD7 loss and TCR clonality. The skin histology — epidermotropic infiltrate of atypical CD4+ T cells with Pautrier microabscesses — is shared with mycosis fungoides; the leukaemic phase is what defines Sézary syndrome. The clinical course is more aggressive than classic MF, and median survival is approximately 3–4 years. Treatment combines extracorporeal photopheresis, systemic agents (bexarotene, mogamulizumab anti-CCR4, romidepsin or vorinostat — HDAC inhibitors, methotrexate, interferon-α), and consideration of allogeneic transplantation in selected patients. CCR4 expression on the malignant clone makes mogamulizumab particularly active.

Distractor analysis. (B) Mycosis fungoides plaque stage without erythroderma or circulating Sézary cells does not meet Sézary syndrome criteria. (C) ATLL would be CD25 POSITIVE (the case is silent on CD25 but CD7 loss and Sézary morphology fit cutaneous T-cell lymphoma) and typically presents with hypercalcaemia and HTLV-1 epidemiology — Caribbean, southwest Japan; flower cells rather than cerebriform Sézary cells. (D) Atopic dermatitis lacks circulating clonal T cells with CD7 loss and Pautrier microabscesses. (E) DRESS is acute drug-induced and reverses with the offending drug; it does not produce a 12-year progression.

Vignette 9. A 16-year-old boy with lymphadenopathy and CD30+ ALK+ lymphoma

A 16-year-old boy presents with a six-week history of fever, night sweats, weight loss, and rapidly enlarging cervical, mediastinal, and axillary lymphadenopathy. CT shows extensive nodal disease and a 7 cm anterior mediastinal mass; PET shows widely FDG-avid disease above and below the diaphragm. Lymph node biopsy shows sheets of large pleomorphic cells with eccentric horseshoe-shaped or "embryo-like" nuclei and abundant cytoplasm, replacing nodal architecture. Immunohistochemistry: CD30 strongly positive, CD45 positive, EMA positive, CD3 positive (cytoplasmic), CD20 negative, ALK positive (cytoplasmic and nuclear pattern), and clonal TCR rearrangement on molecular studies. FISH confirms t(2;5)(p23;q35)/NPM1::ALK. Which of the following is the most appropriate first-line therapy?

- **(A)** Brentuximab vedotin plus CHP (BV-CHP) chemoimmunotherapy.
- **(B)** R-CHOP × 6 cycles.
- **(C)** ABVD chemotherapy with involved-site radiation.
- **(D)** Crizotinib monotherapy as first-line ALK-targeted therapy.
- **(E)** Single-agent brentuximab vedotin without chemotherapy.

Best answer: (A) Brentuximab vedotin plus CHP (BV-CHP) chemoimmunotherapy.

Rationale. The diagnosis is anaplastic large cell lymphoma, ALK-positive, systemic. Morphology (pleomorphic cells with horseshoe "hallmark" nuclei), immunophenotype (CD30 strongly positive, CD45 positive — distinguishing from classical Hodgkin lymphoma; CD3 positive on T-cell origin; EMA positive; ALK positive by IHC with cytoplasmic and nuclear distribution typical of NPM1::ALK), and cytogenetics (t(2;5)/NPM1::ALK in approximately 80% of ALK+ ALCL) are diagnostic. The ECHELON-2 trial established BV-CHP (brentuximab vedotin replacing vincristine in CHOP) as superior to CHOP alone for CD30-positive PTCL including ALCL, and BV-CHP is now first-line standard. ALK-positive ALCL has the most favourable prognosis among ALCL subgroups (5-year overall survival 70–90%); ALK-negative ALCL with DUSP22-IRF4 rearrangement approaches similar outcomes; ALK-negative ALCL with TP63 rearrangement has very poor outcomes. Crizotinib (ALK inhibitor) is active in relapsed ALK-positive ALCL but is not first-line therapy.

Distractor analysis. (B) R-CHOP is for B-cell DLBCL; ALCL is a T-cell lymphoma without CD20 expression and rituximab is irrelevant. (C) ABVD is for Hodgkin lymphoma. (D) Crizotinib monotherapy is not standard first-line for systemic ALK+ ALCL; first-line is chemoimmunotherapy. (E) Single-agent BV is reserved for relapsed disease or for cutaneous ALCL; systemic disease requires combination chemotherapy.

Vignette 10. A 22-year-old man with bilateral cervical lymphadenopathy after a viral illness — the elimination test

A 22-year-old college student presents to student health with three weeks of fatigue, sore throat, and bilateral non-tender cervical lymphadenopathy. He had a febrile pharyngitis two weeks ago that has gradually resolved without treatment. Examination shows multiple non-tender mobile cervical and posterior auricular nodes, none larger than 2 cm; pharyngeal erythema with tonsillar enlargement; mild splenomegaly; no rash, fever, or weight loss. Laboratory studies: haemoglobin 13.8 g/dL, platelets 220,000/µL, white blood cells 14,000/µL with 18% atypical lymphocytes (Downey cells with abundant cytoplasm, irregular nuclear contours, and cytoplasmic vacuolation). Heterophile (Monospot) antibody test is positive; EBV VCA-IgM is positive; LDH 280 U/L (mildly elevated). Which of the following is the most appropriate next step?

- **(A)** Reassure the patient and provide supportive care for infectious mononucleosis; lymph node biopsy is not indicated.
- **(B)** Excisional cervical lymph node biopsy to exclude Hodgkin lymphoma.
- **(C)** Initiate empiric antibiotic therapy for bacterial pharyngitis with persistent lymphadenopathy.
- **(D)** Bone marrow biopsy to exclude an underlying lymphoma.
- **(E)** Start ABVD chemotherapy empirically because of LDH elevation.

Best answer: (A) Reassure the patient and provide supportive care for infectious mononucleosis; lymph node biopsy is not indicated.

Rationale. The clinical picture is classical primary EBV infection (infectious mononucleosis): a young adult with fatigue, pharyngitis, bilateral non-tender symmetrical lymphadenopathy, mild splenomegaly, atypical lymphocytes (Downey cells), positive heterophile antibody, and positive EBV VCA-IgM. The atypical lymphocytes are reactive cytotoxic CD8+ T cells responding to EBV-infected B cells, not malignant cells. Lymph node biopsy in the setting of acute EBV infection can be a diagnostic trap because florid reactive lymph nodes may show large hyperplastic immunoblasts and even occasional Reed-Sternberg–like cells, leading to misdiagnosis as Hodgkin lymphoma. The management is supportive: hydration, NSAIDs for symptom control, avoidance of contact sports for at least 3–4 weeks because of splenic rupture risk, and avoidance of amoxicillin (which produces a characteristic morbilliform rash in EBV infection that can be mistaken for drug allergy). Lymphadenopathy resolves over weeks to months; persistent or progressive adenopathy beyond 6–8 weeks warrants reassessment. The exam-pattern: a young adult with bilateral symmetric lymphadenopathy, atypical lymphocytes, and positive heterophile antibody is mononucleosis — biopsy is the wrong answer.

Distractor analysis. (B) Biopsy in active EBV infection risks misdiagnosis. (C) Bacterial pharyngitis would not produce widespread lymphadenopathy with atypical lymphocytes. (D) Bone marrow biopsy is not indicated; the Heterophile and EBV serology establish the diagnosis. (E) Empiric chemotherapy without a tissue diagnosis would be malpractice and harmful.

14.7 Closing Discriminators

HIGH-YIELD PEARL — Histological transformation of indolent NHL

Indolent B-cell lymphomas — follicular lymphoma, marginal zone lymphomas, and CLL/SLL — can transform to aggressive lymphoma over time. Follicular lymphoma transforms to DLBCL at approximately 2–3% per year; CLL transforms to DLBCL (Richter transformation) in 5–10% over the disease course; MALT lymphoma transforms to DLBCL less commonly. The clinical signature of transformation is uniform: rapid focal nodal growth (often a single dominant node or extranodal mass), B symptoms, and a substantial rise in serum LDH. Imaging may show heterogeneous FDG avidity with focal high-uptake areas. The diagnostic step is a directed excisional biopsy of the most metabolically active lesion (PET-guided), not a repeat marrow biopsy or a generic restaging. Treatment of transformed disease uses DLBCL-directed regimens (R-CHOP or DA-EPOCH-R) with consideration of stem-cell transplant or CAR-T in fit responders. Outcomes are poorer than de novo DLBCL but substantially better than untreated transformation.

HIGH-YIELD PEARL — B symptoms have a defined definition

"B symptoms" in lymphoma staging are tightly defined: unexplained fevers >38.0°C, drenching night sweats, and unintentional weight loss >10% of body weight over the preceding six months. Fatigue, pruritus, and alcohol-induced lymph node pain are not B symptoms (although alcohol-induced pain is a famously specific Hodgkin lymphoma association). B symptoms upstage the patient — Ann Arbour stage IIIA becomes IIIB with B symptoms, with corresponding implications for treatment intensity in cHL and for prognostic scoring (IPI, FLIPI, MIPI) in NHL. The exam pattern: a vignette describing fatigue alone or pruritus alone does NOT meet B-symptom criteria and does not change stage. The diagnostic move when B symptoms are present is to escalate workup (CT chest/abdomen/pelvis, PET, marrow biopsy if not already done) before treatment.

TRAP — Mediastinal mass in a young woman is not always Hodgkin lymphoma

A young to middle-aged woman with an anterior mediastinal mass and B symptoms is the classical Hodgkin lymphoma vignette — but it is also the classical primary mediastinal large B-cell lymphoma (PMBL) vignette. The discriminator is immunohistochemistry. cHL is CD30+, CD15+, CD45−, with dim PAX5 and absent CD20. PMBL is CD20 STRONGLY POSITIVE (a B-cell lymphoma derived from thymic medullary B cells), CD30 weak or partial positive (in approximately 80%), and CD15 negative; it is also frequently positive for MAL, CD23, CD200, and PD-L1. The clinical and imaging features can be similar (large anterior mediastinal mass, superior vena cava syndrome possible, occasional pleural and pericardial effusions). Treatment differs substantially: cHL is treated with ABVD or A+AVD; PMBL is treated with DA-EPOCH-R (which has produced excellent outcomes in PMBL and avoids consolidative radiation in most cases) or R-CHOP plus involved-site radiation. The correct exam answer demands the IHC panel to disambiguate.

IMG-TRAP — "Lymphadenopathy in a young person therefore lymphoma" is wrong

Trainees from settings where infectious lymphadenopathy (tuberculosis, EBV, toxoplasmosis, HIV) and reactive lymphadenitis dominate the differential sometimes overcorrect on USMLE vignettes by reflexively answering "lymphoma" for any cervical lymphadenopathy. The exam-correct discrimination is symmetry, tenderness, and serology. Bilateral symmetric non-tender lymphadenopathy with atypical lymphocytes and positive heterophile is mononucleosis, not Hodgkin lymphoma. Tender, fluctuant, or suppurative nodes with a clear infectious source are reactive lymphadenitis. Painless, asymmetric, firm, progressive, or rubbery nodes — especially with B symptoms or atypical sites (supraclavicular, mediastinal, retroperitoneal) — favour lymphoma and warrant biopsy. The diagnostic threshold for excisional biopsy is generally adenopathy persisting beyond 4–6 weeks of observation in adults, supraclavicular adenopathy at any duration, mediastinal or retroperitoneal disease at any duration, and any lymphadenopathy with B symptoms or unexplained cytopenias.

14.8 Quick Recall

QUICK RECALL — Lymphomas

Hodgkin lymphoma — classical. Reed-Sternberg cells (CD30+, CD15+, CD45−, dim PAX5+); subtypes — nodular sclerosis (most common; young adults; mediastinal; lacunar cells), mixed cellularity (EBV+ ~70%), lymphocyte-rich, lymphocyte-depleted (HIV; worst). ABVD ± radiation for early-stage; N-AVD (nivolumab + AVD) preferred for advanced/bulky per SWOG S1826; BV-AVD and ABVD acceptable alternatives.

NLPBL. Popcorn cells; CD20+, CD45+, CD30−, CD15−. Indolent B-cell lymphoma. Stage IA: observe or radiation. Treated like indolent NHL.

DLBCL. Most common NHL. Hans algorithm → GCB vs ABC. R-CHOP × 6. POLARIX trial: pola-R-CHP for IPI ≥2.

Double-hit lymphoma (DHL). MYC + BCL2 rearrangements by FISH. Very poor with R-CHOP. DA-EPOCH-R or R-CODOX-M/IVAC. Mostly GCB-COO.

Double-expressor lymphoma (DEL). MYC ≥40% + BCL2 ≥50% by IHC. NO gene rearrangement. Intermediate prognosis. R-CHOP or intensified.

Burkitt lymphoma. t(8;14)/MYC::IGH (or t(2;8), t(8;22)). Starry sky; Ki-67 ~100%; BCL2 NEGATIVE; TdT−. Three variants — endemic (jaw, EBV+ >95%), sporadic (abdomen), HIV-associated. DA-EPOCH-R; intrathecal MTX; rasburicase.

Follicular lymphoma. t(14;18)/IGH::BCL2 (~90%). CD20+, CD10+, BCL6+, BCL2+ in follicular pattern. WHO 2022 abolished 1–3A grading. Asymptomatic = observe (GELF criteria). Symptomatic = R-CHOP/R-bendamustine. Maintenance rituximab.

Mantle cell lymphoma. t(11;14)/CCND1::IGH. Cyclin D1+ nuclear. CD5+, CD20 BRIGHT, CD23 NEGATIVE, FMC7+, SOX11+. Older men, GI lymphomatous polyposis. Cytarabine-based induction + autoSCT (younger fit); R-bendamustine (older). BTK inhibitors (acalabrutinib, zanubrutinib; pirtobrutinib for BTK-resistant relapse — ibrutinib withdrawn from US MCL indication Dec 2023) and brexucabtagene autoleucel CAR-T for relapsed disease.

MALT lymphoma. Gastric MALT + H. pylori (no t(11;18)) → triple-therapy eradication first-line. t(11;18)/API2::MALT1 = antibiotic-resistant. Other associations: B. burgdorferi (skin), C. psittaci (ocular), C. jejuni (intestinal IPSID), HCV (splenic MZL).

Waldenström. IgM monoclonal gammopathy + LPL. MYD88 L265P (>90%). CXCR4 ~30% (reduced ibrutinib response). Hyperviscosity → plasmapheresis. BTK inhibitor or rituximab-based.

Mycosis fungoides. CD3+, CD4+, CD7 NEGATIVE epidermotropic infiltrate. Pautrier microabscesses. Patch → plaque → tumour. PUVA, narrowband UVB, brentuximab if CD30+, mogamulizumab.

Sézary syndrome. Erythroderma >80% BSA + circulating cerebriform "Sézary" cells ≥1,000/µL + lymphadenopathy. Leukaemic phase of CTCL. Mogamulizumab + ECP + systemic agents; alloSCT in select.

ATLL. HTLV-1 endemic (SW Japan, Caribbean, parts of Africa). Flower cells. CD3+, CD4+, CD25+, CD7−. Hypercalcaemia (PTHrP, RANKL). Acute, lymphomatous, chronic, smoldering variants. IFN-α + AZT (chronic/smoldering); chemotherapy + mogamulizumab (acute/lymphomatous).

Extranodal NK/T-cell, nasal type. EBV-driven. Midfacial necrosis ("lethal midline granuloma"). CD56+, EBER+, cytotoxic phenotype. SMILE/AspaMetDex + radiation.

AITL. TFH-derived (CD4+, CXCL13+, PD-1+, BCL6+, ICOS+). Polyclonal hypergammaglobulinaemia, autoimmune cytopenias, EBV+ B cells in node. RHOA G17V, TET2, IDH2, DNMT3A mutations. CHOEP + autoSCT; alloSCT if young/fit.

ALCL. CD30 strong+, CD45+, EMA+, T-cell origin. ALK+ (children/young; t(2;5)/NPM1::ALK; favourable). ALK− with DUSP22 (favourable) or TP63 (very poor). BV-CHP first-line per ECHELON-2. Breast implant–associated ALCL: capsulectomy curative.

LCH. CD1a+, S100+, CD207 (Langerin)+; Birbeck granules ("tennis rackets") on EM. BRAF V600E ~50%. Solitary bone lesion → curettage. Multisystem → vinblastine + prednisone; BRAF/MEK inhibition for refractory.

— End of Chapter 14 —

CHAPTER 15

Chapter 15 — Plasma Cell Neoplasms

BIG PICTURE

Plasma cell neoplasms are clonal proliferations of terminally differentiated B cells, unified by a single biochemical signature: monoclonal immunoglobulin (M-protein, paraprotein, or free light chain) circulating in serum, urine, or both. The spectrum is a continuum of risk, not a list of separate diseases. At one end sits monoclonal gammopathy of undetermined significance (MGUS), an asymptomatic finding present in ~3% of people over 50 with a 1% per year risk of progression. At the other end sits multiple myeloma with end-organ damage (CRAB) or biomarkers of malignancy (SLiM), demanding immediate treatment. Smouldering myeloma sits in the middle. Two organising principles unlock the field on every exam. First, the diagnostic threshold is set by the bone marrow plasma cell percentage and the presence or absence of CRAB or SLiM events — not by the size of the M-protein alone. Second, the prognostic threshold is set by FISH cytogenetics on CD138-selected plasma cells: del(17p), t(4;14), and t(14;16) define high-risk myeloma irrespective of stage. Adjacent entities — AL amyloidosis, plasmacytoma, plasma cell leukaemia, POEMS syndrome — are recognised by their characteristic clinical phenotypes layered on top of a small or modest M-protein. The chapter is built to make these distinctions exam-fast and clinically reliable.

MECHANISM HOOK — Why a single monoclonal protein produces such varied disease

A neoplastic plasma cell clone produces an immunoglobulin (or just its light chain) in vast excess. The phenotype that follows depends on what that protein does in tissues. When the M-protein is large and concentrated (especially IgM, a pentamer), it raises serum viscosity and produces hyperviscosity syndrome. When light chains misfold and deposit as antiparallel beta-pleated sheets, they form amyloid fibrils that deposit in the heart, kidney, nerves, and gut — AL amyloidosis. When intact light chains pass freely through the glomerulus and bind Tamm-Horsfall protein in the distal tubule, they precipitate as waxy casts and obstruct the tubule — myeloma cast nephropathy, the dominant renal lesion of multiple myeloma. When clonal plasma cells secrete osteoclast-activating factors (RANKL, MIP-1α) and inhibit osteoblast function via DKK1 and sclerostin, they produce the characteristic punched-out lytic bone lesions and pathological fractures. When neoplastic plasma cells displace normal haematopoiesis, they produce the anaemia of myeloma. The same clone, the same protein, but the destination tissue and the protein behaviour determine the syndrome. Recognising this lets a vignette describing nephrotic-range proteinuria with restrictive cardiomyopathy, an isolated lytic bone lesion, or a hyperviscosity-driven retinal haemorrhage all be traced back to a plasma cell clone — and the next test (SPEP plus immunofixation plus serum free light chain assay) is the same in each case.

15.1 Spectrum and Classification of Plasma Cell Neoplasms

The plasma cell neoplasms form a clinical and biological continuum. Diagnostic thresholds are set by three parameters: the size of the M-protein, the bone marrow clonal plasma cell percentage, and the presence or absence of myeloma-defining events (CRAB end-organ damage or SLiM biomarkers). The 2014 IMWG criteria — refined by IMWG 2021 and aligned with WHO 2022 — are the foundation of every diagnosis in this chapter and should be memorised in their full form before the exam.

Diagnosis	M-protein	BM clonal plasma cells	CRAB / SLiM	Management principle
MGUS	IgG/IgA/IgM <30 g/L; or abnormal FLC ratio without absolute involved FLC ≥100 mg/L	<10%	None	Observation; risk-stratified follow-up; ~1% per year progression
Smouldering myeloma (SMM)	IgG/IgA ≥30 g/L OR urine M-protein ≥500 mg/24h OR (any M-protein with BM PCs 10–59%)	10–59%	None	High-risk SMM (Mayo 20-2-20): consider lenalidomide-based early therapy. Standard-risk: observe.
Multiple myeloma	Any level (or non-secretory variant)	≥10% (or biopsy-proven plasmacytoma)	CRAB or SLiM present	VRd or Dara-VRd induction; ASCT-eligible vs ineligible pathways; maintenance lenalidomide
Plasma cell leukaemia (PCL)	Usually present; aggressive	High; circulating PCs ≥5% of PB WBC (IMWG 2021 / WHO 2022)	Present, often severe	Treat as high-risk MM; ASCT in remission; very poor prognosis
Solitary plasmacytoma (osseous or extramedullary)	Often absent or small	<10% in marrow; lesion biopsy clonal	No systemic CRAB attributable to other lesions	Definitive radiotherapy 40–50 Gy; lifelong surveillance for MM progression

Diagnosis	M-protein	BM clonal plasma cells	CRAB / SLiM	Management principle
AL (light-chain) amyloidosis	Often modest; FLC abnormality common	<10% in pure AL (>10% if coexistent MM)	Tissue amyloid deposition (Congo red apple-green birefringence)	Bortezomib-based induction; daratumumab-CyBorD; risk-adapted ASCT
POEMS syndrome	Lambda-restricted, often small	Usually <5% (often osteosclerotic plasmacytoma)	Polyneuropathy + organomegaly + endocrinopathy + skin changes (Castleman in subset)	Radiotherapy if localised; ASCT or lenalidomide-based therapy if disseminated
Waldenström macroglobulinaemia (LPL with IgM)	IgM (any level)	Lymphoplasmacytic infiltrate (small B cells + plasma cells)	Hyperviscosity, neuropathy, cryoglobulinaemia	See Chapter 14: B-cell NHL — covered as LPL

Table 15.1: The plasma cell neoplasm spectrum. Diagnostic thresholds (IMWG 2014, refined IMWG 2021 / WHO 2022) and management principles. Note: Waldenström macroglobulinaemia is an LPL-class disease with an IgM paraprotein, classified with mature B-cell NHL and detailed in Chapter 14.

HIGH-YIELD PEARL — Waldenström macroglobulinaemia is not IgM myeloma

A patient with an IgM monoclonal paraprotein has either Waldenström macroglobulinaemia (the dominant entity) or, much more rarely, IgM multiple myeloma. The discriminator is the underlying neoplasm. WM is a lymphoplasmacytic lymphoma with a CD20-positive small B-cell infiltrate plus plasmacytoid forms in the marrow; it carries the MYD88 L265P mutation in over 90% of cases. IgM myeloma is a true plasma cell neoplasm with sheets of CD138-positive clonal plasma cells, lytic bone lesions, and a usually MYD88-negative profile. The treatment, biology, and prognosis of the two entities differ fundamentally, and they should never be conflated. Waldenström is detailed in Chapter 14 alongside lymphoplasmacytic lymphoma; this chapter focuses on plasma cell neoplasms proper. The serological clue is the same (IgM M-protein), so the diagnostic move is the bone marrow biopsy with immunophenotyping and MYD88 testing.

15.2 Monoclonal Gammopathy of Undetermined Significance (MGUS)

MGUS is the asymptomatic precursor state of every plasma cell neoplasm. By definition it is detected incidentally — on a screening serum protein electrophoresis ordered for back pain, recurrent infection, neuropathy, or non-specific systemic complaints — in a person with no end-organ damage. Three subtypes are recognised by the immunoglobulin class: non-IgM MGUS (IgG, IgA, or IgD; precursor of myeloma), IgM MGUS (precursor of Waldenström macroglobulinaemia), and light chain MGUS (an abnormal serum FLC ratio with no detectable intact M-protein; precursor of light chain myeloma and AL amyloidosis). The diagnostic criteria require a serum M-protein <30 g/L, clonal bone marrow plasma cells <10%, and the absence of any CRAB end-organ damage or SLiM biomarker.

The annual rate of progression from non-IgM MGUS to multiple myeloma or a related plasma cell neoplasm is approximately 1% per year and does not plateau over time. Three risk factors stratify progression risk: an abnormal serum FLC ratio (outside 0.26–1.65), a non-IgG isotype (IgA or IgD), and an M-protein concentration ≥15 g/L. Patients with all three risk factors have approximately 58% cumulative progression risk at 20 years; patients with none have approximately 5% risk. The Mayo Clinic risk-stratification model uses these three variables to schedule follow-up: low-risk patients can be reassessed every 2–3 years, while high-risk patients warrant 6-monthly review with repeat SPEP, FLC assay, and CBC.

HIGH-YIELD PEARL — When MGUS becomes "monoclonal gammopathy of clinical significance" (MGCS)

A small M-protein with no marrow expansion can still cause organ damage if the protein itself is pathogenic. Examples include monoclonal gammopathy of renal significance (MGRS) — small clones producing nephrotoxic immunoglobulins or light chains that cause proliferative glomerulonephritis with monoclonal immunoglobulin deposits, light chain deposition disease, AL amyloidosis, or fibrillary glomerulonephritis without meeting myeloma criteria — and monoclonal gammopathy of neurological significance (anti-MAG neuropathy, classically with IgM kappa). The exam-relevant point is that the diagnosis "MGUS" does not exclude clinical disease driven by the M-protein. When end-organ damage is present and a small clone is identified, the workup must specifically attribute the lesion to the M-protein (immunofluorescence on renal biopsy showing monoclonal kappa or lambda deposits; nerve conduction with anti-MAG titre) before labelling the patient as MGUS. MGRS in particular requires clone-directed therapy similar to myeloma, despite plasma cell counts <10%.

15.3 Smouldering Multiple Myeloma (SMM)

Smouldering myeloma sits between MGUS and active myeloma. It is defined by a serum M-protein ≥30 g/L (IgG or IgA) or urine M-protein ≥500 mg/24h, OR clonal bone marrow plasma cells of 10–59%, in the absence of any CRAB or SLiM event. The progression rate is approximately 10% per year for the first five years, ~3% per year for the next five, and ~1% per year thereafter — substantially faster than MGUS, with the implication that surveillance must be tighter and that high-risk SMM has emerged as a treatment indication.

The Mayo "20-2-20" model identifies high-risk SMM by three thresholds: bone marrow clonal plasma cells >20%, serum M-protein >2 g/dL, and serum free light chain ratio >20. Patients meeting two or three criteria have approximately 44% progression risk at two years and ~64% at five years (Lakshman et al., BCJ 2018). Two randomised trials (QuiRedex and ECOG E3A06) showed that lenalidomide-based therapy in high-risk SMM delays progression and may improve overall survival, and many guidelines now recommend offering early treatment to high-risk SMM. Standard-risk SMM is observed with 3-monthly clinical review and SPEP/FLC for the first year, then 6-monthly.

HIGH-YIELD PEARL — The MGUS / SMM / MM boundary is dynamic, not static

The 2014 IMWG SLiM update reclassified some patients previously labelled "SMM" as active myeloma requiring immediate therapy. SLiM biomarkers — Sixty percent clonal plasma cells, serum FLC ratio ≥100 (involved/uninvolved) with absolute involved FLC ≥100 mg/L, or MRI showing more than one focal bone lesion ≥5 mm — identify SMM patients with ~80% two-year progression risk to overt myeloma. These patients are now diagnosed and treated as multiple myeloma even without classic CRAB end-organ damage. Vignettes describing "asymptomatic SMM with serum FLC ratio of 250 and a single MRI focal lesion" should not be answered as observation — that patient meets SLiM criteria and is myeloma. The exam-trap is the patient who appears clinically asymptomatic but crosses the SLiM threshold biochemically or radiologically.

15.4 Multiple Myeloma

Clinical features and epidemiology

Multiple myeloma is the second most common haematological malignancy globally and accounts for approximately 1–2% of all cancers and ~10% of haematological cancers. The median age at diagnosis is approximately 65–70 years; cases below age 40 are rare and warrant consideration of an underlying genetic predisposition. African ancestry confers approximately twice the incidence relative to European ancestry. In India, the disease is increasingly recognised, with regional variation in age at presentation skewing somewhat younger than Western series.

The clinical picture is classically built around the CRAB tetrad — hypercalcaemia, Renal impairment, Anaemia, Bone disease — but the underlying mechanisms are unified by the clonal plasma cell expansion and its secreted product. Bone pain (often back, ribs, or pelvis) is the most common presenting complaint, driven by lytic bone lesions, vertebral compression fractures, or pathological fractures. Anaemia (normocytic, normochromic) reflects marrow displacement and inflammatory cytokine effects. Renal impairment has multiple causes: cast nephropathy from light chain precipitation in distal tubules (the dominant mechanism), hypercalcaemia-related dehydration and tubular damage, AL amyloid renal infiltration, light chain deposition disease, and nephrotoxic medications. Hypercalcaemia results from RANKL-driven osteoclast activation and presents with confusion, polyuria, constipation, and renal impairment.

Recurrent bacterial infections — particularly with encapsulated organisms (Streptococcus pneumoniae, Haemophilus influenzae) — reflect functional hypogammaglobulinaemia: although the total immunoglobulin level is high (the M-protein), the polyclonal antibody response is profoundly suppressed. Vaccination against pneumococcus, influenza, and SARS-CoV-2 is important in long-term management. Hyperviscosity is uncommon in IgG and IgA myeloma but can occur with very high M-protein levels (especially IgA, which polymerises) or in IgD myeloma.

Diagnostic criteria — IMWG 2014 SLiM-CRAB

The diagnosis of multiple myeloma requires (1) ≥10% clonal bone marrow plasma cells OR a biopsy-proven plasmacytoma AND (2) at least one myeloma-defining event — either a CRAB criterion (end-organ damage attributable to the plasma cell disorder) or a SLiM biomarker (markers of impending end-organ damage that allow earlier diagnosis and treatment).

FORMULA — IMWG 2014 SLiM-CRAB criteria for active multiple myeloma
REQUIRED — both of the following:
1. Clonal bone marrow plasma cells ≥10% OR biopsy-proven bony or extramedullary plasmacytoma; AND
2. At least one myeloma-defining event — either CRAB or SLiM:

CRAB (end-organ damage attributable to the plasma cell disorder):
C — Hypercalcaemia: serum calcium >0.25 mmol/L (>1 mg/dL) above the upper limit of normal OR >2.75 mmol/L (>11 mg/dL) absolute.

R — Renal insufficiency: creatinine clearance <40 mL/min OR serum creatinine >177 micromol/L (>2 mg/dL), attributable to myeloma.

A — Anaemia: haemoglobin >20 g/L below the lower limit of normal OR <100 g/L.

B — Bone lesions: ≥1 lytic lesion on skeletal radiography, CT, or PET-CT (≥5 mm in size).

SLiM (biomarkers of imminent end-organ damage; >80% two-year progression risk):

S — Sixty percent or more clonal plasma cells in the bone marrow.

Li — Light chain ratio: involved/uninvolved serum FLC ratio ≥100, with absolute involved FLC ≥100 mg/L.

M — MRI: more than one focal bone lesion ≥5 mm in size on whole-body or axial MRI.

Older diagnostic criteria (Durie-Salmon) are no longer in use; IMWG 2014 has fully superseded them.

Laboratory workup — the protein triad

The protein workup of suspected myeloma requires three simultaneous tests: serum protein electrophoresis (SPEP), serum immunofixation electrophoresis (IFE), and serum free light chain (sFLC) assay. The combination has near-100% sensitivity for detecting any monoclonal protein. SPEP detects an M-spike — a tall, narrow peak in the gamma or beta region; quantitation gives the M-protein concentration. IFE identifies the heavy chain class (IgG, IgA, IgM, IgD, or rarely IgE) and the light chain type (kappa or lambda); a heavy/light chain mismatch (e.g. an IgG kappa M-band with isolated lambda free light chain excess) suggests a coexistent second clone or biclonal gammopathy. sFLC quantifies free kappa and free lambda; the kappa/lambda ratio is normally 0.26–1.65 (broadened to 0.37–3.1 in renal impairment because kappa clearance is reduced). Light-chain-only myeloma and AL amyloidosis frequently have negative or barely abnormal SPEP/IFE; the FLC ratio is the single most sensitive test in these cases.

Bone imaging has shifted away from the historical metastatic skeletal survey (plain X-rays). Whole-body low-dose CT (WBLDCT) or whole-body MRI is now standard for newly diagnosed myeloma; PET-CT is increasingly used and is the preferred modality for response assessment and detection of extramedullary disease. The 2014 SLiM update specifically permits MRI-detected focal bone lesions to define active myeloma, reflecting MRI sensitivity for marrow infiltration before lytic destruction is visible on plain films.

Bone marrow morphology and immunophenotype

Bone marrow examination — both aspirate (for cytology, flow cytometry, FISH) and trephine biopsy (for accurate plasma cell quantitation and pattern of infiltration) — is mandatory. The aspirate shows sheets or aggregates of atypical plasma cells, with characteristic morphology: eccentric round-to-oval nuclei, clumped chromatin in a "clock-face" or "cartwheel" pattern, a perinuclear hof (clear zone representing the Golgi apparatus), and deeply basophilic cytoplasm. Variant plasma cell morphologies include multinucleate forms, flame cells (red-stained cytoplasm in IgA myeloma due to glycoprotein content), Mott cells (cytoplasmic Russell bodies — discrete eosinophilic inclusions of immunoglobulin), and grape cells (cells stuffed with multiple Russell bodies). The trephine biopsy quantifies plasma cell percentage more accurately than the aspirate (the aspirate haemodilutes); patterns include interstitial, nodular, and diffuse (sheets effacing normal marrow), with diffuse and nodular patterns conferring a worse prognosis.

Immunohistochemistry on the trephine confirms clonality and identifies plasma cell origin. CD138 is the primary plasma cell marker. CD38 is also positive but less specific (it is also positive on lymphocytes and other cells). Kappa and lambda IHC or in situ hybridisation demonstrates light chain restriction — the sine qua non of a clonal plasma cell population. CD56 is aberrantly expressed in approximately 70% of myeloma cases (negative in normal plasma cells) and is the most useful aberrant marker for flow gating. CD19 is lost in myeloma plasma cells (positive in normal plasma cells); CD20 and cyclin D1 are variably expressed and have prognostic implications in some studies.

Marker	Normal plasma cells	Myeloma plasma cells	Reactive plasmacytosis
CD38	Bright positive	Bright positive (gating)	Bright positive
CD138	Positive	Positive	Positive
CD19	Positive	NEGATIVE (most consistent loss)	Positive
CD45	Positive	Dim or negative	Positive
CD56	Negative	Often positive (aberrant ~70%)	Negative
CD117	Negative	Often positive (especially IgA)	Negative
CD200	Negative or dim	Often positive	Negative
CD81	Positive	Often absent or dim	Positive
Cytoplasmic Ig	Polyclonal (κ + λ)	Monoclonal (κ OR λ — light chain restriction)	Polyclonal (κ + λ)

Table 15.2: Flow cytometry of plasma cells — distinguishing myeloma from reactive plasmacytosis. The diagnostic move is light chain restriction; CD19 loss is the most consistent aberrant marker.

Cytogenetics — high-risk profiles drive treatment

Conventional karyotyping is rarely informative in myeloma because plasma cells have a very low proliferation index. FISH on CD138-selected plasma cells is the standard cytogenetic platform. The cytogenetic profile divides myeloma into hyperdiploid (~50% of cases; trisomies of odd-numbered chromosomes 3, 5, 7, 9, 11, 15, 19, 21; standard-risk) and non-hyperdiploid (with characteristic IGH translocations on chromosome 14q32). Three IGH translocations are routinely tested and define the biological subgroups: t(11;14)/CCND1::IGH (~15%; standard-risk; also produces cyclin D1 expression and can phenotypically mimic mantle cell lymphoma), t(4;14)/FGFR3-MMSET (NSD2)::IGH (~15%; high-risk; bortezomib improves outcomes substantially), t(14;16)/MAF::IGH (~5%; very poor; limited response to current therapy), and the rare t(14;20)/MAFB::IGH (~1%; high-risk).

The three primary high-risk markers are del(17p13.1) (TP53 deletion; ~10% at diagnosis, increasing at relapse), t(4;14), and t(14;16). 1q gain (≥3 copies) and 1q amplification (≥4 copies) are increasingly recognised as adverse prognostic markers and are included in some "double-hit" myeloma schemas: ≥2 high-risk abnormalities concurrent. Triple-hit myeloma (≥3 high-risk abnormalities) carries a particularly dismal prognosis. The IFM/Mayo and the IMWG R2-ISS staging systems both incorporate cytogenetics; del(17p), t(4;14), t(14;16), and 1q gain are the most consistently high-risk markers across schemas.

HIGH-YIELD PEARL — High-risk cytogenetics in myeloma

Three primary high-risk cytogenetic abnormalities define adverse-risk myeloma and must be tested at diagnosis on every patient:

- del(17p13.1) — TP53 deletion. ~10% at diagnosis; rises at relapse. Worst single abnormality. Bortezomib partially overcomes; daratumumab- and pomalidomide-based regimens used.
- t(4;14)(p16;q32) — FGFR3 and MMSET (NSD2) dysregulation. ~15%. Historically poor; outcomes improve substantially with bortezomib-based induction (the rationale for VRd or Dara-VRd in all newly diagnosed myeloma).
- t(14;16)(q32;q23) — MAF translocation. ~5%. Very poor; high-LDH, plasmablastic morphology common; no targeted agent.

Additional adverse markers in widely-used schemas: t(14;20)/MAFB (~1%; very poor); 1q gain (≥3 copies); 1q amplification (≥4 copies); del(1p32) (CDKN2C deletion). Standard-risk myeloma is hyperdiploid (trisomies of odd-numbered chromosomes) without IGH translocations.

Diagnostic move: FISH on CD138-selected plasma cells. Conventional karyotype misses most myeloma cytogenetics because of low plasma cell proliferation.

Risk stratification — R-ISS and the IMWG R2-ISS update

The Revised International Staging System (R-ISS, 2015) integrates the original ISS (based on serum albumin and beta-2 microglobulin) with FISH cytogenetics and serum LDH. The newer R2-ISS (2022) further refines staging by incorporating 1q gain. Both systems are used clinically; R-ISS remains the most widely cited.

R-ISS Stage	Criteria	Median OS
Stage I	ISS Stage I (albumin ≥3.5 g/dL AND beta-2 microglobulin <3.5 mg/L) AND standard-risk cytogenetics by FISH AND normal LDH	Not reached at long follow-up; 5-year OS >80%
Stage II	Neither Stage I nor Stage III	~7 years (median 83 months); 5-yr OS

R-ISS Stage	Criteria	Median OS
		~62%
Stage III	ISS Stage III (beta-2 microglobulin ≥5.5 mg/L) AND (high-risk cytogenetics by FISH: del(17p), t(4;14), or t(14;16); OR elevated LDH)	~29 months

Table 15.3: Revised International Staging System (R-ISS) for newly diagnosed multiple myeloma.

Treatment principles

The modern induction backbone for newly diagnosed myeloma combines a proteasome inhibitor (bortezomib, carfilzomib), an immunomodulatory drug (lenalidomide, pomalidomide), and dexamethasone — VRd or KRd. Adding the anti-CD38 monoclonal antibody daratumumab (Dara-VRd or Dara-KRd) further deepens response and is now standard for transplant-eligible patients on the basis of multiple randomised trials. Autologous stem cell transplantation (ASCT) consolidates response in transplant-eligible patients (typically <70 years and fit) and remains a standard of care; tandem ASCT may be considered in high-risk disease. Lenalidomide maintenance after ASCT improves progression-free and overall survival and is continued indefinitely or until intolerance.

Transplant-ineligible patients — older or unfit patients — receive Dara-Rd or Dara-VRd as induction, with or without subsequent maintenance. Relapsed/refractory myeloma uses sequential triplet and quadruplet regimens, including pomalidomide, carfilzomib, isatuximab, daratumumab, and the BCMA-targeted agents — belantamab mafodotin (BCMA antibody-drug conjugate), idecabtagene vicleucel and ciltacabtagene autoleucel (BCMA CAR-T), and teclistamab and elranatamab (BCMA bispecific T-cell engagers). The therapeutic landscape evolves rapidly; the principle to retain is that triplet therapy is standard, anti-CD38 antibody integration is now early-line, and BCMA-targeted therapies dominate the relapsed-refractory space.

Supportive care is integral. Bisphosphonates (zoledronic acid, pamidronate) or denosumab are given monthly for skeletal protection in any patient with bone disease, irrespective of treatment phase, with attention to renal function and risk of osteonecrosis of the jaw. Antiviral prophylaxis (acyclovir against varicella-zoster reactivation) is mandatory with bortezomib, daratumumab, and BCMA-targeted agents. Pneumococcal and influenza vaccination is recommended. Renal-protective measures (avoidance of NSAIDs, contrast, and aminoglycosides; aggressive hydration in cast nephropathy) and management of hyperviscosity (plasmapheresis if symptomatic) are routine considerations.

15.5 Plasma Cell Leukaemia

Plasma cell leukaemia (PCL) is the most aggressive plasma cell neoplasm, defined by the presence of circulating clonal plasma cells in the peripheral blood at a level ≥5% of total peripheral blood white cells (IMWG 2021 / WHO 2022). The older definition (≥20% PCs of WBC or absolute count ≥2 × 10^9/L) has been formally abandoned because the lower threshold identifies an outcome equivalent group earlier and improves recognition. PCL is divided into primary PCL (de novo presentation; ~60% of cases) and secondary PCL (transformation from preexisting myeloma; ~40%); secondary PCL has even worse outcomes than primary PCL.

Clinically, PCL presents with rapid disease evolution, extensive extramedullary disease, frequent renal failure, hypercalcaemia, anaemia, and B symptoms. The peripheral blood smear shows circulating plasma cells with the classical morphology — eccentric nucleus, perinuclear hof, basophilic cytoplasm — interspersed among the white cells. The cytogenetic profile is enriched for high-risk markers: del(17p), t(14;16), and 1q gain are over-represented compared with myeloma. The phenotype of circulating PCs differs slightly from medullary myeloma: CD56 is more frequently negative in PCL (helping the cells extravasate), while CD20 expression and surface CD45 are more common.

Treatment is patterned on high-risk myeloma and uses early integration of the most active triplet or quadruplet regimens (Dara-VRd, Dara-KRd) followed by autologous stem cell transplantation, ideally tandem ASCT or ASCT followed by allogeneic transplant in fit younger patients. CAR-T therapy and BCMA bispecifics are increasingly used in this aggressive disease. Median overall survival historically was 6–12 months for primary PCL and shorter for secondary PCL; modern therapy has improved median survival to 1–3 years in primary PCL, but prognosis remains the worst of the plasma cell neoplasms.

15.6 Solitary Plasmacytoma

Solitary plasmacytoma is a localised tumour of clonal plasma cells without systemic disease. Two anatomical variants are recognised: solitary plasmacytoma of bone (SPB; the more common form, accounting for ~70%, typically in the axial skeleton — vertebrae, pelvis, ribs) and solitary extramedullary plasmacytoma (EMP; arising in the upper aerodigestive tract — nasopharynx, paranasal sinuses, tonsils, larynx — in 80% of cases, with the remainder distributed across the GI tract, skin, and other sites). Diagnostic criteria require all of: a single biopsy-proven clonal plasma cell tumour, clonal plasma cells <10% on a separate marrow sample, no other myeloma-defining events on imaging, and no CRAB or SLiM features.

Whole-body MRI or PET-CT is essential to exclude additional bone or extramedullary disease before the diagnosis can be made. Because the marrow may show a small accompanying clone (usually <10%), the term "solitary plasmacytoma with minimal marrow involvement" is used when 1–9% clonal plasma cells are present in the marrow without other myeloma-defining events. This intermediate group has a higher progression rate to multiple myeloma than true solitary plasmacytoma.

Treatment is definitive radiation therapy at 40–50 Gy delivered to the lesion plus a margin. Local control is excellent: ~90% for both SPB and EMP. The risk of progression to multiple myeloma is, however, substantial — approximately 50–70% at 10 years for SPB, and 10–30% for EMP. Lifelong follow-up with serial SPEP, FLC assay, and imaging (every 3–6 months in the first 2–3 years, then less frequently) is essential. Surgical excision is sometimes added in EMP for symptom control or when complete resection is feasible.

HIGH-YIELD PEARL — Solitary plasmacytoma vs early myeloma — the imaging move

A patient with a single lytic lesion and clonal plasma cells inside that lesion has either (a) solitary plasmacytoma — if the rest of the workup is negative, or (b) early multiple myeloma — if any second lesion is found on imaging, or any CRAB/SLiM event is present, or marrow shows ≥10% clonal plasma cells. The diagnostic move is whole-body imaging — preferably whole-body MRI or PET-CT, not plain skeletal survey — combined with bone marrow examination and SLiM workup (M-protein quantitation, FLC assay, marrow plasma cell percentage). Vignettes describing "a single bone lesion with biopsy showing 80% plasma cells and CRAB-negative workup with marrow plasma cells of 5%" are solitary plasmacytoma. Vignettes describing "a single bone lesion plus an FLC ratio of 200 plus marrow plasma cells of 12%" are myeloma — the marrow plasma cell threshold (≥10%) and the SLiM biomarker (FLC ratio ≥100) both convert the diagnosis. Treatment differs fundamentally: radiotherapy alone for solitary plasmacytoma; systemic chemoimmunotherapy ± ASCT for myeloma.

15.7 AL (Light-Chain) Amyloidosis

Definition and pathogenesis

AL amyloidosis is a systemic disease in which a small clonal plasma cell or B-cell population produces a free immunoglobulin light chain that misfolds and deposits in tissues as amyloid fibrils. The fibrils are antiparallel beta-pleated sheet structures resistant to proteolysis. Lambda light chains are over-represented (lambda:kappa ~2:1, the inverse of normal serum) and lambda AL is typically more cardiotoxic. The underlying clone is usually small — bone marrow plasma cells <10% in pure AL — and the disease is driven by the pathogenic protein, not by the bulk of the clone. Approximately 10–15% of AL amyloid cases occur on a background of overt multiple myeloma; the term "myeloma with amyloidosis" is used in that setting.

Tissue tropism is determined by the specific light chain and the amyloid fibril composition. Cardiac involvement (~70% of patients) produces restrictive cardiomyopathy with bi-atrial enlargement, granular sparkling appearance on echocardiography, low-voltage QRS on ECG, and elevated cardiac biomarkers (NT-proBNP and troponin) disproportionate to ventricular function. Renal involvement (~70%) presents with nephrotic-range proteinuria, predominantly albumin (a clue distinguishing AL from cast nephropathy, which leaks light chains rather than albumin). Hepatic involvement produces hepatomegaly with elevated alkaline phosphatase. Peripheral and autonomic neuropathy, macroglossia (the textbook clue), periorbital purpura ("raccoon eyes"), gut dysmotility, and factor X deficiency-related bleeding round out the multisystem presentation.

HIGH-YIELD PEARL — Recognising AL amyloid: the four cardinal clues

No single sign is pathognomonic, but several signs in combination are highly suggestive and must trigger evaluation:

- Macroglossia with dental indentations on the tongue margin — present in ~10–20% but pathognomonic when present.
- Periorbital purpura ("raccoon eyes" or "pinch purpura") — bruising around the eyes after minimal trauma; results from amyloid infiltration of small vessels.
- Restrictive cardiomyopathy with low-voltage QRS but increased ventricular wall thickness on echo (the classical "discordance"), elevated NT-proBNP and troponin.
- Nephrotic-range proteinuria with predominantly albumin (vs cast nephropathy where light chains dominate).

Diagnostic move: tissue biopsy with Congo red staining showing apple-green birefringence under polarised light is the gold standard. Abdominal subcutaneous fat aspirate is the least-invasive screening site (sensitivity ~80%); affected organ biopsy (heart, kidney, nerve, gut) confirms organ involvement. Mass spectrometry typing of the amyloid fibril protein is the modern method of choice for distinguishing AL from ATTR (transthyretin), AA (serum amyloid A), and other amyloidoses — this typing changes treatment fundamentally.

Diagnosis and treatment

Diagnosis requires three elements: (1) presence of a monoclonal protein (serum or urine M-protein, abnormal serum FLC ratio, or bone marrow clonal plasma cells); (2) demonstration of amyloid in a biopsied tissue with apple-green birefringence on Congo red; and (3) typing of the amyloid as light chain (AL) using mass spectrometry, immunoelectron microscopy, or immunohistochemistry — typing is critical because ATTR amyloidosis (transthyretin) is increasingly recognised, especially in older patients with cardiac amyloid, and is treated with stabilisers (tafamidis) and silencers (patisiran, inotersen, vutrisiran), not myeloma-directed therapy. The Mayo cardiac staging system uses NT-proBNP and troponin T (or hs-troponin T) thresholds with the difference between involved and uninvolved free light chains (dFLC) added in updated versions, to stratify mortality risk.

Treatment is directed at the underlying clone. Daratumumab plus cyclophosphamide-bortezomib-dexamethasone (Dara-CyBorD) is now the first-line standard for newly diagnosed AL amyloidosis on the basis of the ANDROMEDA trial, which showed substantially deeper haematological responses with daratumumab addition. The aim is rapid haematological response — measured by reduction in dFLC and disappearance of the M-protein on IFE — to halt ongoing amyloid deposition and allow organ recovery. Risk-adapted autologous stem cell transplantation can be considered in carefully selected patients with limited cardiac involvement. Supportive care is critical: management of heart failure, careful diuresis, attention to factor X deficiency before procedures, and avoidance of high-dose corticosteroids in advanced cardiac disease.

15.8 POEMS Syndrome

POEMS syndrome is a rare paraneoplastic disorder driven by an underlying clonal plasma cell neoplasm, typically with a lambda-restricted M-protein. The acronym captures the cardinal features: Polyneuropathy, Organomegaly, Endocrinopathy, Monoclonal protein, and Skin changes. The pathogenic driver is profoundly elevated VEGF, which produces the multisystem clinical picture and is also a useful disease activity marker. The associated clonal plasma cell expansion is typically small (often a discrete osteosclerotic plasmacytoma rather than diffuse marrow involvement), and lambda light chains are nearly universal — kappa POEMS is exceedingly rare and should prompt diagnostic reconsideration.

Diagnostic criteria require both mandatory criteria (peripheral neuropathy, typically demyelinating; clonal plasma cell disorder, typically lambda) plus at least one major criterion (osteosclerotic bone lesion; Castleman disease; elevated VEGF) and at least one minor criterion (organomegaly; extravascular volume overload — oedema, pleural effusion, ascites; endocrinopathy other than diabetes mellitus and hypothyroidism in isolation; skin changes — hyperpigmentation, hypertrichosis, plethora, haemangiomata, glomeruloid angiomata; papilledema; thrombocytosis or polycythaemia).

Treatment depends on whether disease is localised or disseminated. For localised disease (a single osteosclerotic lesion without disseminated disease elsewhere), definitive radiation therapy to the plasmacytoma is highly effective and frequently produces dramatic reversal of neuropathy and other systemic features. For disseminated disease, treatment combines plasma-cell-directed therapy (lenalidomide- or bortezomib-based regimens, often with autologous stem cell transplantation in fit patients) with VEGF-targeted approaches when needed. Bevacizumab (anti-VEGF) has been used historically but with mixed results; the standard now is plasma-cell-directed therapy. Castleman disease coexists in approximately 10–

15% of POEMS cases (some series report up to 30%); its management requires concurrent attention.

HIGH-YIELD PEARL — POEMS lambda restriction and the osteosclerotic clue

POEMS is one of the few clinical scenarios in haematology where a specific light chain restriction (lambda) is nearly diagnostic. A patient with progressive demyelinating peripheral neuropathy, a lambda-restricted small M-protein, and an osteosclerotic bone lesion on plain X-ray or CT has POEMS until proven otherwise. The osteosclerotic plasmacytoma is the structural counterpart of the disease — biopsy shows lambda-restricted clonal plasma cells embedded in dense sclerotic bone, the inverse of the lytic plasmacytoma of myeloma. The exam-significant point is the clue chain: progressive neuropathy + lambda M-protein → request bone imaging looking specifically for osteosclerotic lesions; an isolated osteosclerotic lesion in this context is treated with radiotherapy alone and often produces remarkable clinical recovery.

15.9 Heavy Chain Diseases

Heavy chain diseases are rare lymphoproliferative disorders in which the neoplastic B cells secrete an incomplete immunoglobulin — only the heavy chain, lacking light chain — that does not produce a normal sharp M-spike on SPEP and may be missed by routine workup. Three principal forms are recognised, each with characteristic clinical phenotypes.

Alpha heavy chain disease (Seligmann disease, immunoproliferative small intestinal disease, IPSID) is the most common form globally and is endemic in the Mediterranean, Middle East, and parts of South Asia and Africa. It is associated with chronic Campylobacter jejuni infection and presents as a malabsorption syndrome with diarrhoea, abdominal pain, and weight loss. The duodenum and jejunum show diffuse mucosal infiltration by neoplastic B cells (with plasmacytoid features) producing alpha heavy chain. Early-stage disease responds to antibiotic eradication (tetracyclines or metronidazole) — paralleling the H. pylori-driven gastric MALT model. Advanced disease requires chemotherapy.

Mu heavy chain disease is exceedingly rare, often arising on a background of CLL or related chronic B-cell lymphoproliferative disorder, and manifests with hepatosplenomegaly, vacuolated lymphocytes (or plasmacytoid cells) in the marrow, and a failure to detect any sharp serum M-band despite immunofixation evidence of mu heavy chain. Gamma heavy chain disease (Franklin disease) is also rare; it presents with lymphadenopathy, hepatosplenomegaly, anaemia, and fever and may show a wide M-band on SPEP from the polymerising heavy chain fragments. Treatment of mu and gamma forms is patterned on the underlying lymphoproliferative disorder.

15.10 Translocations and Diagnostic Markers — One-Glance Reference

The cytogenetic and molecular landscape of plasma cell neoplasms is small enough to be memorised on a single page. Hyperdiploid myeloma (~50% of cases; trisomies of odd chromosomes) is standard-risk and dominates the favourable end. The IGH translocations partition the non-hyperdiploid group, with t(11;14) and the rare t(6;14) being standard-risk and t(4;14), t(14;16), t(14;20) being high-risk. Secondary genetic events — del(17p)/TP53, 1q gain, MYC translocations — appear at progression and define adverse risk irrespective of the primary translocation. Outside myeloma, the MYD88 L265P mutation defines Waldenström macroglobulinaemia and IgM MGUS but is absent in IgM myeloma — a critical discriminator. AL amyloidosis is biased to lambda; POEMS is nearly exclusively lambda; light-chain-only myeloma can be either.

Entity	Cytogenetic / molecular hallmark	Diagnostic significance
Hyperdiploid myeloma	Trisomies of odd chromosomes (3, 5, 7, 9, 11, 15, 19, 21)	~50% of MM; standard-risk; favourable outcomes
t(11;14) MM	CCND1::IGH; cyclin D1 overexpression	~15%; standard-risk; venetoclax (BCL2 inhibitor) particularly active
t(4;14) MM	FGFR3 and MMSET (NSD2) dysregulation	~15%; HIGH-RISK; bortezomib partially overcomes — VRd or Dara-VRd induction
t(14;16) MM	MAF::IGH	~5%; VERY POOR; high-LDH, plasmablastic morphology often
t(14;20) MM	MAFB::IGH	~1%; VERY POOR
del(17p13.1)	TP53 deletion	HIGH-RISK; ~10% at diagnosis, rises at relapse; adverse across schemas
1q gain (≥3 copies)	CKS1B amplification	Adverse; included in R2-ISS
Waldenström / LPL	MYD88 L265P (>90%)	Defining mutation; CXCR4 mutations confer reduced ibrutinib response
IgM myeloma	MYD88 usually NEGATIVE	Discriminates from Waldenström; CD138+ plasma cells, lytic bone disease
POEMS	Lambda light chain restriction; high VEGF	Osteosclerotic plasmacytoma + neuropathy; lambda nearly always

Entity	Cytogenetic / molecular hallmark	Diagnostic significance
AL amyloidosis	Lambda over-represented (~2:1 lambda:kappa)	Apple-green birefringence on Congo red; mass spectrometry typing
Cyclin D1+ plasma cell neoplasm	t(11;14)	IHC mimics mantle cell lymphoma but cells are CD138+/CD20− and have plasma cell morphology

Table 15.4: Cytogenetic, molecular, and immunophenotypic markers of plasma cell neoplasms — exam-fast reference.

15.11 Buzzwords and Associations — Vignette Trigger Table

The following table catalogues the most reliable single-line vignette triggers in plasma cell neoplasms. The entity to suspect is in the middle column; the discriminating clue is in the right column. Use this for rapid scanning during exam preparation; the full diagnostic logic is in the body of the chapter.

Vignette buzzword / finding	Diagnosis to trigger	One-line "why"
Older patient, back pain, anaemia, hypercalcaemia, renal failure, M-spike	Multiple myeloma	Classic CRAB tetrad on a plasma cell clone
Punched-out lytic lesions on skull X-ray	Multiple myeloma	RANKL-driven osteoclast activation; bone B of CRAB
Rouleaux on peripheral smear	Monoclonal gammopathy (MM, WM, MGUS, AL)	Paraprotein coats erythrocytes → stacking
Incidental M-spike <30 g/L, no symptoms, marrow PCs <10%, no CRAB	MGUS	1% per year progression; observe with risk stratification
Asymptomatic patient with serum FLC ratio of 200 + 1 MRI focal lesion	Multiple myeloma (SLiM-defined)	SLiM converts apparently SMM into MM requiring treatment
Macroglossia with tooth indentations, periorbital purpura, restrictive cardiomyopathy	AL amyloidosis	Lambda light chain misfolding deposits as amyloid in tissues
Nephrotic-range proteinuria (predominantly albumin) + small M-protein	AL amyloid renal involvement	Glomerular amyloid leaks albumin (vs cast nephropathy: leaks light chains)
Tubular casts on renal biopsy with light-chain immunofluorescence	Myeloma cast nephropathy	Light chains + Tamm-Horsfall in distal tubules → obstruction
Progressive demyelinating neuropathy + lambda M-protein + osteosclerotic bone lesion	POEMS syndrome	High VEGF; nearly always lambda; osteosclerotic plasmacytoma
Circulating plasma cells ≥5% of WBC	Plasma cell leukaemia	IMWG 2021 / WHO 2022 threshold; very poor prognosis
Single lytic bone lesion with biopsy clonal PCs but marrow	Solitary plasmacytoma of bone	Definitive radiotherapy; lifelong surveillance for MM

Vignette buzzword / finding	Diagnosis to trigger	One-line "why"
PCs <10% and no CRAB		progression
Nasopharyngeal mass biopsy showing clonal plasma cells in patient without systemic MM	Solitary extramedullary plasmacytoma	Upper aerodigestive tract is the typical site
IgM M-protein with hyperviscosity + CD20+ small B-cell infiltrate in marrow	Waldenström (Ch 14)	LPL with IgM; MYD88 L265P >90% — NOT IgM myeloma
IgM M-protein with sheets of CD138+ plasma cells and lytic bones	IgM myeloma (rare)	Plasma cell neoplasm with IgM; usually MYD88-negative
Mediterranean / South Asian patient with chronic diarrhoea, malabsorption, alpha heavy chain band	Alpha heavy chain disease (IPSID)	Campylobacter jejuni driven; antibiotics in early disease
Punched-out lesions + flame cells on marrow smear (red-stained PCs)	IgA myeloma	Glycoprotein content of IgA stains the cytoplasm red
Russell bodies / Mott cells on aspirate	Plasma cell neoplasm	Cytoplasmic immunoglobulin inclusions
Marrow PCs 60% with no CRAB and no other myeloma-defining event	Multiple myeloma (SLiM-defined)	S of SLiM: 60% PCs alone defines MM
Sausage-shaped retinal veins on fundoscopy	Hyperviscosity (Waldenström, rarely IgA myeloma)	IgM pentamer; plasmapheresis emergency
Apple-green birefringence on Congo red staining of fat / heart / kidney biopsy	Amyloidosis (AL, ATTR, AA — type by mass spec)	Birefringence is shared; typing distinguishes treatment

Table 15.5: Plasma cell neoplasm vignette triggers — exam-fast clue-to-diagnosis mapping.

15.12 USMLE Vignettes

The following ten vignettes test the highest-yield discriminations in plasma cell neoplasms. Each is built around a common exam pattern: identify the entity, choose the next diagnostic move, or select the correct first-line therapy. The distractors are designed to expose specific cognitive traps in the diagnostic logic.

Vignette 1. A 68-year-old man with the CRAB tetrad

A 68-year-old man presents to his GP with three months of progressive lower back pain unresponsive to analgesics, fatigue, and constipation. Examination shows pallor and a diffusely tender thoracolumbar spine without focal neurological deficit. Laboratory studies: haemoglobin 8.4 g/dL (normocytic, normochromic), platelets 180,000/µL, WBC 6,200/µL with normal differential, corrected calcium 12.1 mg/dL (3.02 mmol/L), creatinine 2.6 mg/dL (rising from baseline 1.0), albumin 2.9 g/dL, total protein 9.4 g/dL, beta-2 microglobulin 6.8 mg/L. SPEP shows a 4.2 g/dL M-spike in the gamma region; immunofixation confirms IgG kappa. Serum FLC: kappa 480 mg/L, lambda 12 mg/L, ratio 40. Urine protein electrophoresis shows Bence-Jones (light chain) protein. Skeletal imaging: whole-body low-dose CT shows multiple punched-out lytic lesions in the skull, spine, pelvis, and proximal femora, with a vertebral compression fracture at T12. Bone marrow: 65% clonal kappa-restricted plasma cells with cartwheel chromatin and perinuclear hof. FISH on CD138-selected plasma cells: t(4;14) positive; del(17p) negative. Which of the following is the most appropriate diagnosis and initial management?

(A) Multiple myeloma, R-ISS Stage III; initiate Dara-VRd induction with bortezomib-based supportive care, bisphosphonate, antiviral prophylaxis, and plan for autologous stem cell transplantation.

(B) Smouldering multiple myeloma; observation with three-monthly review.

(C) MGUS; reassurance and routine annual follow-up.

(D) Solitary plasmacytoma of bone; definitive radiotherapy alone.

(E) Metastatic prostate carcinoma; PSA testing and bone biopsy for confirmation.

Best answer: (A) Multiple myeloma, R-ISS Stage III; initiate Dara-VRd induction with bortezomib-based supportive care, bisphosphonate, antiviral prophylaxis, and plan for autologous stem cell transplantation.

Rationale. The diagnosis meets every IMWG 2014 SLiM-CRAB criterion: clonal marrow plasma cells ≥10% (65%), and multiple CRAB events — hypercalcaemia (12.1 mg/dL), Renal insufficiency (creatinine 2.6 mg/dL), Anaemia (Hb 8.4 g/dL), and Bone lesions (multiple lytic). R-ISS staging: ISS Stage III (B2M 6.8 mg/L) plus high-risk cytogenetics t(4;14) places the patient at R-ISS Stage III with a median OS of approximately 29 months — but bortezomib-based induction substantially overcomes the t(4;14) adverse effect. Dara-VRd (daratumumab + bortezomib + lenalidomide + dexamethasone) is the modern standard induction for transplant-eligible newly diagnosed myeloma. The bortezomib base is particularly important in t(4;14) disease. Supportive care includes monthly zoledronic acid for bone disease, acyclovir prophylaxis (bortezomib and daratumumab both increase varicella-zoster reactivation risk), pneumococcal and influenza vaccination, aggressive hydration with avoidance of NSAIDs and contrast for renal protection, and plasmapheresis if hyperviscosity becomes symptomatic. Following induction, ASCT consolidation and lenalidomide maintenance are standard.

Distractor analysis. (B) SMM requires absence of CRAB and SLiM events — this patient has all four CRAB events. (C) MGUS requires marrow PCs <10% and absent CRAB; both are violated. (D) Solitary plasmacytoma requires only a single lesion with otherwise negative workup — multiple lesions and 65% marrow PCs exclude this. (E) Punched-out lytic lesions are a myeloma pattern; metastatic prostate carcinoma classically produces sclerotic, not lytic, bone lesions.

Vignette 2. A 62-year-old woman with an incidental M-spike

A 62-year-old asymptomatic woman is found to have a total serum protein of 9.0 g/dL on a routine check-up requested for life insurance underwriting. She is well, takes only a vitamin supplement, and has no fatigue, bone pain, recurrent infections, or weight change. Examination is unremarkable. CBC: haemoglobin 13.2 g/dL, platelets 240,000/µL, WBC 5,800/µL with normal differential. Calcium, creatinine, and albumin are normal. SPEP shows a 1.2 g/dL M-spike; IFE confirms IgG kappa. Serum FLC: kappa 22 mg/L, lambda 18 mg/L, ratio 1.22 (normal range 0.26–1.65). Whole-body low-dose CT shows no lytic lesions. Bone marrow biopsy shows 4% clonal kappa-restricted plasma cells with normal trephine architecture. Which of the following is the most appropriate diagnosis and management?

(A) Multiple myeloma; initiate Dara-VRd induction.

(B) Smouldering myeloma; consider lenalidomide-based early therapy.

(C) MGUS, low-risk by Mayo criteria; reassurance and follow-up SPEP plus FLC every 2–3 years.

(D) Solitary plasmacytoma; refer for radiation oncology evaluation.

(E) AL amyloidosis; abdominal fat aspirate for Congo red staining.

Best answer: (C) MGUS, low-risk by Mayo criteria; reassurance and follow-up SPEP plus FLC every 2–3 years.

Rationale. The diagnosis meets every MGUS criterion: M-protein <30 g/L (12 g/L), clonal marrow plasma cells <10% (4%), no CRAB or SLiM event. The Mayo Clinic risk-stratification model uses three variables — abnormal serum FLC ratio (outside 0.26–1.65), non-IgG isotype (IgA or IgD), and M-protein concentration ≥15 g/L. This patient has none of the three — IgG isotype, M-protein 12 g/L, normal FLC ratio — placing her in the low-risk group with approximately 5% cumulative progression risk over 20 years. Surveillance with SPEP and FLC every 2–3 years is appropriate; bone marrow biopsy and imaging do not need routine repetition unless serological monitoring shows rising M-protein, an evolving FLC ratio, or new clinical features. The diagnosis "MGUS" must not be used to dismiss real disease driven by the M-protein (see MGCS pearl in §15.2), so any unexplained renal, neurological, or other end-organ involvement should prompt directed evaluation rather than reassurance.

Distractor analysis. (A) Myeloma requires marrow PCs ≥10% or CRAB/SLiM events — both absent. (B) SMM requires M-protein ≥30 g/L OR marrow PCs 10–59%; neither met. (D) Solitary plasmacytoma requires a biopsy-proven clonal plasma cell tumour at a discrete site — no lesion present. (E) AL amyloidosis would require demonstrated tissue amyloid; no clinical or laboratory clue here.

Vignette 3. A 64-year-old man whose "smouldering myeloma" has crossed the SLiM threshold

A 64-year-old man was diagnosed with smouldering myeloma 14 months ago — IgG lambda M-protein 36 g/L, marrow plasma cells 22%, no CRAB events. He has been observed with three-monthly review. He remains asymptomatic, working full-time, with no bone pain, fatigue, or infections. Repeat workup at 14 months: haemoglobin 13.4 g/dL, platelets 230,000/µL, calcium 9.6 mg/dL, creatinine 1.0 mg/dL. SPEP M-protein 38 g/L; serum FLC: lambda 1,400 mg/L, kappa 6 mg/L, ratio 0.004 (involved/uninvolved lambda:kappa ratio is 233 — well above 100, with absolute involved lambda well above 100 mg/L). Whole-body MRI: two new focal lesions, both >5 mm, in the L2 vertebral body and right ilium. Bone marrow plasma cells now 32%. No lytic lesions on CT. Which of the following is the most appropriate management?

(A) Continue observation with three-monthly review; SLiM criteria require CRAB end-organ damage to trigger treatment.

(B) Reclassify as multiple myeloma based on SLiM biomarkers and initiate Dara-VRd induction with consideration of ASCT.

(C) Add lenalidomide monotherapy as treatment for high-risk smouldering myeloma; defer myeloma-grade therapy until CRAB develops.

(D) Repeat the imaging in 6 months because the lesions are not yet lytic on CT.

(E) Refer for radiation therapy of the L2 lesion as a solitary plasmacytoma.

Best answer: (B) Reclassify as multiple myeloma based on SLiM biomarkers and initiate Dara-VRd induction with consideration of ASCT.

Rationale. This case is the textbook SLiM-converted myeloma. The patient meets two SLiM biomarkers simultaneously — Light chain ratio of 233 (well above the SLiM threshold of 100) with absolute involved lambda free light chain well above 100 mg/L; and MRI showing more than one focal bone lesion ≥5 mm — either of which alone reclassifies SMM as active myeloma requiring immediate treatment. The 2014 IMWG SLiM update was created precisely because patients who cross these biochemical or radiological thresholds have approximately 80% two-year progression risk to classical CRAB-defined myeloma; treating them earlier prevents irreversible end-organ damage. The fact that CT does not yet show lytic lesions is not relevant — MRI sensitivity for marrow infiltration precedes CT-detectable lytic destruction by months to years, and the SLiM criterion specifically incorporates MRI to allow this earlier diagnosis. Initial therapy should be Dara-VRd induction with planned ASCT in the transplant-eligible patient.

Distractor analysis. (A) The SLiM update specifically eliminated the requirement for CRAB end-organ damage when biomarkers cross threshold; this is the central conceptual update of IMWG 2014. (C) High-risk SMM trials used lenalidomide-based therapy in patients without SLiM biomarkers; once SLiM is met, full myeloma-directed triplet/quadruplet therapy is standard. (D) Waiting for "CT-visible lytic disease" defeats the purpose of MRI-based SLiM. (E) The patient has multifocal disease, marrow plasma cells of 32%, and SLiM biomarkers — not solitary plasmacytoma.

Vignette 4. A 58-year-old woman with macroglossia and restrictive cardiomyopathy

A 58-year-old woman presents with six months of progressive exertional dyspnoea, leg oedema, and an enlarging tongue with dental indentations along the lateral margins. She has noted easy bruising around the eyes after sneezing or yawning. Examination: BP 96/62 mmHg, HR 92, JVP elevated, soft heart sounds, hepatomegaly, bilateral pitting oedema, periorbital ecchymoses, and macroglossia. Laboratory studies: haemoglobin 11.0

g/dL, platelets 188,000/µL, calcium 9.4 mg/dL, creatinine 1.4 mg/dL, albumin 2.6 g/dL, urinary protein 8.4 g/24h (predominantly albumin on urine immunofixation), troponin T 0.18 ng/mL, NT-proBNP 9,400 pg/mL. ECG: low-voltage QRS in limb leads. Echocardiography: bi-atrial enlargement, increased LV wall thickness with granular sparkling appearance, restrictive filling pattern, normal ejection fraction. SPEP: small 0.6 g/dL M-spike; IFE: IgG lambda M-protein. Serum FLC: lambda 380 mg/L, kappa 9 mg/L, ratio 0.024. Bone marrow plasma cells 7% (lambda-restricted). Whole-body imaging shows no lytic lesions. Which of the following is the most appropriate next diagnostic step and treatment?

(A) Abdominal subcutaneous fat aspirate with Congo red staining (apple-green birefringence under polarised light) and mass spectrometry typing of the amyloid; if AL confirmed, initiate daratumumab + cyclophosphamide-bortezomib-dexamethasone (Dara-CyBorD).

(B) Diagnose multiple myeloma based on the M-protein and lambda restriction; initiate Dara-VRd induction.

(C) Diagnose transthyretin (ATTR) cardiac amyloidosis; initiate tafamidis without further typing.

(D) Begin diuresis with furosemide and high-dose corticosteroids for presumed nephrotic syndrome of unclear cause; defer further investigation.

(E) Diagnose MGUS and arrange routine SPEP/FLC follow-up in 2 years.

Best answer: (A) Abdominal subcutaneous fat aspirate with Congo red staining (apple-green birefringence under polarised light) and mass spectrometry typing of the amyloid; if AL confirmed, initiate daratumumab + cyclophosphamide-bortezomib-dexamethasone (Dara-CyBorD).

Rationale. The clinical picture is classical multisystem AL amyloidosis. The four cardinal clues are all present: macroglossia with dental indentations (pathognomonic when present, ~10–20% of AL); periorbital purpura ("raccoon eyes"); restrictive cardiomyopathy with low-voltage QRS, increased wall thickness, granular sparkling appearance, and disproportionately elevated NT-proBNP and troponin — the classic ECG-echo discordance of cardiac amyloid; and nephrotic-range proteinuria with predominantly albumin (~albumin-dominant proteinuria distinguishes AL renal involvement from cast nephropathy, where light chains dominate). The lambda-restricted small clone (FLC ratio 0.024 with absolute involved lambda 380 mg/L; marrow plasma cells 7%) is the typical underlying biology. The diagnostic move is tissue confirmation. Abdominal subcutaneous fat aspirate with Congo red is the least invasive screening biopsy (~80% sensitive); affected organ biopsy can confirm if the fat aspirate is negative. Mass spectrometry typing distinguishes AL from ATTR (transthyretin) and from AA (serum amyloid A) — typing is critical because treatment differs fundamentally. Once AL is confirmed, Dara-CyBorD has emerged as the new first-line standard on the basis of the ANDROMEDA trial. ASCT in carefully selected patients with limited cardiac involvement can be considered after induction.

Distractor analysis. (B) Marrow plasma cells <10% and the disease pattern (cardiac/renal infiltrative) point to amyloid, not myeloma. (C) ATTR is possible — especially in older men with cardiac amyloid — but the lambda restriction, periorbital purpura, macroglossia, and large nephrotic range proteinuria all argue against ATTR; mass spectrometry typing is mandatory before treating empirically. (D) High-dose corticosteroids in advanced cardiac amyloidosis can precipitate decompensation; investigation must precede empirical therapy. (E) MGUS does not produce multisystem organ damage attributable to the M-protein; this is monoclonal gammopathy of clinical significance / AL amyloidosis.

Vignette 5. A 56-year-old man with high-risk myeloma and a transplantation question

A 56-year-old previously well man presents with rib pain, anaemia (Hb 9.2 g/dL), normal calcium, and creatinine 1.3 mg/dL. SPEP shows a 5.6 g/dL IgA lambda M-spike. Marrow plasma cells 50%, lambda-restricted. Whole-body imaging shows multiple lytic lesions in ribs, sternum, and pelvis. FISH on CD138-selected plasma cells: t(4;14) positive, 1q gain (3 copies) positive, del(17p) negative. Beta-2 microglobulin 5.8 mg/L, albumin 3.0 g/dL, LDH normal. He has no significant comorbidity, ECOG performance status 1. Which of the following is the most appropriate first-line treatment plan?

(A) Dara-VRd induction × 4–6 cycles, then autologous stem cell transplantation, then lenalidomide maintenance (with bortezomib-containing maintenance considered for high-risk disease).

(B) Lenalidomide-dexamethasone alone, deferring transplant indefinitely.

(C) Allogeneic stem cell transplantation in first remission as standard of care for any high-risk myeloma.

(D) Single-agent BCMA CAR-T therapy as first-line.

(E) High-dose dexamethasone alone with reassessment in 3 months.

Best answer: (A) Dara-VRd induction × 4–6 cycles, then autologous stem cell transplantation, then lenalidomide maintenance (with bortezomib-containing maintenance considered for high-risk disease).

Rationale. The diagnosis is multiple myeloma with two adverse cytogenetic features: t(4;14) (FGFR3-MMSET dysregulation; high-risk) and 1q gain. ISS Stage III is met by B2M ≥5.5 mg/L (here 5.8 mg/L); combined with high-risk cytogenetics, this places the patient at R-ISS Stage III (and Stage IV by R2-ISS). The exam-relevant point about t(4;14) is that bortezomib partially overcomes its adverse effect — this is the original rationale for incorporating bortezomib into all newly diagnosed myeloma induction. Modern induction is Dara-VRd (daratumumab + bortezomib + lenalidomide + dexamethasone), which the GRIFFIN, PERSEUS, and IsKia trials have established as superior to VRd alone. ASCT remains the standard of consolidation for transplant-eligible patients <70 years with adequate organ function. Tandem ASCT can be considered in high-risk disease. Maintenance lenalidomide improves progression-free and overall survival post-ASCT and is continued indefinitely; bortezomib-containing maintenance is often added for high-risk patients including those with t(4;14).

Distractor analysis. (B) Lenalidomide-dexamethasone alone is suboptimal in fit transplant-eligible patients with high-risk disease. (C) Allogeneic transplantation is not standard first-line and carries substantial transplant-related mortality; reserved for highly selected younger patients with very high-risk disease or relapse. (D) BCMA CAR-T is approved for relapsed/refractory disease, not first-line. (E) Steroid monotherapy is inadequate.

Vignette 6. A 51-year-old man with circulating plasma cells

A 51-year-old man presents with two weeks of severe fatigue, fever, and a six-pound weight loss. Examination: pallor, hepatosplenomegaly, and several palpable cervical and inguinal lymph nodes. Laboratory studies: haemoglobin 7.4 g/dL, platelets 78,000/µL, white blood cells 28,000/µL with 24% atypical mononuclear cells with eccentric nuclei, perinuclear pallor, and basophilic cytoplasm — recognisably plasma-cell morphology on the peripheral smear. Calcium 12.4 mg/dL, creatinine 3.2 mg/dL, LDH 1,820 U/L. SPEP: 6.8 g/dL IgG lambda M-spike. Marrow: 80% clonal lambda-restricted plasma cells with anaplastic features, multinucleate forms, and high mitotic activity. FISH: del(17p) and t(14;16) both positive. Whole-body imaging: extensive lytic disease and bilateral pleural effusions with cytology showing clonal plasma cells. Which of the following is the most likely diagnosis?

(A) Plasma cell leukaemia, primary (de novo) — circulating plasma cells ≥5% of WBC by IMWG 2021 / WHO 2022.

(B) Multiple myeloma without leukaemic involvement.

(C) Acute leukaemia with plasmacytoid differentiation.

(D) Reactive plasmacytosis from infection.

(E) Burkitt lymphoma.

Best answer: (A) Plasma cell leukaemia, primary (de novo) — circulating plasma cells ≥5% of WBC by IMWG 2021 / WHO 2022.

Rationale. The diagnosis is primary plasma cell leukaemia. Circulating plasma cells of 24% of total WBC vastly exceeds the IMWG 2021 / WHO 2022 threshold of ≥5% (the older >20% or >2 × 10^9/L threshold has been formally abandoned because the lower threshold identifies an outcome-equivalent group earlier and improves recognition). The cytogenetic profile is enriched for high-risk markers — del(17p) plus t(14;16) is exactly the pattern that drives the very poor prognosis of PCL. Treatment is patterned on high-risk myeloma using early integration of the most active triplet or quadruplet regimens (Dara-VRd, Dara-KRd) followed by autologous stem cell transplantation, ideally tandem ASCT or ASCT followed by allogeneic transplant in fit younger patients. CAR-T therapy and BCMA bispecifics are increasingly used. Prognosis remains the worst of the plasma cell neoplasms despite modern therapy.

Distractor analysis. (B) Conventional MM does not meet the ≥5% peripheral plasma cell threshold. (C) Acute leukaemias have blasts (not plasma cells) and are CD138-negative. (D) Reactive plasmacytosis is polyclonal — kappa-and-lambda IHC would show no light chain restriction; this clone is lambda-restricted. (E) Burkitt has CD20+/CD10+/Ki-67 100% B-cell phenotype, not CD138+ plasma cell phenotype.

Vignette 7. A 49-year-old man with a single bone lesion

A 49-year-old man presents with three months of progressive right-sided lower back pain. Examination is unremarkable. Plain X-ray shows a 4 cm lytic lesion in the right sacrum. CT confirms a single lytic lesion with cortical breakthrough. CT-guided biopsy of the lesion shows sheets of clonal kappa-restricted plasma cells. Workup: haemoglobin 14.2 g/dL, platelets 240,000/µL, calcium 9.5 mg/dL, creatinine 0.9 mg/dL, albumin 4.1 g/dL. SPEP: small 0.4 g/dL IgG kappa M-spike. Serum FLC: kappa 24 mg/L, lambda 18 mg/L, ratio 1.33 (normal). Bone marrow biopsy from the iliac crest: 3% kappa-restricted plasma cells; otherwise normal. Whole-body MRI: only the sacral lesion; no other bone or extramedullary disease. Which of the following is the most appropriate management?

(A) Definitive radiotherapy 40–50 Gy to the sacral lesion plus a margin, followed by lifelong serial SPEP, FLC, and imaging surveillance for progression to multiple myeloma.

(B) Initiate Dara-VRd as for newly diagnosed multiple myeloma.

(C) Surgical en-bloc resection of the sacrum.

(D) Observation alone — the lesion is asymptomatic-equivalent at presentation.

(E) Allogeneic stem cell transplantation.

Best answer: (A) Definitive radiotherapy 40–50 Gy to the sacral lesion plus a margin, followed by lifelong serial SPEP, FLC, and imaging surveillance for progression to multiple myeloma.

Rationale. The diagnosis is solitary plasmacytoma of bone. All criteria are met: a single biopsy-proven clonal plasma cell tumour, marrow clonal plasma cells <10% (3%), no CRAB or SLiM events, and whole-body imaging excluding additional disease. Solitary plasmacytoma is treated with definitive radiotherapy at 40–50 Gy delivered to the lesion plus a margin; local control rates approach 90%. The risk of progression to multiple myeloma is, however, substantial — approximately 50–70% at 10 years for SPB — so lifelong surveillance with serial SPEP, FLC assay, and periodic imaging is essential. The small accompanying serum M-spike (0.4 g/dL) and 3% marrow plasma cells are within the bounds of solitary plasmacytoma — some experts label this "solitary plasmacytoma with minimal marrow involvement" when 1–9% PCs are present, an intermediate risk group with somewhat higher progression rates.

Distractor analysis. (B) Initiating myeloma-grade systemic therapy without meeting myeloma criteria over-treats the patient. (C) Sacral resection is morbid and unnecessary; radiotherapy provides equivalent or better local control. (D) Untreated solitary plasmacytoma will progress to symptomatic disease and seed multiple myeloma; observation is not standard. (E) Allogeneic transplantation is not indicated for solitary plasmacytoma.

Vignette 8. A 47-year-old man with progressive neuropathy and a sclerotic bone lesion

A 47-year-old man presents with eighteen months of progressive distal weakness and numbness affecting both legs and now both hands, with difficulty climbing stairs and frequent falls. He has noted darkening of the skin on his legs and increased body hair. Over the past six months he has developed bilateral lower-extremity oedema and increased abdominal girth. Examination: distal symmetric sensorimotor weakness with absent deep tendon reflexes, hyperpigmented skin with hypertrichosis on the legs, hepatosplenomegaly, ascites, gynaecomastia. CBC: haemoglobin 14.6 g/dL, platelets 580,000/µL (thrombocytosis), WBC 7,400/µL. Calcium and creatinine normal. Nerve conduction study: severe demyelinating sensorimotor polyneuropathy. SPEP: small 0.5 g/dL IgA lambda M-spike. Serum VEGF markedly elevated. CT shows hepatosplenomegaly, ascites, and a single 3 cm sclerotic lesion in the right ilium with surrounding ossification. Iliac biopsy: clonal lambda-restricted plasma cells embedded in dense sclerotic bone. Bone marrow plasma cells 4% (lambda-restricted). Which of the following is the most likely diagnosis and most appropriate first-line therapy?

(A) POEMS syndrome with a localised osteosclerotic plasmacytoma; definitive radiotherapy to the iliac lesion is highly effective and frequently produces dramatic reversal of the neuropathy and systemic features.

(B) Multiple myeloma with peripheral neuropathy as a paraneoplastic phenomenon;

initiate Dara-VRd induction.

(C) Chronic inflammatory demyelinating polyneuropathy (CIDP) unrelated to the M-protein; intravenous immunoglobulin therapy.

(D) Amyloid neuropathy; initiate Dara-CyBorD with cardiac and renal screening.

(E) Waldenström macroglobulinaemia with anti-MAG neuropathy; initiate ibrutinib.

Best answer: (A) POEMS syndrome with a localised osteosclerotic plasmacytoma; definitive radiotherapy to the iliac lesion is highly effective and frequently produces dramatic reversal of the neuropathy and systemic features.

Rationale. The clinical picture is classical POEMS syndrome — Polyneuropathy (severe demyelinating), Organomegaly (hepatosplenomegaly), Endocrinopathy (gynaecomastia from disordered sex steroids), M-protein (small lambda-restricted IgA M-spike), Skin changes (hyperpigmentation, hypertrichosis). Both mandatory criteria are met (peripheral demyelinating neuropathy plus a clonal plasma cell disorder), and major criteria are present (osteosclerotic bone lesion, elevated VEGF), with multiple minor criteria as well (organomegaly, extravascular volume overload, endocrinopathy, skin changes, thrombocytosis). The lambda restriction is nearly universal in POEMS — kappa POEMS is exceedingly rare and should prompt diagnostic reconsideration. The osteosclerotic plasmacytoma — in contrast to the lytic plasmacytoma of myeloma — is the structural counterpart of POEMS. For a single localised osteosclerotic lesion, definitive radiation therapy is the first-line treatment and frequently produces remarkable clinical recovery, including substantial improvement in neuropathy. Disseminated disease requires plasma-cell-directed therapy — lenalidomide- or bortezomib-based regimens with autologous stem cell transplantation in fit patients.

Distractor analysis. (B) Myeloma typically produces lytic, not osteosclerotic, lesions and lacks the systemic POEMS features. Treating with Dara-VRd is reasonable for disseminated POEMS but radiotherapy is preferred for a localised lesion. (C) CIDP is a diagnosis of exclusion when no underlying paraprotein-driven disorder is identifiable; in this patient the lambda M-protein, osteosclerotic lesion, organomegaly, skin changes, and high VEGF point firmly to POEMS. (D) AL amyloid neuropathy typically affects autonomic and small fibres rather than producing severe demyelinating motor neuropathy, and the patient has no cardiac or renal amyloid features. (E) Anti-MAG neuropathy is associated with IgM kappa, not IgA lambda, and lacks the systemic POEMS features.

Vignette 9. A 71-year-old woman with renal failure and a paraprotein — which renal lesion?

A 71-year-old woman with newly diagnosed multiple myeloma (IgG kappa M-protein 5.2 g/dL; marrow plasma cells 35%; multiple lytic lesions; hypercalcaemia and creatinine elevated to 3.4 mg/dL at presentation) is admitted for evaluation of renal failure that has not improved despite hydration and correction of hypercalcaemia. Urine protein quantitation: 4.2 g/24h. Urine immunofixation: predominantly free kappa light chain; minimal albumin. Renal biopsy is performed. Light microscopy: distal tubules contain dense, fractured, eosinophilic casts surrounded by giant-cell reaction; glomeruli appear normal; no Congo red apple-green birefringence. Immunofluorescence: kappa light chain restriction in tubular casts; no glomerular deposits. Which of the following is the most likely diagnosis and the most important therapeutic move?

(A) Myeloma cast nephropathy; rapid reduction of light chain burden through bortezomib-based induction is the most important renal-protective move; supportive care includes aggressive hydration and avoidance of NSAIDs, contrast, and aminoglycosides.

(B) AL amyloid renal involvement; initiate Dara-CyBorD.

(C) Light chain deposition disease (LCDD); initiate myeloma-directed therapy with attention to nodular glomerulopathy.

(D) Hypercalcaemia-related acute tubular necrosis alone; further hydration and bisphosphonate is sufficient.

(E) Diabetic nephropathy unrelated to the myeloma.

Best answer: (A) Myeloma cast nephropathy; rapid reduction of light chain burden through bortezomib-based induction is the most important renal-protective move; supportive care includes aggressive hydration and avoidance of NSAIDs, contrast, and aminoglycosides.

Rationale. The biopsy is diagnostic for myeloma cast nephropathy: distal tubular casts of light chain combined with Tamm-Horsfall protein, with kappa restriction on immunofluorescence and a giant-cell reaction at the cast. Glomerular involvement is absent. The proteinuria is dominantly free light chain (kappa Bence-Jones), with little albumin — this is the discriminator from AL amyloid renal involvement and from light chain deposition disease, both of which produce predominantly albumin-rich (glomerular) proteinuria. The diagnostic clinical clue is the proteinuria pattern: cast nephropathy leaks light chains; amyloid and LCDD leak albumin. Rapid reduction of circulating light chain burden through bortezomib-based induction is the single most important renal-protective intervention; the kidneys can recover function if the light chain insult is interrupted before chronic damage sets in. Supportive measures include aggressive isotonic hydration to flush casts, avoidance of nephrotoxins, and management of hypercalcaemia. Plasmapheresis or extended haemodialysis with high-cut-off dialysers can be considered for very high light chain burden, though randomised data on this intervention are mixed.

Distractor analysis. (B) AL renal involvement would show Congo red birefringence on biopsy and predominantly albumin proteinuria. (C) LCDD shows nodular glomerulosclerosis with linear light chain staining along basement membranes; here the pattern is tubular cast disease, not glomerular deposition. (D) Hypercalcaemic ATN alone would not produce dense tubular casts with giant-cell reaction; light chain casts must be addressed by reducing the clone. (E) No clinical or histological evidence of diabetic disease.

Vignette 10. A 68-year-old man with an IgM paraprotein — myeloma or Waldenström?

A 68-year-old man presents with three months of fatigue and one month of progressive blurred vision. Examination: pallor, hepatosplenomegaly, no significant lymphadenopathy, retinal examination shows tortuous, sausage-shaped retinal veins with scattered haemorrhages. Laboratory studies: haemoglobin 8.6 g/dL, platelets 110,000/μL, WBC 6,400/μL, calcium 9.6 mg/dL, creatinine 1.1 mg/dL, total protein 12.2 g/dL, albumin 3.2 g/dL, serum viscosity 5.2 cP (normal 1.4–1.8). SPEP: 7.4 g/dL M-spike; IFE: IgM kappa. Whole-body imaging shows no lytic bone lesions. Bone marrow biopsy: hypercellular marrow with a paratrabecular and interstitial infiltrate of small lymphocytes admixed with plasmacytoid lymphocytes and mature plasma cells; CD20 strongly positive; CD138 positive on the plasma-cell component; kappa-restricted; MYD88 L265P positive on AS-PCR. Which of the following is the most likely diagnosis and the most appropriate immediate management?

(A) Waldenström macroglobulinaemia (lymphoplasmacytic lymphoma with IgM paraprotein); urgent plasmapheresis for symptomatic hyperviscosity, then BTK inhibitor (ibrutinib or zanubrutinib) or rituximab-based therapy.

(B) IgM multiple myeloma; initiate Dara-VRd induction with ASCT planning.

(C) IgM MGUS; observation with surveillance.

(D) AL amyloidosis with IgM paraprotein; abdominal fat aspirate for Congo red.

(E) Marginal zone lymphoma with IgM paraprotein; rituximab plus bendamustine.

Best answer: (A) Waldenström macroglobulinaemia (lymphoplasmacytic lymphoma with IgM paraprotein); urgent plasmapheresis for symptomatic hyperviscosity, then BTK inhibitor (ibrutinib or zanubrutinib) or rituximab-based therapy.

Rationale. The diagnosis is Waldenström macroglobulinaemia, distinguishable from IgM myeloma by the marrow infiltrate (a CD20-positive small B-cell infiltrate with plasmacytoid forms — a lymphoplasmacytic lymphoma — rather than sheets of CD138-positive plasma cells), the absence of lytic bone disease (myeloma is lytic; WM is not), and the MYD88 L265P mutation (present in >90% of WM, usually absent in IgM myeloma). The retinal findings (sausage-shaped veins, retinal haemorrhages) and elevated serum viscosity (5.2 cP, with a symptomatic threshold around 4 cP) constitute symptomatic hyperviscosity syndrome — an emergency requiring urgent plasmapheresis to rapidly lower IgM levels and viscosity. Definitive treatment after stabilisation uses BTK inhibitors (ibrutinib, zanubrutinib) or rituximab-based regimens (DRC: dexamethasone-rituximab-cyclophosphamide; or BR: bendamustine-rituximab). CXCR4 mutations co-occur in 30–40% of WM and confer reduced ibrutinib response, so CXCR4 testing is increasingly used for treatment selection. Note: although Waldenström is detailed in Chapter 14 alongside lymphoplasmacytic lymphoma, the IgM-myeloma-vs-WM discrimination is core to this chapter on plasma cell neoplasms because IgM myeloma is the rare alternative diagnosis.

Distractor analysis. (B) IgM myeloma would show sheets of CD138-positive plasma cells, lytic bone disease, and usually MYD88-negative profile — the opposite of this case. (C) IgM MGUS requires <10% bone marrow infiltrate and absence of organ damage; this patient has symptomatic hyperviscosity. (D) AL amyloid would show tissue amyloid; not the picture here, although AL amyloid can complicate WM rarely. (E) Marginal zone lymphoma is CD5-/CD10-/CD23- (similar to WM) but lacks the MYD88 L265P mutation and the IgM paraprotein with hyperviscosity is the WM signature.

15.13 Closing Discriminators

HIGH-YIELD PEARL — MGUS vs SMM vs MM at a glance

All three sit on the same continuum and differ only in the size of the M-protein, the marrow plasma cell percentage, and the presence or absence of myeloma-defining events.

- MGUS — M-protein <30 g/L AND marrow plasma cells <10% AND no CRAB or SLiM. Action: observe; risk-stratify by Mayo (FLC ratio, isotype, M-protein concentration).
- SMM — M-protein ≥30 g/L OR marrow plasma cells 10–59%, AND no CRAB or SLiM. Action: observe; offer lenalidomide-based early therapy in high-risk SMM (Mayo 20-2-20).
- MM — Marrow plasma cells ≥10% (or biopsy-proven plasmacytoma) AND at least one CRAB or SLiM event. Action: triplet/quadruplet induction (Dara-VRd standard); ASCT if eligible; lenalidomide maintenance.

Trap: A patient with marrow plasma cells of 65% and no CRAB still meets MM criteria via the SLiM "S" biomarker (≥60% PCs). Do not over-rely on the absence of CRAB end-organ damage.

HIGH-YIELD PEARL — Renal lesions in plasma cell neoplasms — proteinuria pattern is the discriminator

Three principal renal lesions complicate plasma cell neoplasms; each has a characteristic biopsy and proteinuria signature.

- Cast nephropathy (myeloma kidney) — Distal tubular casts of light chain plus Tamm-Horsfall protein; predominantly LIGHT CHAIN proteinuria (Bence-Jones) on urine immunofixation; minimal albumin. Glomeruli are normal. Treatment: rapid clone reduction with bortezomib-based induction; aggressive hydration; nephrotoxin avoidance. The dominant lesion of clinical multiple myeloma.
- AL amyloid renal involvement — Glomerular amyloid deposition (Congo red apple-green birefringence; mass spec confirms AL); predominantly ALBUMIN proteinuria (often nephrotic-range). Treatment: Dara-CyBorD.
- Light chain deposition disease (LCDD) — Nodular glomerulosclerosis with linear monoclonal light chain deposition along glomerular and tubular basement membranes by immunofluorescence (kappa more common than lambda; the inverse of AL); predominantly ALBUMIN proteinuria; Congo red NEGATIVE. Treatment: clone-directed therapy (bortezomib-based).

Diagnostic move: send urine protein electrophoresis with immunofixation to clarify whether albumin or light chain dominates. The biopsy then shows the structural lesion.

HIGH-YIELD PEARL — Macroglossia, neuropathy, lytic vs sclerotic — the discriminating chain

Three syndromes share a paraprotein and a multisystem presentation; the discriminator is the structural pattern.

- Multiple myeloma — Lytic bone lesions; CRAB; ≥10% marrow plasma cells; usually no macroglossia; peripheral neuropathy uncommon at presentation (often bortezomib-induced later).

- AL amyloidosis — Macroglossia, periorbital purpura, restrictive cardiomyopathy, nephrotic-range albuminuria; small clone (<10% PCs); lambda-biased; tissue amyloid on Congo red.
- POEMS syndrome — Demyelinating neuropathy + osteoSCLEROTIC bone lesion (the inverse of myeloma) + organomegaly + endocrinopathy + skin changes; small clone; nearly always lambda; high VEGF.

When neuropathy is the presenting clue, ask three questions: lambda or kappa? lytic or sclerotic? VEGF and CRAB status? POEMS sits in the lambda-sclerotic-high-VEGF corner; AL sits in the lambda-with-tissue-amyloid corner; bortezomib-induced neuropathy is a treatment artefact in established myeloma.

TRAP — IgM paraprotein is not always Waldenström, and not always IgM myeloma

An IgM monoclonal protein has at least four possible underlying neoplasms, and the differential is not optional. Waldenström macroglobulinaemia (lymphoplasmacytic lymphoma with IgM) accounts for the majority and is recognised by the marrow infiltrate of CD20-positive small B cells with plasmacytoid forms and the MYD88 L265P mutation. IgM MGUS is the asymptomatic precursor of WM and is the second most common scenario. Marginal zone lymphoma can produce an IgM paraprotein and overlaps phenotypically with WM (CD5-/CD10-/CD23-) but lacks MYD88 L265P. IgM multiple myeloma is the rare fourth possibility — sheets of CD138-positive clonal plasma cells, lytic bone disease, usually MYD88-negative. The diagnostic move is a properly evaluated bone marrow biopsy with full immunophenotyping and MYD88 testing; the serological clue (IgM M-protein) is the same in all four scenarios but the underlying neoplasm — and therefore the treatment — differs fundamentally.

IMG-TRAP — "Anaemia plus M-spike means myeloma" is wrong without the rest of CRAB

A common reflex is to label any older patient with anaemia and a serum M-spike as multiple myeloma. The IMWG 2014 criteria require at least one CRAB or SLiM event ATTRIBUTABLE to the plasma cell disorder. Anaemia in older patients is multifactorial — iron deficiency (very common in older adults, particularly menstruating women and dietary patterns with limited haem iron), B12 or folate deficiency, anaemia of chronic disease, chronic kidney disease unrelated to myeloma, and myelodysplastic syndromes all coexist with MGUS at high prevalence. Before assigning the anaemia to the M-protein, exclude alternative causes (iron studies, B12, folate, reticulocyte count, peripheral smear, renal function, and, when relevant, marrow morphology for MDS). The clinical sequence is: identify M-protein → quantify clone (marrow PCs, FLC ratio) → test for CRAB and SLiM events → attribute the events to the M-protein only when other causes have been excluded. Failing this step over-treats benign MGUS and under-treats coexistent disease.

15.14 Quick Recall

QUICK RECALL — Plasma Cell Neoplasms

MGUS. M-protein <30 g/L AND marrow PCs <10% AND no CRAB/SLiM. 1% per year progression. Mayo risk stratification: FLC ratio, non-IgG isotype, M-protein ≥15 g/L. Low-risk: 2–3 yr follow-up. High-risk: 6-monthly.

SMM. M-protein ≥30 g/L OR marrow PCs 10–59%, AND no CRAB/SLiM. ~10%/year progression early. Mayo 20-2-20: marrow PCs >20%, M-protein >2 g/dL, FLC ratio >20 → high-risk SMM, consider lenalidomide.

Multiple myeloma. ≥10% clonal marrow PCs (or biopsy-proven plasmacytoma) + ≥1 CRAB or SLiM event. CRAB: hypercalcaemia (>11 mg/dL), Renal (Cr >2 mg/dL), Anaemia (Hb <10 g/dL), Bone lesion. SLiM: 60% PCs; FLC ratio ≥100 with absolute involved FLC ≥100 mg/L; >1 MRI focal lesion ≥5 mm.

Workup triad. SPEP + IFE + sFLC — near-100% sensitivity for any monoclonal protein. WBLDCT or whole-body MRI for bone disease (replaces skeletal survey). PET-CT for response and extramedullary disease.

Marrow morphology. Clock-face chromatin, perinuclear hof, basophilic cytoplasm. Variants: flame cells (IgA), Mott cells (Russell bodies), grape cells. Trephine for accurate quantitation; aspirate haemodilutes.

Flow phenotype. CD138+, CD38 bright+, CD56 often+ (~70%, aberrant), CD117 often+ (esp IgA), CD200 often+, CD45 dim/neg, CD19 NEG (most consistent loss), CD81 dim/absent, monoclonal cytoplasmic Ig (κ or λ). Reactive plasma cells are CD19+, CD56-, polyclonal cytoplasmic Ig.

Cytogenetics. FISH on CD138-selected plasma cells. Standard-risk: hyperdiploid (trisomies of odd chromosomes); t(11;14)/CCND1::IGH (~15%, cyclin D1+). High-risk: del(17p)/TP53, t(4;14)/FGFR3-MMSET, t(14;16)/MAF, t(14;20)/MAFB, 1q gain. ≥2 high-risk = double-hit myeloma.

R-ISS. Stage I: ISS-I + standard cytogenetics + normal LDH (5-yr OS >80%). Stage III: ISS-III + (high-risk cytogenetics OR elevated LDH); median OS ~29 months.

Treatment of newly diagnosed MM. Dara-VRd induction (transplant-eligible) → ASCT → lenalidomide maintenance. Transplant-ineligible: Dara-Rd or Dara-VRd. Relapsed: pomalidomide, carfilzomib, isatuximab, daratumumab, BCMA-targeted (belantamab, ide-cel/cilta-cel CAR-T, teclistamab/elranatamab bispecifics).

Supportive care. Monthly zoledronic acid or denosumab for bone disease. Acyclovir prophylaxis with bortezomib/daratumumab/BCMA-targeted. Pneumococcal/influenza vaccination. Avoid NSAIDs, contrast, aminoglycosides; aggressive hydration in cast nephropathy. Plasmapheresis if hyperviscosity symptomatic.

Plasma cell leukaemia. ≥5% circulating plasma cells of WBC (IMWG 2021/WHO 2022; old ≥20% threshold abandoned). Enriched for del(17p), t(14;16). Treat as high-risk MM; tandem ASCT or ASCT-allo bridge. Worst prognosis in the spectrum.

Solitary plasmacytoma. Single biopsy-proven clonal PC tumour + marrow PCs <10% + no CRAB/SLiM + no other lesion on whole-body MRI/PET. Bone (SPB; axial skeleton) or extramedullary (EMP; upper aerodigestive tract). Definitive radiotherapy 40–50 Gy; ~90% local control. Progression to MM ~50–70% at 10 yr (SPB), ~10–30% (EMP). Lifelong surveillance.

AL amyloidosis. Lambda > kappa (~2:1). Cardiac amyloid: low-voltage QRS + thickened LV + granular sparkling + raised NT-proBNP/troponin. Renal amyloid: nephrotic albuminuria. Macroglossia, raccoon eyes, factor X deficiency. Diagnose: fat aspirate Congo red apple-green birefringence + mass spec typing (distinguish AL/ATTR/AA). Treat: Dara-CyBorD per ANDROMEDA.

POEMS. Polyneuropathy + Organomegaly + Endocrinopathy + M-protein (lambda nearly always) + Skin changes. Major: osteoSCLEROTIC plasmacytoma; Castleman disease; high VEGF. Localised: definitive radiotherapy. Disseminated: lenalidomide-/bortezomib-based ± ASCT.

Heavy chain diseases. Alpha (Seligmann/IPSID): Mediterranean/South Asian; Campylobacter jejuni; small-bowel malabsorption; antibiotics in early disease. Mu: rare, often on CLL background; vacuolated lymphocytes/plasmacytoid cells. Gamma (Franklin): lymphadenopathy, hepatosplenomegaly.

Waldenström (in Ch 14). LPL with IgM. CD20+, CD138 partial; MYD88 L265P >90%. Hyperviscosity → plasmapheresis + BTK inhibitor / rituximab-based therapy. Distinct from IgM myeloma (CD138+, MYD88 usually neg, lytic bones).

— End of Chapter 15 —

CHAPTER 16

Chapter 16 — Haemostasis and Bleeding Disorders

BIG PICTURE

Haemostasis is the controlled physiological response to vascular injury that limits blood loss while preserving vascular patency. The system is built in two layers, and every bleeding disorder maps to one of them. Primary haemostasis is platelet-mediated and produces the initial platelet plug at the site of vessel injury — defects here cause mucocutaneous bleeding (petechiae, purpura, epistaxis, gingival bleeding, menorrhagia, prolonged bleeding from superficial cuts). Secondary haemostasis is the coagulation cascade — sequential serine protease activation generating thrombin, which converts fibrinogen to fibrin and stabilises the plug — defects here cause deep-tissue bleeding (haemarthroses, intramuscular haematomas, retroperitoneal bleeds, intracranial haemorrhage). The bleeding pattern told to you in the vignette is the clue to the layer; the screening coagulation panel (PT, APTT, platelet count, peripheral smear, ± thrombin time) localises the lesion further; and definitive testing (factor assays, vWF studies, mixing studies, ADAMTS13) names the specific defect. Two organising frames unlock the whole field: distinguish primary from secondary by clinical pattern; and within secondary, distinguish prolonged PT (extrinsic / FVII / vit K / liver / warfarin) from prolonged APTT (intrinsic / FVIII–IX–XI–XII / heparin / lupus anticoagulant). Once those frames are second nature, the entire chapter becomes pattern recognition.

MECHANISM HOOK — Why the cell-based model has replaced the textbook intrinsic / extrinsic cascade

The traditional intrinsic/extrinsic cascade (drilled in for decades because it maps cleanly to the APTT and PT) is a useful laboratory abstraction but is biologically misleading. In vivo coagulation does not separate into two parallel pathways. The cell-based model — initiation, amplification, propagation — is the modern framework. Initiation occurs on tissue-factor-bearing cells (subendothelial fibroblasts, activated monocytes) where tissue factor (TF) is exposed on vessel injury and binds plasma FVII, generating small amounts of thrombin (FIIa) via the TF/FVIIa-FX-FIIa axis. Amplification occurs on the activated platelet surface, where thrombin feedback-activates FXI, FVIII, FV, and platelets themselves. Propagation generates the burst of thrombin that converts fibrinogen to fibrin, activates FXIII (cross-linker), and stabilises the clot. Two practical implications follow. First, the laboratory PT and APTT measure isolated portions of the system in vitro and do not reflect in vivo function in real time — viscoelastic tests (TEG, ROTEM) probe whole-blood clot formation in trauma and surgery. Second, the rationale for many therapeutic interventions becomes obvious: recombinant FVIIa (NovoSeven) bypasses inhibitor-blocked FVIII or FIX by directly amplifying thrombin generation; activated prothrombin complex concentrates (FEIBA) similarly bypass inhibitors. Knowing the cell-based model lets you reason about clinical haemostatic emergencies without memorising disconnected facts.

16.1 Normal Haemostasis

Primary haemostasis — vascular and platelet response

Vessel injury exposes subendothelial collagen and tissue factor and triggers immediate reflex vasoconstriction (myogenic spasm + endothelin-1 + thromboxane A2). Within seconds, platelets adhere to exposed collagen — directly via the platelet glycoprotein GPVI and integrin α2β1, and at high shear (arterioles and microcirculation) indirectly via von Willebrand factor (vWF) bridging collagen (vWF A3 domain) to platelet GPIb-IX-V (vWF A1 domain). The vWF–GPIb interaction is the rate-limiting adhesion step at high shear; loss of vWF (von Willebrand disease) or loss of GPIb (Bernard-Soulier syndrome) both produce mucocutaneous bleeding by failing this step.

Adhesion triggers platelet activation: shape change from smooth disc to spiny sphere with pseudopodia; degranulation of alpha granules (vWF, fibrinogen, FV, PF4, PDGF, P-selectin) and dense (delta) granules (ADP, ATP, serotonin, calcium, polyphosphates); and synthesis of thromboxane A2 from arachidonic acid via COX-1. ADP binds platelet P2Y1 and P2Y12 receptors recruiting more platelets — the target of clopidogrel and prasugrel (P2Y12 antagonists) and ticagrelor (reversible P2Y12 antagonist). TXA2 amplifies activation and vasoconstriction — the target of aspirin, which irreversibly acetylates COX-1 for the platelet lifespan (7–10 days). Platelet aggregation requires the integrin GPIIb/IIIa (αIIbβ3) on the activated platelet surface to bind fibrinogen (and vWF) and bridge adjacent platelets. GPIIb/IIIa deficiency or dysfunction is Glanzmann thrombasthenia. Thrombin generated locally feeds back to amplify platelet activation, linking primary and secondary haemostasis.

HIGH-YIELD PEARL — Primary vs secondary haemostasis defects — the bleeding pattern tells you the layer

Primary haemostasis defects (platelet count or function, vWF) produce MUCOCUTANEOUS BLEEDING: petechiae (small flat haemorrhages on gravity-dependent skin and mucosae), purpura, epistaxis, gingival bleeding, menorrhagia, easy bruising, and prolonged bleeding from superficial cuts. Bleeding starts immediately at the time of injury. Bleeding time and PFA-100 closure time are prolonged.

Secondary haemostasis defects (coagulation factor deficiencies — haemophilia, vWD with low FVIII, severe DIC, anticoagulant overdose) produce DEEP-TISSUE BLEEDING: haemarthroses, intramuscular haematomas, retroperitoneal haemorrhage, intracranial bleeding, and post-traumatic delayed bleeding (the platelet plug forms and then fails when fibrin reinforcement does not arrive).

Mixed pattern (mucocutaneous + deep): vWD (loss of platelet adhesion and reduced FVIII carrier), severe DIC, severe liver disease, and complex acquired bleeding states.

When the vignette describes haemarthrosis in a young man, think haemophilia. When it describes petechiae and gum bleeding in a child after viral illness, think ITP. When it describes both bruising and joint bleeds in a girl with menorrhagia, think vWD.

Secondary haemostasis — the coagulation cascade and the cell-based model

The coagulation cascade in laboratory terms separates into the extrinsic pathway (TF + FVII; measured by the prothrombin time, PT), the intrinsic pathway (contact factors XII, XI, IX, VIII;

measured by the activated partial thromboplastin time, APTT), and the common pathway (X, V, II/prothrombin, fibrinogen) that both paths feed into. Thrombin (FIIa) cleaves fibrinogen to fibrin and activates FXIII, which cross-links fibrin to produce a stable clot. The PT measures the extrinsic and common pathway; the APTT measures the intrinsic and common pathway. The cell-based model — initiation on TF-bearing cells, amplification on activated platelets, propagation generating the thrombin burst — is the more biologically accurate framework but the PT and APTT remain the workhorse screening tests because they cleanly localise factor deficiencies.

Test	Pathway tested	Factors required	Prolonged in
PT (prothrombin time)	Extrinsic + common	VII, X, V, II, fibrinogen	FVII deficiency, vitamin K deficiency, warfarin, liver disease (FVII has the shortest half-life — 4–6 h — so PT prolongs first)
APTT (activated partial thromboplastin time)	Intrinsic + common	XII, XI, IX, VIII, X, V, II, fibrinogen	FVIII/IX/XI/XII deficiency, heparin, lupus anticoagulant, vWD with low FVIII
Thrombin time (TT)	Fibrinogen → fibrin	Thrombin + fibrinogen	Hypofibrinogenaemia, dysfibrinogenaemia, heparin, dabigatran, fibrin degradation products
Reptilase time	Fibrinogen → fibrin	Reptilase (snake venom thrombin substitute) + fibrinogen	Hypofibrinogenaemia, dysfibrinogenaemia (NOT prolonged by heparin — discriminator from TT)
Fibrinogen (Clauss)	Quantitative fibrinogen	Functional fibrinogen	Hypofibrinogenaemia (DIC, liver disease, congenital), dysfibrinogenaemia
D-dimer	Cross-linked fibrin breakdown product	Plasmin cleavage of cross-linked fibrin	DIC, VTE, recent surgery/trauma, sepsis, malignancy, pregnancy, advanced age

Table 16.1: The coagulation screening panel — pathway, factors required, and conditions producing prolongation.

Natural anticoagulants and fibrinolysis

Three natural anticoagulant systems prevent unchecked propagation of the coagulation cascade. The protein C / protein S system: thrombin bound to thrombomodulin on intact endothelium activates protein C, which (with its cofactor protein S) inactivates the active forms of FVa and FVIIIa. Antithrombin (AT) inactivates thrombin, FXa, and (less strongly) FIXa, FXIa, and FXIIa; heparin (and the heparan sulfate of intact endothelium) binds AT and accelerates this inactivation by ~1000-fold — this is the mechanism of unfractionated heparin and low-molecular-weight heparin. Tissue factor pathway inhibitor (TFPI) inhibits the TF/FVIIa complex once a small amount of FXa is generated, providing rapid feedback control of the initiation phase.

Fibrinolysis dissolves the clot once vascular repair is complete. Plasminogen, a zymogen, is converted to plasmin by tissue plasminogen activator (tPA, released from endothelium) or urokinase (uPA). Plasmin cleaves fibrin into degradation products (FDPs) including the cross-linked D-dimer fragment. The D-dimer assay is therefore a sensitive marker of recent thrombosis and active fibrinolysis but is not specific (also elevated in surgery, trauma, malignancy, pregnancy, sepsis, and in the elderly). Antifibrinolytic drugs — tranexamic acid and aminocaproic acid — bind plasminogen and block its conversion to plasmin, and are useful adjuncts in surgical and obstetric bleeding, mucosal bleeding in vWD and platelet disorders, and in the management of trauma haemorrhage (the CRASH-2 trial established TXA in this role).

HIGH-YIELD PEARL — Vitamin K, the carboxylation modification, and warfarin

Vitamin K is required for gamma-carboxylation of glutamate residues on the vitamin-K-dependent factors — FII (prothrombin), FVII, FIX, FX, and the natural anticoagulants protein C and protein S. The carboxylated glutamate residues bind calcium, which anchors the factors to phospholipid surfaces. Vitamin K reductase regenerates reduced vitamin K from the oxidised form after each carboxylation cycle.

Warfarin inhibits vitamin K epoxide reductase (VKORC1), depleting reduced vitamin K and producing dysfunctional non-carboxylated factors (PIVKAs — proteins induced by vitamin K absence/antagonism). Because the half-lives differ — FVII (4–6 h, shortest), FIX (24 h), FX (40 h), FII (60 h, longest) and protein C (~8 h), protein S (~30 h) — warfarin produces a transient prothrombotic state on initiation as protein C drops faster than FII. This explains warfarin-induced skin necrosis (typically in patients with underlying protein C deficiency) and the requirement to bridge with parenteral anticoagulant (heparin or LMWH) until INR is therapeutic.

Reversal of warfarin overdose: vitamin K (oral or IV — IV faster but anaphylaxis risk), prothrombin complex concentrate (PCC, contains FII, FVII, FIX, FX) for major bleeding, fresh frozen plasma if PCC unavailable. Andexanet alfa is the specific reversal agent for FXa direct oral anticoagulants (rivaroxaban, apixaban); idarucizumab reverses dabigatran.

16.2 Approach to a Bleeding Patient

The clinical evaluation of bleeding starts with two questions: is the bleeding pattern primary or secondary haemostatic, and is the disorder inherited or acquired? The bleeding history is the single highest-yield part of the workup. Symptoms of mucocutaneous bleeding (epistaxis lasting >10 minutes, gum bleeding with tooth-brushing, easy bruising with bruises >2 cm without recognised trauma, menorrhagia, prolonged bleeding from minor cuts) point to a primary haemostatic defect. Symptoms of deep-tissue bleeding (haemarthroses — particularly of large weight-bearing joints; intramuscular haematomas; retroperitoneal bleeds; intracranial haemorrhage; delayed post-traumatic bleeding) point to a secondary haemostatic defect. Family history (X-linked recessive pattern in haemophilia A and B; autosomal dominant in vWD types 1 and 2 except 2N which is recessive) and challenge history (past dental extractions, surgeries, deliveries, circumcision) clarify whether a defect has been previously unmasked. The ISTH Bleeding Assessment Tool (BAT) is a structured questionnaire that quantifies bleeding severity and is now standard in vWD workup.

The drug and exposure history is critical: aspirin, clopidogrel, prasugrel, and ticagrelor inhibit platelet function; SSRIs cause modest platelet dysfunction; warfarin and DOACs (dabigatran, rivaroxaban, apixaban, edoxaban) interfere with coagulation factors; NSAIDs cause reversible platelet inhibition; certain antibiotics (cephalosporins, beta-lactams) and herbal supplements (ginkgo, ginger, garlic in high doses) can prolong bleeding. Liver disease, kidney disease (uraemic platelet dysfunction), and malignancy (acquired vWF deficiency in MGUS, lymphoma, and Wilms tumour; acquired haemophilia in autoimmune disorders, malignancy, and the postpartum period) all produce acquired bleeding disorders that may present without a personal or family bleeding history.

Examination focuses on the distribution and morphology of skin bleeding (petechiae of dependent skin and mucosae in thrombocytopenia and platelet function disorders; ecchymoses of variable size in primary defects; deep haematomas and joint swelling in secondary defects), splenomegaly (liver disease, hypersplenism, portal hypertension, lymphoproliferative disorders), stigmata of liver disease (jaundice, spider naevi, palmar erythema, caput medusae), and signs of underlying systemic disease (lymphadenopathy, weight loss, masses).

Bleeding pattern	Suggested layer	Differential to consider
Petechiae, gum bleeding, menorrhagia, easy bruising; bleeding immediate at injury	Primary haemostasis	Thrombocytopenia (ITP, drug-induced, infection, BM failure, sequestration), platelet function disorders (vWD, Glanzmann, Bernard-Soulier, storage pool, drug-induced — aspirin/clopidogrel)
Haemarthroses, deep haematomas, intracranial bleed, retroperitoneal; delayed bleeding after injury	Secondary haemostasis	Haemophilia A or B, severe vWD (type 3), rare factor deficiencies, acquired haemophilia, anticoagulant overdose, vitamin K deficiency, severe liver disease

Bleeding pattern	Suggested layer	Differential to consider
Both primary AND secondary features	Mixed	vWD with low FVIII, severe DIC, severe liver disease, snake envenomation, complex acquired states
Cutaneous bleeding without thrombocytopenia and with normal coagulation	Vascular / connective tissue	Senile purpura, steroid-induced vasculopathy, Ehlers-Danlos, scurvy, IgA vasculitis (Henoch-Schönlein), amyloidosis (factor X-related and vascular fragility)

Table 16.2: Clinical bleeding pattern → suggested haemostatic layer → differential diagnosis.

16.3 Lab Approach to a Bleeding Patient — The Screening Panel

Every patient with suspected bleeding undergoes a screening panel: complete blood count with platelet count, peripheral blood smear (to confirm thrombocytopenia, exclude pseudothrombocytopenia from EDTA-induced clumping, and identify schistocytes of microangiopathic haemolytic anaemia), prothrombin time (PT) with INR, activated partial thromboplastin time (APTT), thrombin time (TT) and Clauss fibrinogen if needed, and renal and liver function. The pattern of abnormalities directs the next-tier workup. Bleeding time is now considered insensitive and operator-dependent; the PFA-100 / PFA-200 closure time is preferred where available as an automated screening test for primary haemostatic defects (sensitive to vWD and severe platelet function disorders, less so to mild platelet dysfunction).

FORMULA — Pattern recognition of the screening panel

- Normal PT, normal APTT, low platelets → primary haemostasis defect (thrombocytopenia). Workup: smear, BM if needed, ITP workup, drug history, viral serology.
- Normal PT, normal APTT, normal platelets, mucocutaneous bleeding → vWD or platelet function disorder. Workup: vWF:Ag, vWF:RCo, FVIII:C, multimer; PFA-100; platelet aggregation studies.
- Normal PT, prolonged APTT → intrinsic pathway defect. Workup: mixing study, factor assays (VIII, IX, XI, XII), vWD panel (Type 2N and 3 lower FVIII), heparin, lupus anticoagulant.
- Prolonged PT, normal APTT → FVII deficiency, early vitamin K deficiency, early warfarin therapy, mild liver disease.
- Prolonged PT, prolonged APTT → common pathway defect (FV, FX, FII, fibrinogen), severe liver disease, vitamin K deficiency at full effect, warfarin at therapeutic INR, DIC, supratherapeutic heparin, dabigatran or rivaroxaban / apixaban at peak.
- Prolonged TT with normal reptilase time → heparin or dabigatran. Prolonged TT with prolonged reptilase time → dysfibrinogenaemia or hypofibrinogenaemia.
- Schistocytes on smear + thrombocytopenia + normal coagulation → thrombotic microangiopathy (TTP, HUS, atypical HUS). Workup: ADAMTS13, complement studies.
- Schistocytes + thrombocytopenia + prolonged PT/APTT + low fibrinogen + raised D-dimer → DIC. Treat the underlying trigger.

16.4 Approach to a Prolonged APTT

A prolonged APTT in a bleeding patient signals an intrinsic or common pathway defect; in a patient without bleeding, the same finding may signal a lupus anticoagulant (paradoxically associated with thrombosis, not bleeding) or an FXII deficiency (clinically silent). The discriminating step is the mixing study: 50:50 mix of patient plasma with normal pooled plasma, with the APTT measured immediately and after 1–2 hours of incubation at 37°C.

Mixing study result	Interpretation	Next step
Corrects (APTT normalises	Factor deficiency — patient	Sequential factor assays

Mixing study result	Interpretation	Next step
immediately)	lacks a factor that the normal plasma supplies	for FVIII, IX, XI, XII; vWD panel if FVIII low
Does not correct (immediate)	Inhibitor present (lupus anticoagulant, factor-specific antibody, heparin, DOAC)	Lupus anticoagulant testing (dRVVT + APTT-based); thrombin time + reptilase to exclude heparin/DOAC; factor-specific antibodies if FVIII assay low
Corrects immediately but prolongs after incubation (1–2 h, 37°C)	Time-dependent inhibitor — classic for FVIII inhibitor (acquired haemophilia A) and some FIX inhibitors	Bethesda assay to quantify inhibitor titre; Nijmegen modification for low titres

Table 16.3: Mixing study interpretation in prolonged APTT.

The most common causes of an isolated prolonged APTT in clinical practice are: heparin therapy (UFH; LMWH usually does not prolong APTT meaningfully), lupus anticoagulant (often incidental in young women, in autoimmune disease, in obstetric vignettes), FVIII deficiency in haemophilia A or vWD (especially type 3 and type 2N), FIX deficiency (haemophilia B), FXI deficiency (Ashkenazi Jewish populations), and acquired FVIII inhibitor (older patients, postpartum women, autoimmune disease). FXII deficiency markedly prolongs the APTT but does not cause bleeding — a textbook discriminator from clinically significant intrinsic factor deficiencies.

HIGH-YIELD PEARL — Lupus anticoagulant: prolonged APTT but increased thrombosis risk

A lupus anticoagulant (LA) is an autoantibody against phospholipid-bound proteins (most commonly beta-2 glycoprotein I or prothrombin) that interferes with phospholipid-dependent coagulation reactions in vitro — prolonging the APTT (and dRVVT) — but in vivo paradoxically increases thrombosis risk. The diagnostic move requires (a) a screening test (APTT or dRVVT) showing prolongation; (b) failure to correct on mixing study (immediate); (c) demonstration of phospholipid dependence — the abnormality corrects when excess phospholipid is added (high-phospholipid screen, or hexagonal-phase assay); and (d) exclusion of other inhibitors (no specific factor inhibitor, no heparin/DOAC). The 2023 ISTH guidelines require positive results on two occasions ≥12 weeks apart for a definitive diagnosis. Lupus anticoagulant is part of antiphospholipid syndrome — covered fully in Chapter 17.

16.5 Approach to a Prolonged PT

An isolated prolonged PT (with normal APTT) is most commonly due to FVII deficiency, early warfarin, early vitamin K deficiency, or early liver disease — FVII has the shortest half-life (4–6 h) of all the vitamin K dependent factors, so the PT is the first parameter to prolong in any condition that reduces functional vitamin K dependent factor synthesis. A combined prolonged PT and prolonged APTT signals either (a) a common pathway defect (FX, FV, FII, fibrinogen), (b) advanced or established vitamin K deficiency, established warfarin effect, or established liver disease (where multiple factors are reduced), or (c) DIC (low fibrinogen + raised D-dimer + thrombocytopenia + clinical context).

In suspected liver disease, the picture is often complex because liver synthesises both procoagulant factors (II, V, VII, IX, X, XI, fibrinogen) and natural anticoagulants (protein C, protein S, antithrombin), with FVIII as a notable exception (FVIII rises in chronic liver disease because it is partly synthesised by sinusoidal endothelial cells and is also released from the reticuloendothelial system). The net haemostatic balance is therefore "rebalanced" rather than uniformly hypocoagulable, and traditional PT/INR poorly predicts bleeding risk in cirrhosis. Viscoelastic testing (TEG/ROTEM) gives a more accurate global assessment in liver-related bleeding and is used during liver transplantation.

HIGH-YIELD PEARL — Vitamin K deficiency vs liver disease — the FV discriminator

Both vitamin K deficiency and liver disease prolong PT and APTT and reduce vitamin-K-dependent factors (II, VII, IX, X). The clean discriminator is FV (factor V), which is synthesised by the liver but does NOT require vitamin K for activity. FV is REDUCED in liver disease and NORMAL in vitamin K deficiency.

Practical move: in a patient with prolonged PT/APTT, the response to parenteral vitamin K (10 mg IV; PT/INR rechecked at 24–48 h) discriminates clinically — vitamin K deficiency corrects substantially; liver disease does not.

Common causes of vitamin K deficiency: prolonged broad-spectrum antibiotics (kill gut flora that produce K2), malabsorption (cholestatic liver disease — bile salt deficient absorption; coeliac disease; cystic fibrosis with pancreatic insufficiency; short bowel syndrome), warfarin or "superwarfarin" rodenticide poisoning, and neonatal vitamin K deficiency bleeding (prevented by routine intramuscular vitamin K at birth — a critical nursery practice in India and globally).

16.6 Thrombocytopenia and Immune Thrombocytopenia (ITP)

Approach to thrombocytopenia

Thrombocytopenia is a platelet count <150 × 10^9/L. The clinical bleeding risk is roughly correlated with severity: counts >50 × 10^9/L rarely produce spontaneous bleeding; counts 20–50 × 10^9/L produce easy bruising and minor mucocutaneous bleeding; counts <20 × 10^9/L produce petechiae and mucosal bleeding; counts <10 × 10^9/L carry meaningful risk of spontaneous intracranial haemorrhage. The diagnostic workup begins with a peripheral smear to exclude pseudothrombocytopenia from EDTA-induced platelet clumping (rerun the count on a citrate or heparin tube) and to identify schistocytes (microangiopathic process) or other clues. The differential is broadly divided into reduced production, increased destruction, sequestration, and dilutional thrombocytopenia.

Mechanism	Causes	Discriminating clue
Reduced production	Bone marrow failure (aplastic anaemia), MDS, leukaemia, infiltrative disease (lymphoma, metastatic carcinoma), megaloblastic anaemia (B12/folate), drug-induced marrow suppression (chemotherapy, alcohol), inherited (Fanconi, Wiskott-Aldrich, MYH9-related)	Often pancytopenia; bone marrow biopsy is diagnostic; smear shows other features
Increased destruction (immune)	ITP (primary or secondary — to SLE, lymphoma, viral, drug, post-transplant), neonatal alloimmune thrombocytopenia, post-transfusion purpura, drug-induced (heparin → HIT; quinine; vancomycin)	Isolated thrombocytopenia with normal RBC and WBC; smear shows large young platelets; antiplatelet antibodies are not routinely used (poor sensitivity)
Increased destruction (non-immune)	TTP, HUS, atypical HUS, DIC, mechanical destruction (prosthetic valve, ECMO), preeclampsia/HELLP, malignant hypertension	Schistocytes on smear; MAHA (microangiopathic haemolytic anaemia); Coombs negative; LDH high; haptoglobin low
Sequestration	Hypersplenism (cirrhosis, portal hypertension, lymphoproliferative disorder, chronic haemolytic anaemias, sarcoidosis, infections (EBV, HIV, malaria when present))	Splenomegaly; usually mild thrombocytopenia (rarely below 50 × 10^9/L); other cytopenias common
Dilutional /	Massive transfusion (without platelet	Clinical context

Mechanism	Causes	Discriminating clue
consumption	replacement), massive bleeding with crystalloid resuscitation	
Drug-induced	Heparin (HIT), quinine, sulfonamides, vancomycin, linezolid, GP IIb/IIIa inhibitors (acute), valproate, rifampicin, methotrexate (marrow toxicity)	Drug timing; recovery on withdrawal; specific tests (PF4 antibody for HIT)

Table 16.4: Aetiological framework for thrombocytopenia.

Immune thrombocytopenia (ITP)

Immune thrombocytopenia (ITP, formerly idiopathic thrombocytopenic purpura) is an autoimmune disorder in which IgG antibodies — usually directed against platelet GPIIb/IIIa or GPIb/IX — opsonise platelets for clearance by splenic and hepatic macrophages, accelerated by Fc receptor recognition. The current understanding also recognises antibody-mediated impairment of megakaryocyte maturation and reduced thrombopoietin (TPO) responsiveness, which is the rationale for TPO receptor agonists (eltrombopag, romiplostim, avatrombopag) as second-line therapy.

Primary ITP is diagnosed clinically and by exclusion: isolated thrombocytopenia with otherwise normal blood counts, no schistocytes or other smear abnormality, no clinical or laboratory evidence of another cause (drug, viral hepatitis, HIV, H. pylori, lymphoma, SLE), and no other source. Bone marrow examination is not required in typical adult primary ITP but is performed when atypical features are present (older age, additional cytopenias, palpable splenomegaly, abnormal smear). Children commonly present with acute, post-viral, self-limiting ITP; ~70–80% recover spontaneously within 6 months. Adults more often progress to chronic disease.

FORMULA — ITP treatment ladder (adult primary ITP)

First-line — when treatment is indicated (count <20–30 × 10^9/L or bleeding):

- Corticosteroids: prednisolone 1 mg/kg/day for 2–4 weeks then taper; OR high-dose dexamethasone 40 mg/day × 4 days (single or repeated cycles).
- IVIg 1 g/kg × 1 or 2 days — used when rapid response needed (active bleeding, surgery, pre-procedure).
- Anti-D immunoglobulin (Rh-positive non-splenectomised patients) — historical; less used now.

Second-line — for steroid-dependent or refractory disease:

- TPO receptor agonists: eltrombopag (oral), romiplostim (subcutaneous weekly), avatrombopag (oral). Increase platelet production. Now first or second second-line choice in many guidelines.
- Rituximab — anti-CD20 monoclonal antibody; ~50% response, often transient.
- Splenectomy — historically the second-line standard; ~60–70% durable remission. Less commonly used now given alternatives. Pneumococcal, meningococcal, and

Haemophilus vaccination required pre-splenectomy.

Third-line and refractory — fostamatinib (SYK inhibitor), immunosuppressants (azathioprine, mycophenolate, ciclosporin), combinations.

16.7 Inherited Platelet Function Disorders

Inherited platelet function disorders are uncommon individually but collectively important — they produce mucocutaneous bleeding with normal platelet counts (or mild thrombocytopenia in some) and a normal coagulation panel. The diagnostic workup combines platelet aggregation studies (light transmission aggregometry — gold standard), flow cytometry for specific glycoproteins (CD41/CD61 for GPIIb/IIIa; CD42a/CD42b for GPIb/IX/V), electron microscopy of platelets (for granule disorders), and increasingly next-generation sequencing of platelet disorder gene panels.

Disorder	Defect	Inheritance	Key features and lab
Glanzmann thrombasthenia	GPIIb/IIIa deficiency or dysfunction	Autosomal recessive	Mucocutaneous bleeding from infancy; normal platelet count and morphology; aggregation absent to ADP, collagen, epinephrine, thrombin, but PRESERVED to ristocetin (vWF-mediated); flow cytometry confirms loss of CD41/CD61
Bernard-Soulier syndrome	GPIb/IX/V complex deficiency	Autosomal recessive	Mucocutaneous bleeding; LARGE platelets (giant platelets) on smear; mild to moderate thrombocytopenia; aggregation NORMAL to ADP/collagen/epinephrine/thrombin but ABSENT to ristocetin (no vWF binding); flow cytometry confirms loss of CD42a/CD42b
Storage pool disease (delta and alpha)	Reduced dense or alpha granule content	Autosomal dominant or recessive	Mild to moderate mucocutaneous bleeding; aggregation may show absent secondary wave; electron microscopy is the diagnostic gold standard. Hermansky-Pudlak (delta SPD + albinism + pulmonary fibrosis) and Chédiak-Higashi (delta SPD + giant granules +

Disorder	Defect	Inheritance	Key features and lab
			immunodeficiency) are syndromic forms
MYH9-related disorders	Mutations in non-muscle myosin heavy chain 9	Autosomal dominant	Macrothrombocytopenia (large platelets, low count); Döhle-like inclusions in neutrophils; spectrum from May-Hegglin anomaly to Sebastian, Fechtner, Epstein syndromes; sensorineural deafness, nephritis, cataracts in some
Wiskott-Aldrich syndrome	WAS gene mutation	X-linked recessive	Eczema + immunodeficiency (recurrent infections) + microthrombocytopenia (small platelets, low count). Lymphoma and autoimmunity in survivors. Stem cell transplant curative
Aspirin-like defect / COX-1 deficiency	Reduced thromboxane synthesis	Variable	Aggregation absent to arachidonic acid; reduced response to ADP and epinephrine

Table 16.5: Inherited platelet function disorders — exam-relevant features.

HIGH-YIELD PEARL — Glanzmann vs Bernard-Soulier — the ristocetin discriminator

Both Glanzmann thrombasthenia and Bernard-Soulier syndrome produce mucocutaneous bleeding from infancy with normal coagulation and an apparently normal platelet count (Bernard-Soulier may show mild thrombocytopenia and giant platelets). Platelet aggregation studies discriminate them cleanly:

- Glanzmann thrombasthenia — GPIIb/IIIa deficiency. Aggregation is ABSENT in response to all physiological agonists (ADP, collagen, epinephrine, thrombin) because all converge on GPIIb/IIIa for the final aggregation step. Aggregation is PRESERVED in response to ristocetin (which depends on vWF–GPIb agglutination, not aggregation through GPIIb/IIIa).
- Bernard-Soulier syndrome — GPIb/IX/V deficiency. Aggregation is NORMAL to ADP, collagen, epinephrine, thrombin (these still converge on intact GPIIb/IIIa) but is ABSENT to ristocetin (no GPIb to interact with vWF).

Mnemonic: Glanzmann = no aggregation EXCEPT ristocetin works; Bernard-Soulier = ristocetin DOES NOT work (everything else does).

16.8 Thrombotic Microangiopathies — TTP, HUS, and atypical HUS

Thrombotic microangiopathies (TMAs) are a group of disorders defined by microvascular thrombosis, microangiopathic haemolytic anaemia (MAHA — schistocytes on the peripheral smear, raised LDH, low haptoglobin, indirect hyperbilirubinaemia, negative direct antiglobulin test), thrombocytopenia, and end-organ ischaemia. The three principal entities — thrombotic thrombocytopenic purpura (TTP), Shiga-toxin-mediated haemolytic uraemic syndrome (STEC-HUS), and atypical HUS — share this triad but differ fundamentally in mechanism and treatment.

Feature	TTP	STEC-HUS (typical)	Atypical HUS (aHUS)
Mechanism	ADAMTS13 deficiency (severe, <10%) — autoimmune (acquired, ~95%) or hereditary (Upshaw-Schulman, ~5%) — leads to ultra-large vWF multimers and platelet aggregation	Shiga toxin from E. coli O157:H7 (or O104:H4) damaging endothelium and triggering microthrombosis	Dysregulation of complement alternative pathway — mutations in CFH, CFI, MCP, C3, CFB, or autoantibodies to factor H
Trigger / context	Often idiopathic; HIV, autoimmune disease, pregnancy, drugs (clopidogrel, ticlopidine, calcineurin inhibitors), malignancy	Bloody diarrhoea (3–10 days prior) from contaminated food (uncooked beef, unpasteurised dairy); childhood predominance	Often idiopathic; triggered by infection, pregnancy, drugs in genetically susceptible individual
Predominant organ injury	Neurological (confusion, focal deficits, seizures, coma) > cardiac > renal — kidney often spared	Renal failure (often dialysis-dependent acutely); central neurological less common	Renal failure dominant; extrarenal involvement (heart, brain, GI) possible
Diagnostic test	ADAMTS13 activity <10%; PLASMIC score (clinical + lab) ≥6 supports TTP	Stool culture or PCR for STEC; serology for E. coli O157	Complement C3 may be low; genetic testing for complement mutations; exclude TTP and STEC-HUS first
Treatment	Plasma exchange (PEX) urgently — DAILY until platelets recover and LDH normalises; corticosteroids; rituximab; caplacizumab (anti-vWF nanobody) accelerates response	Supportive care — hydration, dialysis as needed; antibiotics WORSEN outcomes (release more toxin); eculizumab in severe / atypical features	Eculizumab (anti-C5 monoclonal antibody) — definitive therapy; lifelong; meningococcal vaccination required first; ravulizumab is the long-acting alternative

Feature	TTP	STEC-HUS (typical)	Atypical HUS (aHUS)
Mortality (untreated)	>90%; with PEX, <10–20%	~5% in childhood typical disease; higher in adult E. coli O104:H4	Historically high; eculizumab transformed outcomes

Table 16.6: Distinguishing TTP, STEC-HUS, and atypical HUS — mechanism, diagnosis, and treatment.

HIGH-YIELD PEARL — The TTP pentad is mostly historical — the diagnostic move is ADAMTS13

The classical "pentad" of TTP — fever, neurological symptoms, renal failure, MAHA, thrombocytopenia — is now considered an incomplete and late presentation. Most patients with TTP have only MAHA + thrombocytopenia and need treatment urgently before the full pentad develops.

Modern diagnostic move: any patient with MAHA + thrombocytopenia without an alternative cause has TTP until proven otherwise. The PLASMIC score (PLAtelet count, haemolysis, Active malignancy, Stem cell or solid organ transplant, MCV, INR, Creatinine) ≥6 has high sensitivity and specificity for severe ADAMTS13 deficiency and is widely used to support empirical PEX initiation.

Send blood for ADAMTS13 activity AND inhibitor testing BEFORE starting plasma exchange (which will replace ADAMTS13 and confound the result). Initiate PEX without waiting for the result — TTP mortality without PEX exceeds 90%, and the test typically takes >24 hours. Caplacizumab (anti-vWF A1 domain nanobody) is now added to PEX in many centres on the basis of the HERCULES trial, accelerating platelet recovery and reducing TTP-related death and refractoriness.

16.9 von Willebrand Disease

von Willebrand disease (vWD) is the most common inherited bleeding disorder, affecting approximately 1% of the general population by laboratory criteria, although clinically significant disease is much rarer (~1 in 10,000). vWF has two essential haemostatic roles: it bridges platelets to subendothelial collagen at the site of vascular injury (via GPIb-IX-V binding) — failure of which causes mucocutaneous bleeding — and it is the carrier protein for FVIII in plasma, stabilising it against degradation — failure of which causes a secondary FVIII deficiency that can mimic haemophilia A. Classification is by quantitative vs qualitative defects, divided into types 1, 2, and 3.

Type	Defect	Inheritance	Frequency	Diagnostic features
Type 1	Partial quantitative deficiency of vWF — vWF:Ag <30 IU/dL per 2021 ASH/ISTH/NHF/WFH guidelines (values 30–50 IU/dL with bleeding are now classified as "low VWF")	Autosomal dominant	70–80% of vWD	vWF:Ag and vWF:RCo (or vWF:GPIbM) reduced proportionally; vWF:RCo / vWF:Ag ratio >0.7; multimer pattern normal; FVIII may be reduced proportionally
Type 2A	Loss of high-molecular-weight (HMW) multimers — defective synthesis or increased clearance	Autosomal dominant	~10–15%	vWF:RCo / vWF:Ag ratio <0.7; HMW multimers absent on gel; FVIII near-normal
Type 2B	Gain-of-function: increased affinity of vWF for platelet GPIb	Autosomal dominant	~5%	Enhanced ristocetin-induced platelet aggregation (RIPA) at LOW-DOSE ristocetin; mild thrombocytopenia (vWF binds platelets in vivo and clears them); HMW multimers depleted in plasma but present in platelet lysates; DDAVP CONTRAINDICATED (worsens thrombocytopenia)
Type 2M	Decreased vWF binding to GPIb without loss of HMW multimers	Autosomal dominant	~5%	Low vWF:RCo / vWF:Ag ratio; multimer pattern NORMAL (the discriminator from 2A);

Type	Defect	Inheritance	Frequency	Diagnostic features
				some 2M variants have mutations affecting collagen binding (vWF:CB)
Type 2N (Normandy)	Decreased vWF binding to FVIII	Autosomal recessive	~1%	Low FVIII:C (often 5–30%) with normal vWF:Ag and vWF:RCo; mimics mild haemophilia A. Diagnostic: vWF:FVIIIB (FVIII binding capacity) assay
Type 3	Complete or near-complete absence of vWF	Autosomal recessive	<5%	Severe disease from infancy; vWF:Ag and vWF:RCo undetectable; very low FVIII (typically <5%, often 1–5% — often haemarthroses similar to severe haemophilia)

Table 16.7: Classification of von Willebrand disease — types, defects, and diagnostic features.

Diagnostic workup begins with screening tests: bleeding history (ISTH-BAT score), CBC and smear, PFA-100 closure time (prolonged in vWD; sensitive but not specific), APTT (may be prolonged when FVIII is reduced), and vWF:Ag, vWF:RCo (ristocetin cofactor activity, the functional measure) or the modern equivalent vWF:GPIbM, and FVIII:C. The vWF:RCo / vWF:Ag ratio discriminates type 1 (>0.7, proportional reduction) from type 2 (<0.7, disproportionate functional loss). Second-tier tests include vWF multimer analysis by agarose gel (loss of HMW multimers in 2A and 2B; normal in 2M and 1), low-dose RIPA (enhanced in 2B), vWF collagen binding assay (vWF:CB), and vWF:FVIIIB binding assay (low in 2N — diagnostic). Genetic testing of the VWF gene confirms type 2B and 2N and characterises type 3.

Treatment principles divide into desmopressin-responsive vs concentrate-requiring patients. Desmopressin (DDAVP) releases endogenous vWF from endothelial Weibel-Palade bodies and produces a 3- to 5-fold rise in vWF:Ag for 6–12 hours. It is effective in most type 1 patients and many type 2A and 2M patients. A DDAVP trial should be performed in advance of clinical need to document the individual patient response, because not all type 1 patients respond. DDAVP is CONTRAINDICATED in type 2B (worsens thrombocytopenia) and ineffective in type 3. Hyponatraemia and seizures (from antidiuretic effect) are risks of repeated DDAVP doses, especially in young children. vWF-containing factor concentrates (Humate-P, Wilate, Voncento — recombinant vWF/FVIII) are used in patients unresponsive to DDAVP, in type 3, in type 2B, and for major surgery in any type. Tranexamic acid (oral or IV, 25 mg/kg up to 1 g 8-hourly) is a useful adjunct for mucosal bleeding in vWD and for menorrhagia.

HIGH-YIELD PEARL — vWD type 2N vs mild haemophilia A — the diagnostic move

that changes treatment

Type 2N vWD (Normandy variant) and mild haemophilia A both present with isolated low FVIII:C (often 5–30%), normal vWF:Ag and vWF:RCo, prolonged APTT, and bleeding pattern dominated by deep-tissue bleeding. The two conditions are biologically distinct and require different treatment:

- Mild haemophilia A — X-linked recessive; family history follows X-linkage; treatment is FVIII concentrate (recombinant or plasma-derived).
- Type 2N vWD — autosomal recessive; family history follows autosomal pattern (affected siblings of either sex); treatment is vWF-containing concentrate (Humate-P; recombinant vWF) — pure FVIII concentrates do not help because the FVIII has no carrier protein in vivo and is rapidly degraded.

Diagnostic discriminator: vWF:FVIIIB assay (vWF–FVIII binding capacity) — markedly reduced in type 2N, normal in haemophilia A. Genetic testing of the VWF gene confirms 2N. Always check vWF:FVIIIB in any patient with apparent mild haemophilia A who is female, has an unusual family history, or is unresponsive to FVIII concentrate.

16.10 Haemophilia A and B

Haemophilia A (FVIII deficiency) and Haemophilia B (FIX deficiency, also known as Christmas disease, after the first patient described) are X-linked recessive disorders of secondary haemostasis. Haemophilia A occurs in approximately 1 in 5,000 male births worldwide; Haemophilia B in approximately 1 in 30,000 male births. Approximately 30% of cases are de novo mutations with no family history. Female carriers are usually asymptomatic but have a 50% chance of transmitting the mutation to each son and 50% chance of producing a carrier daughter; lyonisation (skewed X-inactivation) occasionally produces symptomatic female carriers.

Severity	FVIII or FIX activity	Bleeding pattern
Severe	<1%	Spontaneous haemarthroses (especially knee, ankle, elbow), intramuscular haematomas, intracranial haemorrhage; presents in infancy or early childhood with first walking, dental eruption, or circumcision
Moderate	1–5%	Bleeding after minor trauma; occasional spontaneous haemarthrosis; often presents later in childhood
Mild	5–40%	Bleeding only after significant trauma, surgery, or dental work; may not be diagnosed until adulthood (e.g., tonsillectomy or hernia repair)

Table 16.8: Severity classification of haemophilia A and B.

The clinical hallmark of haemophilia is haemarthrosis — bleeding into a synovial joint. Repeated joint bleeds produce haemophilic arthropathy: synovitis, cartilage damage, joint deformity, and ultimately joint destruction. The "target joint" concept (a joint with three or more spontaneous bleeds in 6 months) signals the need to intensify factor prophylaxis. Intracranial haemorrhage is the leading cause of death in untreated severe haemophilia and a major cause of disability when survived. Intramuscular haematomas in iliopsoas, gastrocnemius, or forearm flexor compartments can produce compartment syndrome (Volkmann ischaemic contracture in the forearm). Haematuria and oropharyngeal bleeding are also common.

Diagnostic workup: prolonged APTT, normal PT, normal platelet count and morphology, and specific factor assay (FVIII:C or FIX:C) confirms the diagnosis and quantifies severity. Mixing study corrects in factor deficiency; failure to correct (immediate or delayed) signals an inhibitor. Inhibitor testing (Bethesda or Nijmegen-modified assay) is essential at diagnosis and during treatment because 20–30% of severe haemophilia A patients develop FVIII inhibitors during treatment, and inhibitors fundamentally change management.

FORMULA — Treatment of haemophilia A and B

Factor replacement — calculate dose by patient weight and target factor level:

- Haemophilia A (FVIII): 1 IU/kg of FVIII raises plasma level by ~2%. Target levels: 30–50% for joint bleeds, 50–80% for muscle bleeds, 80–100% for intracranial / life-threatening bleeds and major surgery. Half-life ~12 h; dose every 12 h initially.
- Haemophilia B (FIX): 1 IU/kg of FIX raises plasma level by ~1%. Target levels as for FVIII. Half-life ~24 h; dose every 24 h.
- Extended half-life (EHL) products (PEGylated, Fc fusion, albumin fusion) reduce dosing frequency to twice-weekly or weekly.

Prophylaxis — primary prophylaxis (started before second joint bleed in severe disease) prevents arthropathy and is now standard of care globally; access varies.

Non-factor therapy — emicizumab (Hemlibra) is a bispecific antibody that mimics FVIIIa by bridging FIXa and FX, allowing weekly or fortnightly subcutaneous prophylaxis; effective even in patients with FVIII inhibitors; transformed haemophilia A care.

Inhibitor management — bypassing agents: recombinant FVIIa (NovoSeven), activated prothrombin complex concentrate (FEIBA). Immune tolerance induction (ITI) with daily high-dose factor over 6–24 months can eradicate inhibitors. Emicizumab is now used widely as prophylaxis in inhibitor patients.

Gene therapy — etranacogene dezaparvovec (haemophilia B) and valoctocogene roxaparvovec (haemophilia A) are AAV-based one-time gene therapies now approved with substantial sustained factor expression in many recipients. Long-term durability and access remain evolving.

Adjuncts — DDAVP can be used in mild haemophilia A (raises FVIII 3–5×); tranexamic acid for mucosal bleeding (avoid in haematuria — clot retention).

16.11 Rare Coagulation Factor Deficiencies

Rare factor deficiencies — FXI, FVII, FXIII, fibrinogen abnormalities, FV, FX, prothrombin (FII), and combined deficiencies — collectively account for less than 5% of inherited coagulation disorders. They are recognised by characteristic patterns on the screening panel combined with clinical phenotype.

Deficiency	Inheritance	Screening panel pattern	Clinical features
FXI deficiency (haemophilia C)	Autosomal recessive — particularly common in Ashkenazi Jewish populations (~8%)	Prolonged APTT, normal PT	Variable bleeding — surgery and trauma-induced rather than spontaneous; correlation between factor level and bleeding is poor
FXII / prekallikrein / HMWK deficiency	Autosomal recessive	Prolonged APTT, normal PT	NO bleeding — clinically silent. Discriminator from clinically significant intrinsic factor deficiency

Deficiency	Inheritance	Screening panel pattern	Clinical features
FVII deficiency	Autosomal recessive	Prolonged PT, normal APTT	Mucocutaneous and joint bleeding; severity correlates with FVII level; treatment with recombinant FVIIa or FVII concentrates
FXIII deficiency	Autosomal recessive	PT and APTT NORMAL — diagnostic trap	Delayed umbilical stump bleeding (classical neonatal presentation), recurrent miscarriage, intracranial haemorrhage. Diagnose: clot solubility in 5M urea or factor XIII activity assay
Fibrinogen disorders	Autosomal recessive (afibrinogenaemia, hypofibrinogenaemia); autosomal dominant (dysfibrinogenaemia)	Prolonged PT, APTT, TT (with prolonged reptilase time — discriminates from heparin)	Bleeding pattern variable. Dysfibrinogenaemia may produce thrombosis as well as bleeding
FX, FV, FII (prothrombin), combined V+VIII	Autosomal recessive	Prolonged PT and APTT	Variable bleeding patterns; combined V+VIII deficiency is due to LMAN1 or MCFD2 mutations affecting factor secretion

Table 16.9: Rare coagulation factor deficiencies — exam-relevant features.

HIGH-YIELD PEARL — FXIII deficiency: bleeding with NORMAL screening tests

FXIII (the fibrin-stabilising factor) cross-links fibrin monomers into the mature stable clot. The PT and APTT measure clot formation (thrombin generation and fibrin polymerisation) and are NORMAL in FXIII deficiency because clot formation occurs — only clot stability is impaired.

The classical neonatal presentation is delayed umbilical stump bleeding 1–3 weeks after birth. Older patients present with delayed post-traumatic bleeding (initial clot forms, then breaks down hours later), recurrent miscarriage (FXIII is required for placental implantation), and intracranial haemorrhage.

Diagnostic move: clot solubility test in 5M urea or 1% monochloroacetic acid (a normal clot is stable; the FXIII-deficient clot dissolves within 24 hours) is a classical screen; specific FXIII activity assay confirms. Treatment: FXIII concentrate — Corifact/Fibrogammin P (plasma-derived) or Tretten/catridecacog (recombinant FXIII-A subunit); long half-life (~7 days) allows monthly or 4-weekly prophylaxis.

Vignettes describing "delayed umbilical stump bleeding in a neonate with normal PT and APTT" or "recurrent miscarriage with normal coagulation panel" are testing FXIII deficiency.

16.12 Disseminated Intravascular Coagulation and Acquired Bleeding States

Disseminated intravascular coagulation (DIC)

DIC is an acquired syndrome characterised by systemic activation of the coagulation cascade, leading to widespread microvascular thrombosis (with secondary multi-organ failure) AND simultaneous consumption of platelets, coagulation factors, and fibrinogen (with secondary bleeding). It is always a manifestation of an underlying disease — never a primary diagnosis. The triggering condition must be identified and treated; without resolution of the trigger, DIC continues regardless of supportive measures.

Trigger category	Examples
Sepsis	Gram-negative septicaemia (commonest), gram-positive sepsis, severe viral infection (dengue, severe COVID-19), severe malaria (especially falciparum); ~50% of DIC cases
Obstetric	Placental abruption, amniotic fluid embolism, retained products of conception, severe preeclampsia / HELLP, acute fatty liver of pregnancy
Malignancy	Acute promyelocytic leukaemia (APL — characteristic at diagnosis and during induction; tretinoin-treated has lower DIC), mucin-secreting adenocarcinomas (pancreatic, gastric, prostate), other solid and haematological malignancies
Trauma / surgery / shock	Severe trauma (especially head injury — brain tissue rich in tissue factor), massive crush injury, major burns, post-cardiopulmonary bypass
Other	Snake envenomation (Russell's viper, Echis), severe hepatic failure, transfusion reactions, transplant rejection, severe pancreatitis, vascular malformations (Kasabach-Merritt phenomenon)

Table 16.10: Triggers of disseminated intravascular coagulation. Sepsis dominates the differential globally.

Diagnosis is made by combining the clinical context (a recognised trigger) with the laboratory pattern: thrombocytopenia, prolonged PT and APTT, low fibrinogen (Clauss assay; <1.5 g/L is consumptive), markedly raised D-dimer (and FDPs), and schistocytes on the peripheral smear. The ISTH DIC scoring system uses platelet count, PT prolongation, fibrinogen, and D-dimer to categorise overt vs non-overt DIC; a score ≥5 is consistent with overt DIC. Some triggers produce predominantly thrombotic DIC (cancer, especially adenocarcinoma) and others produce predominantly haemorrhagic DIC (obstetric, APL); the picture depends on the balance of consumption vs activation.

Management has two axes. The primary intervention is treatment of the underlying trigger — antibiotics and source control in sepsis; delivery of the placenta in placental abruption or

HELLP; ATRA in APL; surgical control in trauma; antivenom in envenomation. Without addressing the trigger, supportive measures fail. The secondary axis is haemostatic support guided by the dominant clinical picture: in bleeding DIC, replace platelets to >50 × 10^9/L (>100 in CNS bleeding), fresh frozen plasma to correct PT/APTT, and cryoprecipitate or fibrinogen concentrate to maintain fibrinogen >1.5 g/L (>2 g/L in obstetric DIC). In thrombotic DIC with active microthrombosis, low-dose heparin or LMWH may be used cautiously when bleeding risk is acceptable. Antifibrinolytic agents (tranexamic acid) are generally avoided in DIC because they may exacerbate microvascular thrombosis — though they are used selectively in obstetric haemorrhage with concurrent fibrinolytic activity.

HIGH-YIELD PEARL — APL and DIC: the early-treatment imperative

Acute promyelocytic leukaemia (APL; AML with t(15;17)/PML::RARA) is associated with severe DIC at diagnosis and during the first days of induction therapy, because the APL blasts release tissue factor and annexin II–mediated tPA activation, simultaneously driving consumptive coagulopathy and primary fibrinolysis. Early intracranial haemorrhage is the leading cause of death in APL — and this risk is highest in the first 24–72 hours, before disease control is achieved.

The clinical imperative: when APL is even suspected (young patient with pancytopenia, atypical promyelocytes with bundles of Auer rods or "faggot cells", DIC), all-trans retinoic acid (ATRA) must be started EMPIRICALLY before molecular confirmation. ATRA differentiates the APL blasts and rapidly resolves the coagulopathy. Concurrent platelet support (target >50 × 10^9/L, often >100), cryoprecipitate or fibrinogen concentrate (target fibrinogen >1.5 g/L), and fresh frozen plasma are given aggressively. Arsenic trioxide is added in standard-risk APL on the basis of the Lo-Coco trial. The exam-significant point: never wait for molecular confirmation in suspected APL — start ATRA on clinical suspicion.

Other acquired bleeding states

Liver disease produces complex haemostatic dysfunction — reduced synthesis of multiple procoagulant factors (II, V, VII, IX, X, XI, fibrinogen) and natural anticoagulants (protein C, S, antithrombin), with FVIII paradoxically elevated. The result is a "rebalanced" haemostasis — not uniformly hypocoagulable, despite the prolonged PT/INR. Bleeding risk in cirrhosis is poorly predicted by PT/INR; viscoelastic testing is more informative. Vitamin K deficiency (covered in §16.5) presents with prolonged PT initially, followed by prolonged APTT as longer-half-life factors fall. Acquired vWF deficiency (in lymphoproliferative disorders, MGUS, severe aortic stenosis — Heyde syndrome — and in mechanical circulatory support devices like LVADs) presents as new mucocutaneous bleeding in adults; vWF studies show pattern resembling type 2A. Acquired haemophilia A (autoantibody to FVIII, occurring in autoimmune disease, malignancy, postpartum, idiopathic) is a potentially catastrophic disorder with extensive bruising and bleeding; mortality up to 20% without prompt diagnosis. Treatment is bypassing agents (rFVIIa, FEIBA) for active bleeding plus immunosuppression (steroids + cyclophosphamide or rituximab) to eradicate the inhibitor.

16.13 Buzzwords and Associations — Vignette Trigger Table

Single-line cues that should prompt specific diagnostic reflexes in haemostasis.

Vignette buzzword / finding	Diagnosis to trigger	One-line "why"
Toddler boy, spontaneous knee swelling and pain, X-linked family history	Haemophilia A or B	Severe FVIII or FIX deficiency presenting with first ambulation
Young woman, heavy menses, easy bruising, family history of bleeding	von Willebrand disease (Type 1)	Most common inherited bleeding disorder; mucocutaneous + family history
Mild thrombocytopenia + enhanced ristocetin-induced aggregation at low dose	Type 2B vWD	vWF gain-of-function for GPIb; DDAVP CONTRAINDICATED
Child with petechiae 1–4 weeks after viral illness; isolated thrombocytopenia	ITP, post-viral	70–80% spontaneous recovery in 6 months
Mucocutaneous bleeding from infancy; aggregation absent EXCEPT to ristocetin	Glanzmann thrombasthenia	GPIIb/IIIa deficiency
Mucocutaneous bleeding + giant platelets + mild thrombocytopenia + absent ristocetin response	Bernard-Soulier syndrome	GPIb/IX/V deficiency
Delayed umbilical stump bleeding; PT and APTT NORMAL	FXIII deficiency	Clot solubility test in 5M urea is the screen
Schistocytes + thrombocytopenia + neuro symptoms + AKI/fever (any combination)	TTP — empirically start PEX	ADAMTS13 <10%; PLASMIC ≥6 supports empirical treatment
Child with bloody diarrhoea 5 days ago + AKI + schistocytes + thrombocytopenia	STEC-HUS (E. coli O157:H7)	Antibiotics WORSEN; supportive care + dialysis
Adult with new severe bruising, prolonged APTT not correcting on incubated mixing study	Acquired haemophilia A (FVIII inhibitor)	Bethesda assay confirms; bypassing agents + immunosuppression
Young woman with prolonged APTT, no bleeding, recurrent miscarriage	Lupus anticoagulant / APLAS	Mixing does not correct; phospholipid-dependent

Vignette buzzword / finding	Diagnosis to trigger	One-line "why"
Promyelocytes with bundles of Auer rods (faggot cells) + DIC + low fibrinogen	Acute promyelocytic leukaemia (APL)	Start ATRA empirically; do not wait for molecular confirmation
Placental abruption + bleeding + low fibrinogen + raised D-dimer	Obstetric DIC	Deliver placenta; replace fibrinogen aggressively
Sepsis + low platelets + prolonged PT/APTT + low fibrinogen + raised D-dimer + schistocytes	Septic DIC	Treat the source; supportive blood products as needed
Heparin therapy day 5–10 + new thrombocytopenia (≥50% drop) + new venous or arterial thrombosis	Heparin-induced thrombocytopenia (HIT)	4Ts score; PF4 ELISA; serotonin release confirms; STOP heparin, start alternative anticoagulant (argatroban, fondaparinux)
Severe aortic stenosis + GI angiodysplasia bleeding	Heyde syndrome (acquired type 2A vWF deficiency)	High shear cleaves HMW multimers; resolves with valve replacement
Cirrhosis + bleeding; PT prolonged but bleeding worse than expected	Liver disease "rebalanced" haemostasis	TEG/ROTEM more informative than INR
Patient on warfarin + prolonged PT/INR + bleeding	Warfarin reversal	Vitamin K + PCC (4-factor preferred) for major bleeding
Patient on dabigatran + bleeding	Dabigatran reversal	Idarucizumab (specific anti-dabigatran Fab fragment)
Snake bite + bleeding from gums and venepuncture sites; prolonged PT/APTT and low fibrinogen	Russell's viper or Echis envenomation	Polyvalent antivenom + supportive blood products

Table 16.11: Haemostasis vignette triggers — exam-fast clue-to-diagnosis mapping.

16.14 USMLE Vignettes

Ten vignettes covering the highest-yield discriminations in haemostasis. Each tests a specific cognitive trap.

Vignette 1. An 18-month-old boy with a swollen knee

An 18-month-old boy is brought to the paediatric emergency department with a swollen, painful, warm right knee. He had been crawling and bumped his knee on the floor 24 hours earlier. There is no fever or systemic illness. His maternal uncle died as a young adult from "a bleeding problem after a tooth extraction." Examination: hot, tense, painful right knee with limited range of motion; no other joint involvement. Laboratory studies: haemoglobin 11.0 g/dL, platelet count 280,000/μL, peripheral smear normal. PT 12 seconds (control 11), APTT 78 seconds (control 30), thrombin time 14 seconds (normal). Mixing study: APTT corrects to 32 seconds immediately and remains normal after incubation. Factor assays: FVIII:C 0.8% (severe deficiency), FIX:C 95%, FXI 100%, FXII 100%, vWF:Ag 110%. Which of the following is the most appropriate diagnosis and immediate management?

(A) Haemophilia A, severe (FVIII:C <1%); FVIII concentrate 25 IU/kg IV (target FVIII ~50% for haemarthrosis), then prophylaxis programme to prevent recurrent joint bleeds.

(B) Haemophilia B, severe; FIX concentrate.

(C) Septic arthritis; joint aspirate, blood culture, IV antibiotics.

(D) Type 3 von Willebrand disease; vWF-containing concentrate.

(E) Reactive synovitis; rest, ice, and NSAIDs.

Best answer: (A) Haemophilia A, severe (FVIII:C <1%); FVIII concentrate 25 IU/kg IV (target FVIII ~50% for haemarthrosis), then prophylaxis programme to prevent recurrent joint bleeds.

Rationale. The clinical picture is severe haemophilia A presenting with first joint bleed at the start of ambulation. The X-linked family history (maternal uncle) confirms the inheritance pattern. The screening panel — prolonged APTT correcting on immediate mixing study (factor deficiency, not inhibitor), normal PT, normal platelets, normal vWF — and the specific factor assay (FVIII:C 0.8%) make the diagnosis. Severe haemophilia A is defined by FVIII:C <1%; clinical haemarthroses begin when the child becomes ambulant. Acute haemarthrosis treatment requires immediate FVIII replacement to ~40–50% (25 IU/kg IV; 1 IU/kg raises plasma FVIII by ~2%), with redosing every 12 h until clinical resolution. Joint rest, ice, and analgesia are adjuncts; NSAIDs are AVOIDED because of platelet inhibition. After the acute episode, prophylaxis (regular FVIII or extended half-life FVIII or emicizumab) should be initiated to prevent recurrent bleeds and target-joint development. Inhibitor screening (Bethesda assay) is performed at baseline and periodically because 20–30% of severe haemophilia A patients develop FVIII inhibitors during treatment.

Distractor analysis. (B) Haemophilia B has the same APTT-prolonging pattern but FIX:C is the deficient factor; FVIII is reduced here. (C) Septic arthritis is the differential for any single hot joint but does not explain the prolonged APTT and X-linked family history; the bleeding picture comes first. (D) Type 3 vWD would show very low vWF:Ag (this patient has 110%) and reduced FVIII as a secondary consequence. (E) Reactive synovitis would not explain the coagulation abnormality.

Vignette 2. A 16-year-old girl with menorrhagia and easy bruising

A 16-year-old girl is referred for evaluation of heavy menstrual bleeding requiring tampon plus pad, with passage of clots, lasting 8–10 days each cycle. She also bruises easily, has frequent epistaxis, and bled excessively after a dental extraction at age 12. Her mother had similar problems and required transfusion after delivery. Examination: scattered bruises on extremities; otherwise normal. Laboratory studies: haemoglobin 9.4 g/dL, MCV 76 fL, ferritin 8 ng/mL (iron deficiency from chronic blood loss), platelets 220,000/µL, normal smear. PT 12 s, APTT 38 s (slightly prolonged), thrombin time normal. PFA-100: closure time prolonged on both collagen-ADP and collagen-epinephrine cartridges. vWF:Ag 25%, vWF:RCo 20%, ratio 0.80, FVIII:C 30%. vWF multimer analysis: full range of multimers, all reduced. Which of the following is the most appropriate diagnosis and management?

(A) von Willebrand disease, Type 1; iron repletion, tranexamic acid for menses, and DDAVP trial in clinic to confirm response — DDAVP for procedures and bleeding episodes if responsive.

(B) Type 2B vWD; vWF-containing concentrate; DDAVP contraindicated.

(C) Type 3 vWD; vWF-containing concentrate; DDAVP ineffective.

(D) Mild haemophilia A; FVIII concentrate.

(E) Idiopathic menorrhagia; oral contraceptive pill alone.

Best answer: (A) von Willebrand disease, Type 1; iron repletion, tranexamic acid for menses, and DDAVP trial in clinic to confirm response — DDAVP for procedures and bleeding episodes if responsive.

Rationale. The clinical picture is Type 1 vWD: lifelong mucocutaneous bleeding (menorrhagia, epistaxis, easy bruising, prolonged dental bleeding), autosomal dominant family history, and proportionate reduction of vWF:Ag (25%, below the 2021 ASH/ISTH/NHF/WFH Type 1 threshold of <30 IU/dL) and vWF:RCo (20%) with a normal vWF:RCo / vWF:Ag ratio of 0.80 (>0.7) and a full multimer pattern at reduced concentration. FVIII is reduced proportionally as a secondary consequence. Treatment combines (i) iron repletion (chronic blood loss has produced iron-deficiency anaemia); (ii) tranexamic acid (oral 1–1.5 g 8-hourly during menses); (iii) DDAVP trial in advance of clinical need to document the individual response — if responsive, DDAVP (intranasal or IV) can cover procedures and bleeding episodes; (iv) hormonal therapy (combined OCP, progestin IUD) may help heavy menstrual bleeding; (v) vWF concentrates if DDAVP fails, for major surgery, or in type 3 disease.

Distractor analysis. (B) Type 2B has reduced HMW multimers, enhanced low-dose RIPA, and mild thrombocytopenia — not seen here. (C) Type 3 has UNDETECTABLE vWF:Ag and very low FVIII (often <10%); the mild reduction here excludes it. (D) Mild haemophilia A is X-linked, would not explain the menorrhagia, and would have normal vWF:Ag/RCo. (E) Treating only the menses misses the underlying vWD diagnosis.

Vignette 3. A 24-year-old woman with mild thrombocytopenia and bleeding — the DDAVP trap

A 24-year-old woman is referred for preoperative evaluation prior to a planned cholecystectomy. She has a history of easy bruising and menorrhagia. CBC: platelet count 110,000/µL (mildly reduced), normal Hb and WBC. PT 12 s, APTT 36 s, vWF:Ag 60%, vWF:RCo 28%, ratio 0.47 (<0.7 — disproportionate functional loss), FVIII:C 65%. vWF multimer analysis: HMW multimers reduced in plasma; preserved in platelet lysates.

Low-dose ristocetin (0.5 mg/mL) induced platelet aggregation (RIPA): markedly enhanced response. Which of the following is the most appropriate management?

(A) Type 2B von Willebrand disease — DDAVP is CONTRAINDICATED. Cover surgery with vWF-containing concentrate (Humate-P / Wilate / Voncento); platelet transfusion if needed.

(B) Type 1 vWD; DDAVP intranasally pre-procedure.

(C) ITP; corticosteroids and IVIg before surgery.

(D) Heparin-induced thrombocytopenia; argatroban.

(E) Type 2A vWD; DDAVP.

Best answer: (A) Type 2B von Willebrand disease — DDAVP is CONTRAINDICATED. Cover surgery with vWF-containing concentrate (Humate-P / Wilate / Voncento); platelet transfusion if needed.

Rationale. The diagnostic profile is classical Type 2B vWD: vWF:RCo / vWF:Ag ratio <0.7 (functional loss disproportionate to antigen), HMW multimers depleted in plasma but preserved in platelet lysates (the discriminator from Type 2A, where multimers are absent in both), enhanced RIPA at low-dose ristocetin (the key functional finding — gain-of-function of vWF for GPIb, leading to increased platelet binding in vivo and the secondary mild thrombocytopenia), and mild thrombocytopenia (~110,000/µL). DDAVP is CONTRAINDICATED in Type 2B because it releases more abnormal vWF, which binds platelets and worsens thrombocytopenia, paradoxically increasing bleeding risk. The exam trap is to default to DDAVP for any "mild" vWD without testing for Type 2B with multimer analysis and low-dose RIPA. Procedures in Type 2B vWD are covered with vWF-containing factor concentrates (Humate-P, Wilate, Voncento, recombinant vWF), with platelet transfusion as needed for active bleeding.

Distractor analysis. (B) Type 1 has proportionate reduction (ratio >0.7) and preserved multimers — this case has neither. (C) ITP would not have the abnormal vWF profile. (D) HIT requires heparin exposure and the 4Ts pattern. (E) Type 2A also has reduced HMW multimers but no platelet binding gain-of-function and no thrombocytopenia; DDAVP can be used in 2A.

Vignette 4. A 6-year-old girl with petechiae two weeks after a viral illness

A 6-year-old girl is brought in with petechiae over both legs and trunk and gum bleeding while brushing teeth. She had a febrile upper respiratory illness three weeks ago that resolved spontaneously. She is otherwise well, attending school, with normal growth and development. Examination: scattered petechiae on legs, trunk, and oral mucosa; no lymphadenopathy or hepatosplenomegaly; otherwise normal. Laboratory studies: haemoglobin 12.4 g/dL, white blood cells 7,200/µL with normal differential, platelets 12,000/µL. Peripheral smear: occasional large platelets (young, large platelets typical of accelerated turnover); no schistocytes; normal red and white cell morphology. PT 12 s, APTT 30 s, fibrinogen normal. ANA, HIV, hepatitis C: negative. Which of the following is the most appropriate management?

(A) Diagnose primary immune thrombocytopenia (post-viral); given platelets <20,000/µL with mucosal bleeding, treat with corticosteroids OR IVIg; consider observation alone if no significant bleeding.

(B) Bone marrow biopsy is required before any treatment to exclude leukaemia.

(C) Splenectomy.

(D) Platelet transfusion alone.

(E) Heparin for suspected DIC.

Best answer: (A) Diagnose primary immune thrombocytopenia (post-viral); given platelets <20,000/µL with mucosal bleeding, treat with corticosteroids OR IVIg; consider observation alone if no significant bleeding.

Rationale. The clinical picture is classical paediatric primary immune thrombocytopenia (ITP) following a recent viral infection. The criteria are met: isolated thrombocytopenia (no anaemia, no leukocyte abnormality, no schistocytes, normal coagulation), no organomegaly or lymphadenopathy, no clinical or serological evidence of secondary cause (normal ANA, negative HIV and HCV). Bone marrow biopsy is NOT required in typical paediatric ITP; it is reserved for atypical features (additional cytopenias, organomegaly, abnormal smear). 70–80% of paediatric ITP recovers spontaneously within 6 months. Treatment indications in paediatric ITP are bleeding (not just platelet count alone). For platelets <20,000 with mucosal bleeding, first-line options are corticosteroids (prednisolone 2–4 mg/kg/day for 2–4 weeks then taper) OR IVIg 1 g/kg (rapid effect, fewer steroid side-effects). Anti-D Ig is an alternative in Rh-positive non-splenectomised children but used less now. Observation is reasonable in mild bleeding with platelets >20,000.

Distractor analysis. (B) Bone marrow biopsy is not required in typical childhood ITP; the smear and clinical picture are sufficient. (C) Splenectomy is reserved for chronic refractory disease, not first-line. (D) Platelet transfusion alone is ineffective in ITP because transfused platelets are also destroyed; reserved for life-threatening bleeding alongside specific therapy. (E) DIC requires evidence of consumptive coagulopathy (low fibrinogen, raised D-dimer, prolonged PT/APTT) — none present here.

Vignette 5. A 38-year-old woman with confusion, fever, and a low platelet count

A 38-year-old woman is admitted with three days of progressive confusion, fever, and bruising. Her husband reports she has been increasingly forgetful and is now intermittently disoriented. She has no significant past medical history and is on no medications. Examination: temperature 38.4°C, BP 142/88, pulse 102, alert but confused; scattered ecchymoses; no focal neurological deficit; no significant lymphadenopathy or hepatosplenomegaly. Laboratory studies: haemoglobin 8.2 g/dL, MCV 92 fL, reticulocyte count elevated, platelets 14,000/µL, white blood cells 9,800/µL. Peripheral smear: numerous schistocytes (>5 per high-power field), polychromasia, no spherocytes. LDH 1,840 U/L, total bilirubin 4.2 mg/dL (predominantly indirect), haptoglobin <10 mg/dL, direct antiglobulin test negative. PT 13 s, APTT 32 s, fibrinogen 280 mg/dL (normal), D-dimer mildly elevated. Creatinine 1.4 mg/dL. Urinalysis: trace protein, no haematuria. PLASMIC score: 7. Which of the following is the most appropriate immediate management?

(A) Send blood for ADAMTS13 activity and inhibitor testing, then INITIATE PLASMA EXCHANGE THE SAME DAY without waiting for the result; add corticosteroids; consider caplacizumab and rituximab.

(B) Eculizumab for atypical haemolytic uraemic syndrome.

(C) Empirical antibiotics for sepsis-associated DIC; supportive care.

(D) Corticosteroids alone; platelet transfusion to raise count above 50,000.

(E) Wait for ADAMTS13 result before initiating any specific therapy.

Best answer: (A) Send blood for ADAMTS13 activity and inhibitor testing, then INITIATE PLASMA EXCHANGE THE SAME DAY without waiting for the result; add corticosteroids; consider caplacizumab and rituximab.

Rationale. The clinical picture is acquired immune-mediated TTP. The key elements are microangiopathic haemolytic anaemia (schistocytes, raised LDH, low haptoglobin, indirect hyperbilirubinaemia, negative DAT), thrombocytopenia, neurological involvement (confusion), mild renal impairment, fever, and a normal coagulation panel (DIC excluded by normal fibrinogen and only mildly raised D-dimer). The classical pentad — fever + neuro symptoms + renal failure + MAHA + thrombocytopenia — is mostly historical; modern diagnosis requires only MAHA + thrombocytopenia without an alternative cause to start treatment urgently. The PLASMIC score (≥6 supports severe ADAMTS13 deficiency) is 7 here. ADAMTS13 activity will likely be <10% with an inhibitor present. Plasma exchange is the cornerstone — it removes the inhibitor and replaces ADAMTS13. Without PEX, mortality exceeds 90%; with PEX, mortality drops to <10–20%. PEX must be initiated the same day as suspicion arises; ADAMTS13 testing takes >24 h and PEX cannot wait. Corticosteroids (prednisolone 1 mg/kg or pulsed methylprednisolone) are added. Caplacizumab (anti-vWF A1 nanobody) accelerates platelet recovery and reduces TTP-related mortality and refractoriness — added to PEX in many centres. Rituximab is added for refractory disease or to prevent relapse in confirmed autoimmune TTP. Platelet transfusion is AVOIDED in TTP unless life-threatening bleeding is present (may worsen microvascular thrombosis).

Distractor analysis. (B) Atypical HUS is a complement-mediated TMA primarily affecting the kidney; this patient's neurological dominance with mild renal involvement and adult onset fits TTP better. Eculizumab is reserved when ADAMTS13 is ≥10% and complement disease is suspected. (C) DIC requires consumptive coagulopathy (low fibrinogen, raised D-dimer, prolonged PT/APTT); none present. (D) Corticosteroids alone are inadequate without PEX. (E) Waiting for ADAMTS13 risks fatal delay; the PLASMIC score and clinical pattern justify empirical PEX.

Vignette 6. A 5-year-old boy with bloody diarrhoea and acute kidney injury

A 5-year-old boy is admitted with one day of progressive lethargy, oliguria, and pallor. Five days previously he had developed bloody diarrhoea, which has now resolved, after a family barbeque where undercooked beef was served. His older sister had similar diarrhoea but no further symptoms. Examination: pallor, mild abdominal tenderness, otherwise unremarkable; alert and oriented. Laboratory studies: haemoglobin 6.8 g/dL, MCV 88 fL, platelets 38,000/µL, reticulocytes 6%, white blood cells 14,200/µL. Peripheral smear: schistocytes, polychromasia, no spherocytes, occasional helmet cells. LDH 1,420 U/L, total bilirubin 2.4 mg/dL, haptoglobin <10 mg/dL, DAT negative. Creatinine 3.8 mg/dL (baseline normal), urea 78 mg/dL, urinalysis with proteinuria and red blood cell casts. PT, APTT, fibrinogen all normal. Stool PCR positive for Shiga-toxin-producing Escherichia coli O157:H7. Which of the following is the most appropriate management?

(A) Supportive care — careful intravenous fluid resuscitation, correction of electrolyte abnormalities, dialysis if needed, transfusion as needed; AVOID antibiotics (worsen outcomes by lysing bacteria and releasing more Shiga toxin).

(B) Plasma exchange for thrombotic thrombocytopenic purpura.

(C) Eculizumab as first-line for typical (Shiga toxin–mediated) HUS.

(D) Empirical broad-spectrum antibiotics for invasive Shigella-like infection.

(E) Anti-motility agents (loperamide) for symptomatic relief.

Best answer: (A) Supportive care — careful intravenous fluid resuscitation, correction of electrolyte abnormalities, dialysis if needed, transfusion as needed; AVOID antibiotics (worsen outcomes by lysing bacteria and releasing more Shiga toxin).

Rationale. The clinical picture is classical Shiga-toxin-producing E. coli (STEC) haemolytic uraemic syndrome — a child with bloody diarrhoea (resolved) followed in 3–10 days by MAHA, thrombocytopenia, and acute kidney injury. The triad of MAHA + thrombocytopenia + AKI in the post-diarrhoeal context is HUS. Stool PCR confirms STEC O157:H7. Treatment is supportive: careful fluid resuscitation (avoiding overload that worsens AKI), management of electrolyte derangements (hyperkalaemia, hyperphosphataemia, metabolic acidosis), red cell transfusion for symptomatic anaemia (target Hb >7 g/dL), and dialysis when indicated for AKI. Antibiotics WORSEN outcomes in STEC-HUS — multiple observational studies and a meta-analysis show that antibiotic exposure increases progression to HUS in children with STEC diarrhoea, possibly by inducing bacterial lysis and increased toxin release. Anti-motility agents are similarly avoided because they prolong intestinal transit and toxin exposure. Plasma exchange is not effective in typical STEC-HUS (the mechanism is toxin-driven endothelial injury, not ADAMTS13 deficiency). Eculizumab is reserved for atypical HUS (complement-mediated) or severe refractory STEC-HUS in selected patients. Most children recover renal function with supportive care; ~5% mortality; some develop chronic kidney disease.

Distractor analysis. (B) PEX is for TTP (severe ADAMTS13 deficiency); not effective in typical STEC-HUS. (C) Eculizumab is for atypical HUS (complement-mediated), not first-line for STEC-HUS. (D) Antibiotics worsen STEC-HUS. (E) Anti-motility agents prolong toxin exposure and worsen outcomes.

Vignette 7. A 28-year-old woman in obstructed labour with placental abruption and bleeding

A 28-year-old G3P2 woman at 38 weeks gestation is admitted in labour with severe abdominal pain and vaginal bleeding. She has hypertension (BP 168/110) and protein on urine dipstick. Ultrasound: extensive placental abruption. After delivery of a stillborn infant, she develops profuse vaginal bleeding, oozing from venepuncture sites, and haematuria. Vital signs: BP 86/54, pulse 132, oxygen saturation 94%. Examination: pallor, oozing from IV sites, scattered petechiae. Laboratory studies (drawn during resuscitation): haemoglobin 6.4 g/dL, platelets 38,000/µL (was 220,000/µL on admission), peripheral smear with schistocytes. PT 28 s (control 12), APTT 76 s (control 30), thrombin time 32 s, Clauss fibrinogen 0.7 g/L (normal 2–4), D-dimer markedly elevated. ISTH DIC score: 7 (overt DIC). Which of the following is the most appropriate management?

(A) Treat the trigger (uterotonics, surgical control of haemorrhage, evacuate retained products if present) AND replace fibrinogen aggressively (cryoprecipitate or fibrinogen concentrate; target fibrinogen >2 g/L in obstetric DIC), platelet transfusion (target >50 × 10^9/L), fresh frozen plasma to correct PT/APTT, packed red cells, tranexamic acid 1 g IV (WOMAN trial).

(B) Heparin to interrupt the consumptive coagulopathy.

(C) Plasma exchange for TTP.

(D) Recombinant FVIIa empirically without correction of fibrinogen.

(E) Observation only — DIC will self-resolve once the placenta is delivered.

Best answer: (A) Treat the trigger (uterotonics, surgical control of haemorrhage, evacuate retained products if present) AND replace fibrinogen aggressively (cryoprecipitate or fibrinogen concentrate; target fibrinogen >2 g/L in obstetric DIC), platelet transfusion (target >50 × 10^9/L), fresh frozen plasma to correct PT/APTT, packed red cells, tranexamic acid 1 g IV (WOMAN trial).

Rationale. The clinical picture is severe obstetric DIC from placental abruption complicated by preeclampsia. The diagnostic features — thrombocytopenia, prolonged PT and APTT, very low fibrinogen (0.7 g/L), markedly raised D-dimer, schistocytes — meet the ISTH overt DIC criteria. The principles of management are simultaneous: (1) treat the underlying trigger — uterotonics (oxytocin, then ergometrine, carboprost, misoprostol), surgical haemostasis, B-Lynch suture, internal iliac artery ligation, or hysterectomy if conservative measures fail; (2) replace coagulation factors with cryoprecipitate or fibrinogen concentrate (fibrinogen <1 g/L and obstetric haemorrhage demand aggressive replacement to >2 g/L), fresh frozen plasma, platelets, and red cells; (3) tranexamic acid 1 g IV (the WOMAN trial established TXA in postpartum haemorrhage, reducing maternal mortality from bleeding when given within 3 hours of bleeding onset). The MOET / OBLS protocols and obstetric early warning scores guide local practice. Heparin is GENERALLY AVOIDED in haemorrhagic DIC because it worsens bleeding; reserved for thrombotic DIC (e.g., adenocarcinoma). rFVIIa is a last-resort option after correction of fibrinogen, platelets, and core temperature.

Distractor analysis. (B) Heparin in actively bleeding DIC worsens bleeding. (C) TTP requires MAHA + thrombocytopenia without low fibrinogen — this case has consumptive coagulopathy, not TMA. (D) rFVIIa requires adequate fibrinogen, platelets, and temperature for efficacy; using it without correction is ineffective. (E) Observation in active obstetric DIC is fatal.

Vignette 8. A 22-year-old woman with pancytopenia, bruising, and atypical promyelocytes

A 22-year-old woman presents with two weeks of progressive fatigue, fever, and easy bruising, and one day of gum bleeding. Examination: pallor, petechiae, ecchymoses, oral mucosal bleeding, no organomegaly. Laboratory studies: haemoglobin 7.4 g/dL, platelets 18,000/µL, white blood cells 38,000/µL with 78% atypical cells. Peripheral smear: large hypergranular cells with bilobed or kidney-shaped nuclei, abundant azurophilic granules, and bundles of Auer rods (faggot cells). PT 22 s, APTT 48 s, fibrinogen 0.9 g/L, D-dimer markedly elevated, schistocytes occasional on smear. Immunophenotyping (preliminary, on flow): blasts CD34 negative, HLA-DR negative, CD117 bright, CD33 bright, CD13 positive. Cytogenetics and PML::RARA RT-PCR results are pending. Which of the following is the most appropriate immediate management?

(A) Initiate ATRA (all-trans retinoic acid) IMMEDIATELY on clinical suspicion, before molecular confirmation; aggressive platelet (target >30–50 × 10^9/L), cryoprecipitate / fibrinogen concentrate (target fibrinogen >1.5 g/L), and FFP support; arsenic trioxide added once standard-risk APL is confirmed.

(B) Wait for the PML::RARA RT-PCR result before starting ATRA; supportive care in the interim.

(C) Standard "7+3" induction (cytarabine + daunorubicin) for AML.

(D) Heparin infusion to interrupt the consumptive coagulopathy.

(E) Plasma exchange for thrombotic thrombocytopenic purpura.

Best answer: (A) Initiate ATRA (all-trans retinoic acid) IMMEDIATELY on clinical suspicion, before molecular confirmation; aggressive platelet (target >30–50 × 10^9/L), cryoprecipitate / fibrinogen concentrate (target fibrinogen >1.5 g/L), and FFP support; arsenic trioxide added once standard-risk APL is confirmed.

Rationale. The clinical picture is acute promyelocytic leukaemia (APL; AML-M3 in older nomenclature, or AML with t(15;17) / PML::RARA in WHO 2022). The diagnostic clues are the morphology (hypergranular promyelocytes with bundles of Auer rods — "faggot cells"), the immunophenotype (CD34 negative, HLA-DR negative, CD117+, CD33 bright — distinguishes APL from typical AML which is CD34+/HLA-DR+), and the dramatic DIC at presentation (low platelets, low fibrinogen, raised D-dimer, prolonged PT/APTT). APL blasts release tissue factor and annexin II–mediated tissue plasminogen activator, simultaneously driving consumptive coagulopathy and primary fibrinolysis. Early intracranial haemorrhage is the leading cause of death in APL — and risk is highest in the first 24–72 hours. The clinical imperative is to start ATRA EMPIRICALLY on clinical suspicion (without waiting for PML::RARA molecular confirmation, which can take 24–48 hours). ATRA differentiates the APL blasts within days and resolves the coagulopathy. Aggressive haemostatic support — platelet transfusion to target >30–50 × 10^9/L (some guidelines >50), cryoprecipitate or fibrinogen concentrate to target fibrinogen >1.5 g/L, and FFP to correct PT/APTT — is given concurrently. Arsenic trioxide is added once the diagnosis is confirmed as standard-risk APL (Lo-Coco trial: ATRA + ATO is curative in ~95% of standard-risk APL without traditional chemotherapy).

Distractor analysis. (B) Waiting for confirmation risks fatal intracranial haemorrhage; the morphology and immunophenotype are sufficient to start ATRA. (C) Standard 7+3 in APL is associated with a high early death rate from DIC; ATRA is the disease-defining treatment. (D) Heparin in APL DIC is generally avoided because of dominant haemorrhagic features. (E) TTP requires MAHA without low fibrinogen; APL DIC has consumptive coagulopathy.

Vignette 9. A 32-year-old woman with two miscarriages and a prolonged APTT

A 32-year-old woman is referred for evaluation of three consecutive first-trimester miscarriages and an isolated prolonged APTT noted on routine pre-procedural workup before a planned cholecystectomy. She has had no spontaneous bleeding. Examination is unremarkable. Laboratory studies: haemoglobin 13.2 g/dL, platelets 178,000/µL, normal smear. PT 12 s, APTT 52 s (control 30), thrombin time normal. Mixing study: APTT does NOT correct on immediate mix (53 s vs expected 36 s). Thrombin time and reptilase time normal (excludes heparin and dabigatran). dRVVT prolonged with high screen-to-confirm ratio; lupus anticoagulant confirmed; anti-cardiolipin IgG and anti-beta-2 glycoprotein I IgG both elevated. Which of the following is the most likely diagnosis and most appropriate management?

(A) Antiphospholipid syndrome (lupus anticoagulant + recurrent pregnancy loss + persistent antibodies on confirmation); refer for haematology and rheumatology assessment, plan low-molecular-weight heparin + low-dose aspirin during a future pregnancy; do NOT defer the cholecystectomy on the basis of the APTT alone (the in-vitro prolongation does not predict bleeding).

(B) Acquired haemophilia A; corticosteroids and bypassing agents.

(C) FXII deficiency; reassurance only.

(D) Low-molecular-weight heparin overdose; reverse with protamine.

(E) Defer cholecystectomy indefinitely until APTT normalises.

Best answer: (A) Antiphospholipid syndrome (lupus anticoagulant + recurrent pregnancy loss + persistent antibodies on confirmation); refer for haematology and rheumatology assessment, plan low-molecular-weight heparin + low-dose aspirin during a future pregnancy; do NOT defer the cholecystectomy on the basis of the APTT alone (the in-vitro prolongation does not predict bleeding).

Rationale. The diagnostic picture is antiphospholipid syndrome (obstetric form). The criteria are met: (i) clinical — three unexplained consecutive first-trimester miscarriages (the obstetric criterion: three or more <10 weeks, OR one or more ≥10 weeks, OR one premature birth before 34 weeks due to placental insufficiency); (ii) laboratory — lupus anticoagulant (mixing study fails to correct, dRVVT confirms phospholipid dependence) AND anti-cardiolipin IgG AND anti-beta-2 glycoprotein I IgG, with definitive diagnosis requiring confirmation by repeat antibody testing ≥12 weeks apart. The in-vitro APTT prolongation is a paradoxical laboratory artefact; lupus anticoagulant patients tend to thrombosis, NOT bleeding, in vivo. The cholecystectomy can proceed safely because the bleeding risk is not increased by the APTT prolongation; thromboprophylaxis is the priority. Future pregnancy management is LMWH + low-dose aspirin (the standard combination since the Greer/Empson/Rai trials). APLAS is covered comprehensively in Chapter 17.

Distractor analysis. (B) Acquired haemophilia A would have severe spontaneous bleeding (this patient has none), and the inhibitor would specifically deplete FVIII (the case shows lupus anticoagulant, not FVIII-specific antibody). (C) FXII deficiency causes prolonged APTT without bleeding but does not cause recurrent miscarriage and would not show lupus anticoagulant on confirmatory testing. (D) No history of LMWH exposure. (E) Cancelling surgery on the basis of an APTT that does not predict bleeding is a clinical error.

Vignette 10. A 71-year-old man with new severe bruising and a prolonged APTT

A 71-year-old man with no past medical history of bleeding is admitted with two weeks of progressive extensive bruising over the trunk and limbs, including a large flank haematoma. He had no preceding trauma. He takes no anticoagulants or antiplatelet agents. Examination: extensive deep ecchymoses, a 10 × 8 cm right flank haematoma, no joint swelling, no lymphadenopathy or hepatosplenomegaly. Laboratory studies: haemoglobin 7.8 g/dL, platelets 240,000/µL, normal smear. PT 12 s, APTT 78 s (control 30), thrombin time normal. Mixing study: APTT corrects to 38 s IMMEDIATELY (close to normal range), but on incubation at 37°C for 2 h prolongs to 65 s (TIME-DEPENDENT inhibitor). FVIII:C 4% (markedly reduced); FIX, FXI, FXII normal; vWF:Ag and vWF:RCo normal. Bethesda assay: FVIII inhibitor titre 22 BU. Which of the following is the most likely diagnosis and most appropriate management?

(A) Acquired haemophilia A (autoantibody to FVIII); urgent treatment with bypassing agents (recombinant FVIIa or activated prothrombin complex concentrate / FEIBA) for active bleeding; immunosuppression (corticosteroids + cyclophosphamide OR rituximab) to eradicate the inhibitor.

(B) Inherited mild haemophilia A presenting in old age; FVIII concentrate.

(C) Lupus anticoagulant; aspirin.

(D) Type 3 von Willebrand disease; vWF concentrate.

(E) Vitamin K deficiency; oral vitamin K.

Best answer: (A) Acquired haemophilia A (autoantibody to FVIII); urgent treatment with bypassing agents (recombinant FVIIa or activated prothrombin complex concentrate / FEIBA) for active bleeding; immunosuppression (corticosteroids + cyclophosphamide OR rituximab) to eradicate the inhibitor.

Rationale. The diagnosis is acquired haemophilia A — an autoantibody (autoimmune inhibitor) directed against FVIII, producing severe bleeding in a previously haemostatically normal patient, typically older or postpartum. The diagnostic chain is decisive: (i) prolonged APTT with normal PT and platelet count; (ii) mixing study correcting immediately but prolonging on incubation (TIME-DEPENDENT inhibitor — the kinetic signature of FVIII inhibitors); (iii) low FVIII:C with otherwise normal coagulation factors; (iv) Bethesda assay confirms inhibitor titre and quantifies severity. Mortality of acquired haemophilia A is up to 20% if untreated; aggressive management is required. Acute bleeding is treated with bypassing agents — recombinant FVIIa (NovoSeven) or activated prothrombin complex concentrate (FEIBA) — which generate thrombin without FVIII. Some guidelines now use emicizumab in this context. Immunosuppression to eradicate the inhibitor combines corticosteroids with cyclophosphamide or rituximab; complete remission is achieved in most patients within months. Underlying associations include autoimmune disease (RA, SLE), malignancy (lymphoproliferative, solid), pregnancy and postpartum (younger women), and idiopathic; investigate for underlying cause once acute treatment is established.

Distractor analysis. (B) Inherited haemophilia A presents in childhood with X-linked family history; new severe bleeding in a 71-year-old with no prior bleeding history is acquired. (C) Lupus anticoagulant produces APTT prolongation that does NOT correct on mixing (immediate or delayed) and is not associated with severe spontaneous bleeding. (D) Type 3 vWD presents in childhood with very low vWF:Ag — this patient has normal vWF. (E) Vitamin K deficiency prolongs PT (and APTT later); this patient has isolated APTT prolongation with low FVIII.

16.15 Closing Discriminators

HIGH-YIELD PEARL — Primary vs secondary bleeding pattern — the bleeding tells you the layer

Bleeding immediately at the time of injury, mucocutaneous distribution (petechiae, gum bleeding, menorrhagia, easy bruising, prolonged epistaxis, prolonged bleeding from superficial cuts) → primary haemostasis defect (platelet count or function, vWF). Bleeding time / PFA-100 prolonged.

Bleeding delayed after injury (the platelet plug forms then fails when fibrin reinforcement does not arrive), deep-tissue distribution (haemarthroses, intramuscular haematomas, retroperitoneal, intracranial) → secondary haemostasis defect (coagulation factor deficiency). PT and/or APTT prolonged.

Mixed pattern (mucocutaneous + deep) → vWD (loss of platelet adhesion + reduced FVIII), severe DIC, severe liver disease, complex acquired states.

Bleeding pattern + screening panel + family history together resolve >90% of bleeding disorders before specific factor assays are sent.

HIGH-YIELD PEARL — DDAVP contraindications across vWD subtypes

DDAVP releases endogenous vWF from endothelial Weibel-Palade bodies, producing a 3- to 5-fold rise in vWF:Ag for 6–12 hours. Use depends critically on vWD subtype:

- Type 1 — DDAVP usually effective. Always perform an in-clinic DDAVP trial in advance to document the individual patient response (not all type 1 patients respond).
- Type 2A — DDAVP often partially effective; use guided by trial response.
- Type 2B — DDAVP CONTRAINDICATED. Releasing more abnormal gain-of-function vWF binds platelets and worsens thrombocytopenia, paradoxically increasing bleeding risk. Use vWF-containing concentrate.
- Type 2M — DDAVP usually effective but variable; trial first.
- Type 2N — DDAVP transiently raises vWF and FVIII but the released vWF still cannot bind FVIII; useful for minor procedures, not for major surgery — use vWF concentrate.
- Type 3 — DDAVP INEFFECTIVE (no endogenous vWF stores to release). Use vWF concentrate.

Other DDAVP cautions: hyponatraemia and seizures from antidiuretic effect (limit fluids; especially in young children); avoid repeated dosing within 24–48 hours; avoid in the elderly with cardiovascular comorbidity.

HIGH-YIELD PEARL — Mixing study decision tree for prolonged APTT

A prolonged APTT in a bleeding patient (or one that needs explanation) is resolved by the 50:50 mixing study with NORMAL pooled plasma, with timing matters:

- CORRECTS immediately → factor deficiency. Send sequential factor assays (FVIII, IX, XI, XII) and a vWD panel if FVIII is reduced.
- DOES NOT correct immediately → immediate-acting inhibitor. Most commonly LUPUS ANTICOAGULANT (test with dRVVT and confirm phospholipid dependence). Also: heparin (TT prolonged, reptilase normal — discriminates), DOAC (drug history; specific

anti-Xa or anti-IIa assays), or factor-specific antibody.

- CORRECTS immediately but PROLONGS on incubation (1–2 h, 37°C) → TIME-DEPENDENT INHIBITOR. The kinetic signature of FVIII inhibitor (acquired haemophilia A) and some FIX inhibitors. Quantify with Bethesda assay (Nijmegen modification for low titres).

Always run TT and reptilase time alongside any unexplained APTT prolongation: TT prolonged + reptilase normal = heparin; TT prolonged + reptilase prolonged = dysfibrinogenaemia or hypofibrinogenaemia.

HIGH-YIELD PEARL — DIC vs TTP vs HELLP vs liver disease — discriminators

Four conditions can produce thrombocytopenia + coagulopathy in the unwell hospitalised patient. The discriminator lies in fibrinogen, D-dimer, ADAMTS13, and clinical context.

- DIC — Low fibrinogen, very high D-dimer, prolonged PT and APTT, schistocytes; ALWAYS has an underlying trigger (sepsis, obstetric, malignancy, trauma). ISTH score ≥5 = overt DIC. Treat the trigger; replace components.
- TTP — MAHA + thrombocytopenia + neuro/renal involvement; FIBRINOGEN AND COAGULATION ARE NORMAL (the discriminator from DIC); ADAMTS13 <10%. PLASMIC ≥6 supports empirical PEX.
- HELLP (preeclampsia) — Pregnancy-associated; Haemolysis + Elevated Liver enzymes + Low Platelets; LDH raised, AST/ALT raised, schistocytes; coagulation usually normal unless overlapping DIC. Treat: deliver the fetus.
- Liver disease — Prolonged PT, prolonged APTT (variable), thrombocytopenia (hypersplenism), but FVIII often elevated (paradoxical) and natural anticoagulants reduced; haemostasis "rebalanced". TEG/ROTEM more informative than INR. Discriminator from vitamin K deficiency: FV is reduced in liver disease, normal in vitamin K deficiency.

Send the right test: fibrinogen + D-dimer (DIC); ADAMTS13 + PLASMIC (TTP); LFTs in pregnancy (HELLP); FV in unclear liver/coagulopathy.

IMG-TRAP — Tropical-anchor bias on USMLE thrombocytopenia vignettes

The trap. IMGs trained in tropical settings often default to dengue, falciparum malaria, tuberculosis, or visceral leishmaniasis when faced with thrombocytopenia or DIC, because that is the dominant pattern in their daily case mix. USMLE vignettes are written from a US epidemiological frame: the high-yield answer key is ITP (idiopathic or post-viral, especially in children), drug-induced thrombocytopenia (heparin/HIT, quinine, vancomycin, sulfa, linezolid), TTP (severe ADAMTS13 deficiency), STEC-HUS (post-bloody-diarrhoea in a child), DIC (sepsis, APL, obstetric emergencies), and the inherited disorders (vWD, Glanzmann, Bernard–Soulier, haemophilia).

The rule. Even when a USMLE stem mentions recent travel or tropical exposure, find the unique discriminator before reaching for an infection-driven explanation. Schistocytes plus neurological signs in a young woman = TTP (not malaria). Bloody diarrhoea then thrombocytopenia and AKI in a child = STEC-HUS (not dengue). New thrombocytopenia 5–10 days after surgery on heparin = HIT (not TB). Faggot cells with DIC at induction = APL (not severe sepsis). Travel exposure is usually a red herring on the exam; the morphology, timing, drug history, or coagulation discriminator picks the answer.

16.16 Quick Recall

QUICK RECALL — Haemostasis and Bleeding Disorders

Primary haemostasis = platelet plug (vWF–GPIb adhesion, ADP/TXA2 activation, GPIIb/IIIa-fibrinogen aggregation). Defects → mucocutaneous bleeding.

Secondary haemostasis = coagulation cascade. Cell-based model: initiation (TF + FVII), amplification (thrombin feedback on platelets), propagation (thrombin burst → fibrin → FXIII cross-link). Defects → deep-tissue bleeding.

PT measures extrinsic + common (FVII shortest half-life — first to fall). APTT measures intrinsic + common. TT measures fibrinogen → fibrin (heparin and dabigatran prolong; reptilase corrects for heparin/DOAC).

Natural anticoagulants: protein C/S (inactivate FVa, FVIIIa via thrombin-thrombomodulin); antithrombin (inactivates IIa and Xa; heparin accelerates 1000×); TFPI.

Vitamin K dependent factors: II, VII, IX, X + protein C, S. Warfarin → PIVKAs. FVII shortest half-life. Reversal: vitamin K + PCC.

DOAC reversal: idarucizumab (dabigatran); andexanet alfa (rivaroxaban, apixaban).

Thrombocytopenia: production (BM failure, MDS, leukaemia, infiltrative, B12/folate); destruction immune (ITP, drug, viral); destruction non-immune (TTP, HUS, DIC); sequestration (hypersplenism); dilutional (massive transfusion).

ITP: diagnosis of exclusion. First-line: corticosteroids OR IVIg. Second-line: TPO agonists (eltrombopag, romiplostim, avatrombopag), rituximab, splenectomy. Paediatric: 70–80% spontaneous resolution in 6 months.

Inherited platelet function disorders. Glanzmann (GPIIb/IIIa def): aggregation absent EXCEPT to ristocetin. Bernard-Soulier (GPIb def): giant platelets, mild thrombocytopenia, ABSENT response to ristocetin only.

TMA. TTP: ADAMTS13 <10%; PLASMIC ≥6 supports empirical PEX. Pentad historical; MAHA + thrombocytopenia is enough. STEC-HUS: bloody diarrhoea, AKI, supportive care, AVOID antibiotics. Atypical HUS: complement dysregulation, eculizumab.

vWD. Type 1 (70–80%; partial quantitative; AD; DDAVP often works). Type 2A (HMW multimers absent in plasma and platelets). Type 2B (gain-of-function for GPIb; mild thrombocytopenia; DDAVP CONTRAINDICATED). Type 2M (multimers preserved, function low). Type 2N (FVIII binding defect; mimics mild haemophilia A; AR). Type 3 (severe; AR; DDAVP ineffective).

Haemophilia A (FVIII; XLR; 1 in 5,000 male births) and B (FIX; 1 in 30,000). Severity: <1% severe (haemarthroses), 1–5% moderate, 5–40% mild. Modern care: prophylaxis, EHL products, emicizumab, gene therapy. Inhibitors: 20–30% of severe HA; bypassing agents (rFVIIa, FEIBA), ITI, emicizumab.

Rare factor deficiencies. FXI (Ashkenazi). FXII (silent — APTT prolonged but no bleeding). FVII (PT prolonged). FXIII (PT and APTT NORMAL; delayed umbilical bleeding; clot solubility in 5M urea). Fibrinogen (TT and reptilase prolonged).

DIC. Triggers: sepsis (50%), obstetric (abruption, AFE, HELLP), APL, mucinous adenocarcinoma, trauma, snake bite. Diagnosis: thrombocytopenia + low fibrinogen + raised D-dimer + prolonged PT/APTT. ISTH score ≥5 = overt DIC. Treat the trigger; replace components in haemorrhagic DIC; cautious heparin in thrombotic DIC. APL: start ATRA empirically.

Acquired haemophilia A. Older or postpartum patient with new severe bleeding. Mixing corrects immediately, prolongs on incubation (TIME-DEPENDENT inhibitor). Bypassing agents + immunosuppression.

Lupus anticoagulant: prolonged APTT, fails immediate mix, phospholipid-dependent. Paradoxically thrombotic. Part of APLAS (Ch 17).

— End of Chapter 16 —

CHAPTER 17

Chapter 17 — Thrombosis, Thrombophilia, and Anticoagulation

BIG PICTURE

Thrombosis is the formation of an intravascular clot in the wrong place at the wrong time. It is the mirror image of bleeding — the same haemostatic system, the same coagulation factors, the same platelets — tipped toward thrombus formation rather than haemorrhage. Three clinical questions organise the entire chapter. First, was the thrombosis provoked (by surgery, immobilisation, hospitalisation, hormone therapy, malignancy, pregnancy) or unprovoked? An unprovoked thrombosis at a young age, at an unusual site (cerebral venous, splanchnic, retinal), or with a strong family history demands a thrombophilia workup. Second, is the underlying defect inherited (Factor V Leiden, prothrombin G20210A, antithrombin / protein C / protein S deficiency) or acquired (antiphospholipid syndrome, malignancy-associated, oestrogen-related, pregnancy, myeloproliferative neoplasm, paroxysmal nocturnal haemoglobinuria, inflammatory bowel disease)? Third, what anticoagulant is appropriate now and for how long — and how is it monitored, reversed, and adjusted in special situations (renal impairment, pregnancy, cancer, the perioperative period)? The clinical task is rarely diagnostic puzzle-solving; it is matching the right drug to the right patient for the right duration.

MECHANISM HOOK — Virchow's triad and the modern molecular update

Rudolf Virchow's 1856 triad — endothelial injury, stasis, and hypercoagulability — remains the conceptual backbone of thrombosis. Every thrombotic mechanism reduces to one or more of these three categories. Endothelial injury exposes subendothelial collagen and tissue factor, triggering platelet adhesion and the coagulation cascade — the mechanism in atherosclerotic plaque rupture (arterial thrombi), trauma, surgery, central venous catheters, and antiphospholipid antibodies (which activate endothelium). Stasis allows local accumulation of activated coagulation factors and prevents their dilution into the circulating pool — the mechanism in immobilisation, prolonged travel, atrial fibrillation, surgical positioning, varicose veins, and venous compression by tumour. Hypercoagulability shifts the balance of pro- and anti-coagulant proteins toward thrombosis — the mechanism in inherited thrombophilias (Factor V Leiden, prothrombin G20210A, deficiencies of antithrombin / protein C / protein S), in pregnancy and oestrogen therapy (raised fibrinogen, FVII, FVIII, vWF; reduced protein S), in malignancy (Trousseau's syndrome — adenocarcinoma–driven hypercoagulability, especially pancreatic, gastric, and ovarian), and in inflammation (raised fibrinogen, FVIII, and reduced protein C / S in active inflammation). The molecular update of the triad recognises that thrombi differ by site: arterial thrombi (white thrombi, platelet-rich, formed under high shear) drive myocardial infarction and stroke and are treated with antiplatelet therapy; venous thrombi (red thrombi, fibrin- and erythrocyte-rich, formed under low shear and stasis) drive deep vein thrombosis and pulmonary embolism and are treated with anticoagulation. The clinical exam-trap to retain: Virchow's triad explains the pathogenesis; the site (arterial vs venous) drives the choice between antiplatelet and anticoagulant therapy.

17.1 Approach to Thrombosis

The clinical approach to thrombosis begins by classifying the event as provoked or unprovoked, identifying the site (arterial, venous, or microvascular), and judging whether a thrombophilia workup will alter management. Provoked thrombosis (surgery within 3 months, hospitalisation with significant immobility, hormonal therapy, pregnancy and the puerperium, active malignancy, major trauma) is treated for a defined course (usually 3 months) with anticoagulation continued only as long as the provoking factor persists. Unprovoked thrombosis — particularly at a young age (<50 years), at unusual sites (cerebral venous sinus, splanchnic — portal/hepatic/mesenteric, renal, retinal), with strong family history, or as recurrent disease — warrants thrombophilia evaluation and often indefinite anticoagulation given high recurrence risk (~10% per year unprovoked vs <3% per year for provoked).

FORMULA — When to test for thrombophilia

Testing is appropriate when the result will change management — duration of anticoagulation, family screening, or counselling for special situations. Testing is generally indicated in:

- Unprovoked VTE in a patient <50 years.
- VTE at an unusual site (cerebral venous sinus, splanchnic — portal/hepatic/mesenteric, renal, retinal, upper limb without catheter).
- Recurrent VTE without provoking factor.
- Strong family history of VTE in first-degree relatives.
- Recurrent pregnancy loss or late fetal loss (suggests APLAS).
- Warfarin-induced skin necrosis (suggests protein C or protein S deficiency).
- Neonatal purpura fulminans (suggests homozygous protein C or protein S deficiency).
- Heparin resistance — apparent failure to anticoagulate with adequate UFH dosing (suggests antithrombin deficiency).

Testing is generally NOT indicated in: typical provoked VTE in older patients, isolated provoked DVT in the context of clear surgical/hospital risk factors, asymptomatic family screening of children, or routine pre-operative screening.

Critical timing: do NOT test antithrombin, protein C, protein S during acute thrombosis (consumption produces falsely low levels), on UFH (antithrombin consumed), on warfarin (protein C and S falsely low — vitamin K dependent), on DOACs (interfere with chromogenic assays — varies by reagent), or during pregnancy / OCP use (protein S physiologically low). Wait at least 2 weeks after stopping anticoagulation; preferably 4–6 weeks. APLAS testing must be on two occasions ≥12 weeks apart.

17.2 Inherited Thrombophilia

Inherited thrombophilias are a small group of conditions that increase lifetime VTE risk by raising the procoagulant signal or reducing natural anticoagulant function. Five classical entities account for the majority of identifiable inherited thrombophilia: Factor V Leiden (the most common, especially in European populations), prothrombin G20210A, antithrombin deficiency (the rarest but clinically the strongest), protein C deficiency, and protein S deficiency. The MTHFR C677T polymorphism (and elevated homocysteine) is no longer considered a meaningful inherited thrombophilia in the absence of severe hyperhomocysteinaemia and is removed from most modern thrombophilia panels.

Condition	Defect	Population prevalence	VTE risk increase
Factor V Leiden	Point mutation R506Q in factor V — eliminates the APC cleavage site, so activated FV (FVa) is resistant to APC inactivation	3–8% of European populations; rare in African and Asian populations	Heterozygous: 3–8 fold; homozygous: 50–80 fold
Prothrombin G20210A	Point mutation in 3' UTR of prothrombin gene; raised plasma prothrombin levels	1–3% of European populations	2–5 fold; modestly higher in homozygotes (rare)
Antithrombin deficiency	Type I (quantitative — reduced AT antigen and activity); Type II (qualitative — normal antigen, reduced activity)	0.02–0.2%	10–50 fold (HIGHEST risk among inherited thrombophilias); presents with severe early-onset VTE
Protein C deficiency	Reduced PC activity (Type I quantitative or Type II qualitative)	0.2–0.5%	5–10 fold; warfarin-induced skin necrosis risk; homozygous → neonatal purpura fulminans
Protein S deficiency	Reduced free protein S (Type I, II, or III)	0.1–1%	5–10 fold; same warfarin skin necrosis risk; homozygous → neonatal purpura fulminans
Dysfibrinogenaemia (rare)	Functionally abnormal fibrinogen	<0.01%	Variable — bleeding, thrombosis, or both

Condition	Defect	Population prevalence	VTE risk increase
Elevated factor VIII	Persistently raised FVIII (genetic + acquired contributors)	~10% have raised FVIII >150%	~2–6 fold; not routinely tested but clinically meaningful

Table 17.1: Inherited thrombophilia — classical entities, defects, prevalence, and VTE risk magnitude.

Factor V Leiden and APC resistance

Factor V Leiden is the most common inherited thrombophilia in European populations. The arginine-to-glutamine substitution at position 506 (R506Q) eliminates one of the activated protein C cleavage sites on factor V, rendering the activated form (FVa) resistant to APC inactivation. The functional consequence is sustained thrombin generation. The screening test is the activated protein C resistance assay — a modified APTT measured with and without addition of APC; the ratio of APTT-with-APC to APTT-without-APC is reduced (typically <2.0–2.5, depending on the assay). Confirmatory testing is by PCR for the F5 R506Q mutation. Heterozygotes have approximately 5% lifetime VTE risk in the absence of additional risk factors but rise sharply with co-existing factors (oestrogen, pregnancy, surgery). Homozygotes have 50- to 80-fold relative risk. The clinical practical point: heterozygous Factor V Leiden alone is rarely an indication for indefinite anticoagulation after a single provoked VTE, but it raises the threshold for hormonal contraception in unaffected family members.

HIGH-YIELD PEARL — Warfarin-induced skin necrosis: the protein C / S signature

Warfarin-induced skin necrosis classically appears between days 3 and 6 of warfarin initiation, typically in fatty areas (breast, thighs, abdomen, buttocks). The mechanism is a TRANSIENT hypercoagulable state: warfarin depletes the natural anticoagulants protein C (half-life ~6–8 h) and protein S (~30 h) BEFORE it depletes the procoagulant factors II (~60 h), IX (~24 h), and X (~40 h). Patients with underlying protein C or protein S deficiency have low baseline anticoagulant function; warfarin pushes them into severe transient hypercoagulability with microvascular thrombosis and skin necrosis.

Prevention: ALWAYS bridge warfarin with parenteral anticoagulant (UFH, LMWH, or fondaparinux) for 5 days AND until the INR is therapeutic for at least 24 hours — and start warfarin at modest doses, not loading doses, in patients with known protein C or S deficiency.

When this picture is present in a vignette — necrotic skin lesions days 3–7 after starting warfarin in an adult — think protein C deficiency. In a neonate with massive purpura fulminans within hours of birth, think homozygous (or compound heterozygous) protein C or S deficiency — a haematological emergency requiring protein C concentrate (Ceprotin — plasma-derived zymogen) and lifelong anticoagulation.

Antithrombin deficiency — testing and pitfalls

Antithrombin deficiency is the rarest but clinically strongest inherited thrombophilia, with 10- to 50-fold VTE risk and frequent presentation in adolescence or young adulthood. Type I (quantitative) deficiency reduces both AT antigen and activity; Type II (qualitative) deficiency reduces activity with normal antigen. Type II is further subclassified by mutation site: reactive site (RS — high thrombotic risk), heparin-binding site (HBS — homozygous form is severe, heterozygous milder), or pleiotropic. The functional assay (chromogenic; AT incubated with excess heparin and thrombin or FXa, residual protease activity measured) is the screening test of choice and detects both Type I and Type II deficiency. The antigenic assay distinguishes Type I (low) from Type II (normal). The diagnostic move on a prolonged thromboembolism workup is the functional AT assay first.

AT deficiency may also present clinically as heparin resistance — apparent failure to achieve a therapeutic APTT despite escalating UFH doses. Heparin acts by accelerating AT-mediated thrombin and FXa inactivation by ~1000-fold; with insufficient AT, heparin has no co-factor to bind. Suspected heparin resistance demands AT measurement, with consideration of recombinant antithrombin replacement (Atryn, Thrombate) or LMWH (less AT-dependent in some settings) or argatroban (direct thrombin inhibitor, AT-independent).

TRAP — Do NOT test thrombophilia during acute thrombosis or on anticoagulation

The single most common error in thrombophilia workup is testing in the wrong situation. The following timing rules are absolute:

- ANTITHROMBIN — falsely low during acute thrombosis (consumption), on UFH (heparin–AT complex consumed), and (variably) on DOACs (interfere with chromogenic assays).
- PROTEIN C and PROTEIN S — falsely low on warfarin (vitamin K dependent), in pregnancy (especially second/third trimester for protein S), on oestrogen-containing oral contraceptives (lower protein S), and during acute illness or thrombosis.
- LUPUS ANTICOAGULANT — falsely positive or falsely negative on heparin and DOACs (interfere with phospholipid-dependent assays); cardiolipin and beta-2 GPI ELISAs are NOT affected by anticoagulants.
- FACTOR V LEIDEN and PROTHROMBIN G20210A — these are GENETIC tests (PCR for fixed mutations) and are NOT affected by anticoagulation, illness, or pregnancy. They can be tested at any time.

Practical move: test the genetic markers (FVL, PT G20210A) acutely if needed; defer the protein assays (AT, PC, PS, lupus anticoagulant) until at least 2–4 weeks after stopping anticoagulation. APLAS antibodies must be confirmed on two occasions ≥12 weeks apart.

17.3 Antiphospholipid Syndrome

Antiphospholipid syndrome (APS, sometimes APLAS) is an acquired autoimmune thrombophilia defined by vascular thrombosis (venous, arterial, or microvascular) and/or characteristic obstetric morbidity in the presence of persistent antiphospholipid antibodies (aPL). The name is misleading: aPL do not bind phospholipids directly but bind protein cofactors — most importantly beta-2 glycoprotein I (β2GPI) and prothrombin — that are themselves complexed with phospholipid surfaces on activated cells. Pathogenesis combines endothelial activation (upregulation of tissue factor and adhesion molecules), platelet activation, complement activation, monocyte activation, and interference with natural anticoagulant pathways (impaired protein C activation, displacement of annexin V).

Classification — the Sydney (revised Sapporo) criteria

Diagnosis requires AT LEAST ONE clinical criterion AND AT LEAST ONE laboratory criterion, with laboratory criteria confirmed on TWO occasions at least 12 weeks apart. The 12-week rule eliminates transient positivity from infections, drugs, and acute illness.

Clinical criteria (≥1)	Laboratory criteria (≥1, confirmed ≥12 weeks apart)
Vascular thrombosis: ≥1 episode of arterial, venous, or small-vessel thrombosis confirmed by imaging or histopathology, in any tissue or organ	Lupus anticoagulant: positive on ≥2 occasions ≥12 weeks apart, detected per ISTH guidelines (screening + mixing + phospholipid confirmation; exclusion of factor inhibitors)
Obstetric morbidity: (a) ≥1 unexplained fetal death ≥10 weeks of a morphologically normal fetus; OR (b) ≥1 premature birth <34 weeks due to severe preeclampsia, eclampsia, or placental insufficiency; OR (c) ≥3 unexplained consecutive spontaneous abortions <10 weeks (after exclusion of anatomical, hormonal, and chromosomal causes)	Anti-cardiolipin antibodies (aCL): IgG and/or IgM, MEDIUM or HIGH titre (>40 GPL or MPL units, or >99th percentile), on ≥2 occasions ≥12 weeks apart
	Anti-beta-2 glycoprotein I antibodies (anti-β2GPI): IgG and/or IgM, >99th percentile, on ≥2 occasions ≥12 weeks apart

Table 17.2: Sydney (revised Sapporo) criteria for antiphospholipid syndrome.

Triple positivity (lupus anticoagulant + anti-cardiolipin + anti-β2GPI all present at high titre) confers the highest thrombotic risk and the strongest indication for indefinite anticoagulation after a first thrombotic event. Single antibody positivity at low titre carries lower risk and may not justify lifelong therapy, particularly when only weakly clinical (e.g. one early miscarriage). Lupus anticoagulant is the strongest single laboratory predictor of thrombosis among the three. APS may be primary (no underlying autoimmune disease) or secondary (most often to systemic lupus erythematosus).

Catastrophic antiphospholipid syndrome (CAPS)

CAPS is the rare, life-threatening variant of APS, characterised by simultaneous multi-organ thrombosis (≥3 organ systems) developing rapidly (over <1 week), histopathological evidence of small-vessel thrombosis, and confirmed antiphospholipid antibody positivity. Triggers include infection, surgery, medication non-adherence, malignancy, and pregnancy. Mortality is approximately 30–50% even with treatment. Management combines anticoagulation (heparin), high-dose corticosteroids, plasma exchange, and IVIg as the standard "triple therapy"; rituximab and eculizumab (anti-C5) are added in refractory cases. CAPS is included in the differential for any patient with rapid multi-organ failure of unclear cause and a known or newly suspected antiphospholipid profile.

Treatment of APLAS

Treatment of APS-related VTE has three main components. For patients with venous thromboembolism, warfarin is the established standard with a target INR of 2.0–3.0 indefinitely after a first unprovoked event in confirmed APS. The 2018 TRAPS trial and subsequent studies have shown that DOACs (specifically rivaroxaban) are INFERIOR to warfarin in triple-positive APS — with significantly more arterial thrombotic events on rivaroxaban — and DOACs are NOT recommended in triple-positive APS or in those with a history of arterial events. DOACs may be considered in single-positive APS without arterial events on shared decision-making. For arterial events (stroke, MI), antiplatelet therapy (aspirin) ± anticoagulation is added depending on the site and recurrence risk. For pregnancy in APS, low-molecular-weight heparin plus low-dose aspirin (75–100 mg) is standard and is continued through pregnancy and into the postpartum period (typically 6 weeks postpartum for prophylaxis; longer if there is a personal thrombotic history).

17.4 Acquired Thrombophilia and Other Hypercoagulable States

Several acquired and clinical states substantially raise VTE risk and frequently dominate the differential in real-world thrombosis. They are recognised by clinical context rather than by laboratory testing of inherited markers.

State	Mechanism	Clinical relevance
Active malignancy (Trousseau's syndrome)	Mucin-producing adenocarcinomas (pancreatic, gastric, ovarian, colorectal, lung) release tissue factor and procoagulant mucins; chemotherapy adds endothelial injury and immobilisation	Cancer-associated thrombosis is common (up to 20% of cancer patients); LMWH historically preferred over warfarin (CLOT trial); apixaban and edoxaban now non-inferior to LMWH in selected patients (Caravaggio, Hokusai-Cancer); avoid in luminal GI/GU cancers due to bleeding risk
Pregnancy and the puerperium	Physiological hypercoagulability: raised fibrinogen, FVII, FVIII, vWF; reduced free protein S; venous stasis from gravid uterus; endothelial injury at delivery	VTE risk ~5× non-pregnant baseline; highest risk in immediate postpartum period (~6 weeks); LMWH is the anticoagulant of choice (does not cross placenta; warfarin teratogenic; DOACs not used)
Oestrogen-containing contraception / hormone therapy	Raised prothrombin, FVIII, fibrinogen; reduced protein S; modest reduction in tissue factor pathway inhibitor	Increases VTE risk ~3–5×; risk additive with FVL or PT G20210A heterozygosity
Myeloproliferative neoplasms (MPNs)	JAK2 V617F driver mutation produces hypercoagulability via leukocyte activation, platelet dysfunction, and altered erythrocyte rheology	Polycythaemia vera and essential thrombocythaemia present with arterial and venous thrombosis (especially splanchnic — Budd-Chiari, portal vein); always test JAK2 in unprovoked splanchnic thrombosis even with normal counts
Paroxysmal nocturnal haemoglobinuria (PNH)	PIG-A mutation; loss of GPI-anchored CD55 and CD59; complement-mediated platelet and erythrocyte activation	Thrombosis at unusual sites (Budd-Chiari, cerebral venous, splanchnic) is the leading cause of death in untreated PNH; eculizumab transformed prognosis; flow cytometry with FLAER for diagnosis (covered in Ch 13)

State	Mechanism	Clinical relevance
Heparin-induced thrombocytopenia (HIT)	IgG antibodies against PF4–heparin complexes activate platelets via FcγRIIa; paradoxically thrombotic despite thrombocytopenia	Develops 5–10 days after heparin exposure; 4Ts score (Thrombocytopenia, Timing, Thrombosis, oTher causes) ≥4 prompts testing; PF4 antibody ELISA + serotonin release assay (functional confirmation); STOP heparin, start non-heparin anticoagulant (argatroban, fondaparinux, bivalirudin)
Inflammatory bowel disease	Inflammation-driven raised fibrinogen, FVIII, reduced protein C/S; immobility	VTE risk 2–3× general population; venous thromboprophylaxis during admission and active flares
Nephrotic syndrome	Urinary loss of antithrombin; raised fibrinogen and FVIII; platelet activation	Renal vein thrombosis and DVT/PE; prophylaxis when albumin <2.0–2.5 g/dL
Severe COVID-19 / sepsis-associated coagulopathy	Endothelial injury, complement activation, NET formation, immobilisation	Macrovascular and microvascular thrombosis; anticoagulant prophylaxis and therapeutic dosing (INSPIRATION, REMAP-CAP, ATTACC trials guide intensity)

Table 17.3: Acquired hypercoagulable states — mechanism and clinical relevance.

17.5 Laboratory Workup of Thrombophilia

When thrombophilia testing is clinically indicated (per the formula in §17.1), the panel is structured to maximise diagnostic yield while minimising false-positive results from preanalytical interference. The standard panel comprises the genetic markers (Factor V Leiden by APC resistance assay or PCR; prothrombin G20210A by PCR), the natural anticoagulant proteins (antithrombin functional and antigenic; protein C functional; protein S free antigen and functional), and the antiphospholipid antibody panel (lupus anticoagulant by dRVVT; anti-cardiolipin IgG and IgM; anti-β2GPI IgG and IgM). Homocysteine is no longer routine in most modern panels.

FORMULA — Interpreting the thrombophilia panel

Step 1. Confirm the timing rules: ≥2–4 weeks after stopping anticoagulation; not during acute thrombosis or pregnancy; not on UFH (AT) or warfarin (PC, PS, LA) or DOACs (LA and chromogenic AT/PC variably affected). If acute testing is required, run the genetic markers (FVL, PT G20210A) only.

Step 2. Interpret the functional assays in context. Low antithrombin + on UFH = consumption artefact, not deficiency. Low protein C or S + on warfarin = expected, not deficiency. Low protein S + pregnancy = physiological. Confirm any abnormal protein assay on a repeat sample at least 6 weeks later off any confounding agent.

Step 3. Distinguish Type I from Type II deficiency. Both functional and antigenic low = Type I (quantitative). Functional low with antigenic normal = Type II (qualitative).

Step 4. Confirm APLAS antibodies on 2 occasions ≥12 weeks apart. Triple positivity (LA + aCL + anti-β2GPI) = highest thrombotic risk and warrants warfarin (NOT DOACs — TRAPS trial).

Step 5. Decide whether the result will change management. In a young patient with unprovoked VTE planned for indefinite anticoagulation, identifying the specific defect rarely changes drug choice (warfarin or DOAC for non-APLAS) but informs family screening and counselling for pregnancy/contraception. In APLAS, the result drives drug choice: warfarin for triple positive; LMWH + aspirin in pregnancy.

Step 6. In family screening, test relatives only if a specific abnormality is identified in the proband and if knowledge will change the relative's management (typically: avoid oestrogen-containing contraception in heterozygous Factor V Leiden carriers; thromboprophylaxis around surgery / pregnancy / immobilisation in known carriers).

17.6 Heparins and Heparin-Induced Thrombocytopenia

Heparins are sulphated glycosaminoglycans that anticoagulate by binding antithrombin and accelerating its inactivation of thrombin (FIIa) and FXa by approximately 1000-fold. Three preparations are clinically important: unfractionated heparin (UFH), low-molecular-weight heparins (LMWHs — enoxaparin, dalteparin, tinzaparin, nadroparin), and the synthetic pentasaccharide fondaparinux. The pharmacological differences drive the clinical choices.

Property	Unfractionated heparin (UFH)	LMWH (enoxaparin, dalteparin)	Fondaparinux
Mean molecular weight	15,000 Da (heterogeneous chains)	4,000–5,000 Da	1,728 Da (synthetic pentasaccharide)
Mechanism	AT-mediated inhibition of both thrombin and FXa (1:1)	AT-mediated inhibition with FXa preference (~3:1 anti-Xa:anti-IIa)	AT-mediated FXa inhibition only (no anti-IIa activity)
Route	IV (continuous infusion preferred for therapeutic anticoagulation) or subcutaneous	Subcutaneous (once or twice daily)	Subcutaneous (once daily)
Monitoring	APTT (target 1.5–2.5× baseline) or anti-Xa level (target 0.3–0.7 U/mL)	Routine monitoring not required; anti-Xa level useful in pregnancy, renal impairment, extremes of body weight	Routine monitoring not required
Half-life	~1 hour (dose-dependent; longer at higher doses)	~4–6 hours	~17 hours
Renal clearance	Largely non-renal	Renal (~40%) — accumulate in renal impairment; dose reduce CrCl <30 mL/min	Renal — contraindicated CrCl <30 mL/min
Reversal	Protamine (1 mg per 100 IU UFH within last hour) — full reversal	Protamine partially reverses (~60–70% of anti-Xa effect)	Protamine does NOT reverse; activated PCC may help in major bleeding
HIT risk	~1–3% (highest of the three; especially in surgical / cardiac patients)	~0.1–1% (much lower than UFH)	Very rare; fondaparinux has been used to treat HIT

Table 17.4: Heparins — pharmacology, monitoring, and reversal.

Heparin-induced thrombocytopenia (HIT)

Heparin-induced thrombocytopenia (HIT) is an immune-mediated, paradoxically PRO-thrombotic complication of heparin exposure. IgG antibodies against complexes of platelet factor 4 (PF4) and heparin bind FcγRIIa on platelets, producing massive platelet activation, procoagulant microparticle release, and thrombin generation. The result is thrombocytopenia (typically a 50% drop from baseline platelet count) AND thrombosis (venous more than arterial; deep vein, pulmonary embolism, limb ischaemia, stroke, MI, skin necrosis at heparin injection sites).

Timing is characteristic: HIT develops 5–10 days after first heparin exposure (or within 24 hours if prior recent exposure has primed an immune response). The clinical recognition uses the 4Ts score: Thrombocytopenia magnitude (>50% drop or nadir 20–100,000), Timing (5–10 days from exposure, or rapid in re-exposure), Thrombosis (new thrombosis or skin necrosis), and other Causes excluded. A 4Ts score ≥4 prompts immediate cessation of all heparin (UFH and LMWH; even heparin flushes count), and initiation of a non-heparin anticoagulant. Laboratory confirmation uses PF4 antibody ELISA (highly sensitive, less specific) followed by a functional confirmatory test (serotonin release assay or HIPA — heparin-induced platelet activation), the latter being the gold standard.

FORMULA — Management of HIT

- STOP all heparin (UFH, LMWH, heparin flushes, heparin-coated catheters).
- Start a NON-HEPARIN anticoagulant immediately — argatroban (direct thrombin inhibitor; metabolised hepatically; no renal adjustment), bivalirudin (direct thrombin inhibitor; partly renal), or fondaparinux (off-label in HIT but widely used; pentasaccharide does not cross-react with PF4 antibodies in most patients). DO NOT use warfarin alone in acute HIT — protein C falls faster than the procoagulant factors, worsening the prothrombotic state and risking warfarin-induced limb gangrene.
- Wait for platelet count recovery (>150,000/µL) before transitioning to oral anticoagulation; bridge with the non-heparin anticoagulant during warfarin initiation.
- Document HIT in the medical record permanently — heparin must be avoided in future, including in cardiac surgery (use bivalirudin or argatroban for cardiopulmonary bypass).
- Treatment duration: at least 4 weeks for "isolated" HIT (thrombocytopenia without thrombosis); 3 months for HIT with thrombosis.

17.7 Warfarin

Warfarin (and other coumarin derivatives — acenocoumarol, phenprocoumon) is an oral vitamin K antagonist (VKA). Warfarin inhibits the enzyme vitamin K epoxide reductase (VKORC1), which regenerates reduced vitamin K from the oxidised form after each gamma-carboxylation cycle. Without reduced vitamin K, the vitamin-K-dependent factors (II, VII, IX, X) and natural anticoagulants (protein C and protein S) cannot be carboxylated and circulate as functionally inactive PIVKAs (proteins induced by vitamin K antagonism/absence). The half-lives of these factors differ — FVII shortest (~6 h), FIX (~24 h), FX (~40 h), FII longest

(~60 h), protein C ~8 h, protein S ~30 h — explaining the transient hypercoagulable state on warfarin initiation that produces warfarin-induced skin necrosis in protein C/S deficient patients.

Warfarin is monitored by the International Normalised Ratio (INR), a standardised PT measurement. Therapeutic targets: INR 2.0–3.0 for most indications (atrial fibrillation, VTE, biological prosthetic valves, APS without arterial events); INR 2.5–3.5 for mechanical mitral valves and triple-positive APS in some guidelines. The drug has narrow therapeutic index, multiple drug interactions (CYP2C9 metabolism — antibiotics, amiodarone, and many others potentiate; rifampicin, carbamazepine, and others reduce effect), and dietary interactions (vitamin K-rich foods — green leafy vegetables — moderately reduce effect, but consistency rather than avoidance is the practical advice). Pharmacogenetic variation (CYP2C9 and VKORC1 polymorphisms) accounts for substantial inter-patient dose variability, particularly across populations of South Asian and East Asian ancestry, where CYP2C9 and VKORC1 polymorphism distributions differ from European populations and average therapeutic doses tend to be lower.

FORMULA — Warfarin reversal by INR and bleeding context

- INR therapeutic to <4.5, no bleeding → continue warfarin or skip a dose; recheck INR; resume at adjusted dose.
- INR 4.5–10, no bleeding → withhold 1–2 doses; small dose oral vitamin K (1–2.5 mg) optional; recheck INR.
- INR >10, no bleeding → withhold warfarin; oral vitamin K 2.5–5 mg; recheck INR daily until therapeutic.
- Any INR with major or life-threatening bleeding → withhold warfarin; IV vitamin K 5–10 mg (slow infusion to avoid anaphylaxis); 4-FACTOR PROTHROMBIN COMPLEX CONCENTRATE (PCC; contains FII, FVII, FIX, FX) preferred over fresh frozen plasma for major bleeding (faster, smaller volume, avoids volume overload). Dose: typically 25–50 IU/kg of PCC. FFP is acceptable if PCC unavailable but is volume-rich and slower.
- Pre-procedure reversal — depends on urgency. Elective: hold warfarin 5 days, bridge with LMWH if high thrombotic risk. Urgent (within 24 h): oral vitamin K 2.5 mg. Emergent: IV vitamin K + PCC.
- Bridging in atrial fibrillation: routine bridging is NOT recommended for most non-mechanical-valve AF (BRIDGE trial showed bridging increases bleeding without reducing thrombosis); reserved for high CHA2DS2-VASc with recent stroke or mechanical valves.

17.8 Direct Oral Anticoagulants (DOACs)

Direct oral anticoagulants (DOACs, formerly NOACs) inhibit specific coagulation factors directly without requiring antithrombin as a cofactor. Two mechanistic classes are in clinical use: the direct factor Xa inhibitors (rivaroxaban, apixaban, edoxaban, betrixaban) and the direct thrombin inhibitor dabigatran. They have largely replaced warfarin for most indications because of fixed-dose prescribing (no INR monitoring), fewer drug-drug and drug-food interactions, and a more favourable bleeding profile (especially less intracranial bleeding) in major randomised trials.

Drug	Mechanism	Half-life	Renal clearance	Reversal agent
Dabigatran	Direct thrombin (FIIa) inhibitor	12–17 h	~80% renal; avoid CrCl <30	Idarucizumab (Praxbind) — humanised monoclonal antibody Fab fragment that specifically binds dabigatran
Rivaroxaban	Direct FXa inhibitor	5–13 h	~33% renal; caution CrCl <30; avoid <15	Andexanet alfa (Andexxa) — recombinant inactive FXa decoy; OR 4-factor PCC (off-label, off-label dose 50 IU/kg)
Apixaban	Direct FXa inhibitor	~12 h	~25% renal; can be used in dialysis patients (off-label) with apixaban dose reduction	Andexanet alfa OR 4-factor PCC
Edoxaban	Direct FXa inhibitor	10–14 h	~50% renal; avoid CrCl <30 or >95	Andexanet alfa OR 4-factor PCC

Table 17.5: Direct oral anticoagulants — mechanism, pharmacokinetics, and reversal.

DOAC selection in clinical practice depends on indication, renal function, body weight, and bleeding risk. For atrial fibrillation, all four DOACs have been shown non-inferior or superior to warfarin in pivotal trials; apixaban has the lowest major bleeding profile and is often preferred in elderly patients. For acute VTE, all four are non-inferior to warfarin with reduced bleeding; apixaban and rivaroxaban allow single-drug oral therapy from day one (with a higher loading dose for the first 7–21 days), whereas dabigatran and edoxaban require an initial 5–10 days of parenteral anticoagulation. For cancer-associated thrombosis, the Caravaggio (apixaban) and Hokusai-Cancer (edoxaban) trials demonstrated non-inferiority to LMWH for most cancers, but increased GI bleeding in luminal GI cancers; LMWH remains preferred in luminal GI / GU cancers and in poor-risk patients. DOACs are CONTRAINDICATED in mechanical heart valves (RE-ALIGN trial — dabigatran inferior to warfarin), in moderate-to-severe mitral stenosis, and in triple-positive APS (TRAPS trial — rivaroxaban inferior to warfarin). DOACs are not recommended in pregnancy or breastfeeding.

17.9 Treatment of Venous Thromboembolism

Acute VTE (deep vein thrombosis, pulmonary embolism) is treated in three phases. Initial therapy (first 5–10 days) controls clot propagation and stabilises the patient. Long-term therapy (3 months minimum) prevents recurrence. Extended (or indefinite) therapy is considered for unprovoked VTE, recurrent VTE, or persistent strong risk factor — with shared decision-making weighing recurrence risk against bleeding risk.

Clinical scenario	Recommended initial / long-term anticoagulation	Duration
Provoked VTE (surgery, trauma, hospitalisation, hormone, pregnancy)	Apixaban or rivaroxaban (single-drug from day 1, with loading dose); OR LMWH bridge to warfarin; OR LMWH bridge to dabigatran/edoxaban	3 months (or until provoking factor resolves, whichever is longer)
First unprovoked VTE	Same as provoked initially; reassess at 3 months for indefinite therapy based on bleeding risk and patient preference	3 months minimum; consider indefinite if bleeding risk acceptable (HERDOO2 score; D-dimer testing post-treatment)
Recurrent unprovoked VTE	Indefinite anticoagulation	Indefinite
Active cancer-associated VTE	LMWH preferred (CLOT trial historically); apixaban or edoxaban non-inferior in most cancers (Caravaggio, Hokusai-Cancer); avoid in luminal GI / GU cancers — bleeding risk	Throughout active cancer (often indefinite)
Pregnancy-associated VTE	LMWH (does not cross placenta; warfarin teratogenic in 1st trimester and fetotoxic later; DOACs not used)	Throughout pregnancy + 6 weeks postpartum (minimum 3 months total)
Antiphospholipid syndrome (any thrombosis)	WARFARIN target INR 2.0–3.0 (NOT DOACs in triple-positive APS — TRAPS trial)	Indefinite for confirmed APS
Catheter-related upper limb DVT	Anticoagulate; remove catheter only if non-functional or infection or recurrent thrombosis on therapeutic anticoagulation	3 months (longer if catheter remains)
Extensive ileofemoral DVT in young patient	Standard anticoagulation; consider catheter-directed thrombolysis (CDT)	As above

Clinical scenario	Recommended initial / long-term anticoagulation	Duration
	or pharmacomechanical thrombectomy (CaVenT, ATTRACT trials — selected patients only) to reduce post-thrombotic syndrome	
Massive pulmonary embolism (haemodynamic instability, RV strain)	Systemic thrombolysis (alteplase 100 mg over 2 h or weight-based); surgical or catheter-directed embolectomy in selected patients	Standard anticoagulation thereafter

Table 17.6: Treatment of VTE by clinical scenario.

17.10 Buzzwords and Associations — Vignette Trigger Table

Single-line cues that should prompt specific diagnostic reflexes in thrombosis and anticoagulation.

Vignette buzzword / finding	Diagnosis to trigger	One-line "why"
Young adult, unprovoked DVT or PE, family history of VTE	Inherited thrombophilia (most likely Factor V Leiden in European populations)	Most common inherited thrombophilia; APC resistance assay or PCR
Skin necrosis days 3–6 of warfarin therapy	Warfarin-induced skin necrosis (protein C or S deficiency)	Transient hypercoagulability from rapid PC/PS depletion before procoagulants
Neonate with massive purpura fulminans within hours of birth	Homozygous or compound heterozygous protein C or S deficiency	Protein C concentrate (Ceprotin — plasma-derived zymogen) is life-saving
Adolescent or young adult with severe early VTE; heparin appears ineffective at high doses	Antithrombin deficiency	Heparin needs AT cofactor; without enough AT, heparin fails
Recurrent first-trimester miscarriages + lupus anticoagulant	Antiphospholipid syndrome (obstetric form)	LMWH + low-dose aspirin in subsequent pregnancies
Triple-positive APLAS (LA + aCL + anti-β2GPI) with arterial thrombosis	Confirmed APS — use WARFARIN, not DOAC	TRAPS trial: rivaroxaban inferior to warfarin in triple-positive APS
Heparin therapy day 5–10 + platelet drop ≥50% + new thrombosis	Heparin-induced thrombocytopenia (HIT)	4Ts ≥4 → STOP heparin, start argatroban / fondaparinux; PF4 ELISA + SRA
Pancreatic adenocarcinoma + migratory superficial thrombophlebitis	Trousseau's syndrome	LMWH historically preferred; apixaban / edoxaban now options for non-luminal cancers
Splanchnic thrombosis (Budd-Chiari, portal vein) with normal blood counts	JAK2 V617F testing	Latent MPN; JAK2 positive even before counts rise
Splanchnic thrombosis + intravascular haemolysis + cytopenias + thrombosis at unusual site	Paroxysmal nocturnal haemoglobinuria (PNH)	FLAER on granulocytes / monocytes; eculizumab transformed prognosis

Vignette buzzword / finding	Diagnosis to trigger	One-line "why"
Major bleeding on dabigatran	Idarucizumab (Praxbind)	Specific Fab antibody fragment for dabigatran reversal
Major bleeding on rivaroxaban or apixaban	Andexanet alfa (Andexxa) OR 4-factor PCC	Andexanet — recombinant inactive FXa decoy
Mechanical mitral valve patient on dabigatran with stroke	STOP dabigatran, switch to warfarin (target INR 2.5–3.5)	RE-ALIGN: dabigatran inferior to warfarin in mechanical valves
Pregnant woman with prior unprovoked DVT	LMWH antepartum + 6 weeks postpartum	Warfarin teratogenic 1st trimester and fetotoxic later; DOACs not used
Patient on warfarin with INR 12 and active GI bleed	Hold warfarin; IV vitamin K + 4-factor PCC	PCC faster than FFP; smaller volume; preferred for major bleeding
Patient on warfarin scheduled for elective surgery in 5 days	Hold warfarin 5 days; bridge with LMWH only if high thrombotic risk	BRIDGE trial: routine bridging in AF without mechanical valves increases bleeding
Multi-organ thrombosis developing over <1 week with confirmed aPL antibodies	Catastrophic APS (CAPS)	Anticoagulation + corticosteroids + plasma exchange + IVIg "triple therapy"
Cancer patient with luminal GI tumour and acute DVT	LMWH preferred over DOAC	Apixaban/edoxaban have higher GI bleeding in luminal cancers (Caravaggio, Hokusai-Cancer subgroups)
Renal vein thrombosis + nephrotic syndrome + serum albumin <2.0	Nephrotic-syndrome-associated thrombophilia	Urinary AT loss; raised fibrinogen and FVIII; anticoagulate
First-line VKA-independent treatment of VTE with same-day oral therapy from day 1	Apixaban (10 mg BD × 7 days, then 5 mg BD) or rivaroxaban (15 mg BD × 21 days, then 20 mg OD)	Single-drug oral therapy without parenteral lead-in

Table 17.7: Thrombosis and anticoagulation vignette triggers — exam-fast clue-to-diagnosis mapping.

17.11 USMLE Vignettes

Ten vignettes covering the highest-yield discriminations in thrombosis and anticoagulation.

Vignette 1. A 28-year-old man with unprovoked DVT and a family history

A 28-year-old previously healthy man presents with a swollen, painful left calf for three days. He had no recent surgery, hospitalisation, immobilisation, long-distance travel, or trauma. He is on no medications. His mother had a "leg clot" in her thirties and his maternal uncle had a pulmonary embolism at age 35. Examination: tender, swollen left calf with positive Homan's sign; otherwise normal. Doppler ultrasound of the left lower limb confirms occlusive deep venous thrombosis extending from the popliteal to the femoral vein. CBC normal. Therapeutic anticoagulation is started with apixaban 10 mg twice daily. After 7 days, a thrombophilia screen is sent. Activated protein C resistance ratio: 1.6 (low; consistent with APC resistance). PCR confirms heterozygous Factor V R506Q (Factor V Leiden). Antithrombin functional 95% (normal); protein C functional 110%; protein S free antigen 78%; lupus anticoagulant negative. Which of the following is the most appropriate ongoing management?

(A) Continue apixaban for at least 3 months, then reassess for indefinite therapy on bleeding risk and patient preference; counsel against oestrogen-containing contraception in unaffected female first-degree relatives; offer first-degree relative testing if results would change their contraception or pregnancy management.

(B) Stop anticoagulation at 6 weeks because a heritable defect explains the thrombosis.

(C) Switch to warfarin indefinitely because DOACs are inferior in inherited thrombophilia.

(D) Lifelong full-dose anticoagulation regardless of preference because heterozygous Factor V Leiden mandates indefinite therapy.

(E) Switch to LMWH indefinitely because oral anticoagulants are not effective in heritable thrombophilia.

Best answer: (A) Continue apixaban for at least 3 months, then reassess for indefinite therapy on bleeding risk and patient preference; counsel against oestrogen-containing contraception in unaffected female first-degree relatives; offer first-degree relative testing if results would change their contraception or pregnancy management.

Rationale. Heterozygous Factor V Leiden is the most common inherited thrombophilia in European-ancestry populations, with a 3- to 8-fold relative risk of first VTE. The clinical decision after a first unprovoked VTE in a young patient with heterozygous FVL is to complete the standard 3-month treatment course and then reassess for indefinite anticoagulation balancing recurrence risk against bleeding risk and patient preference. Heterozygous FVL alone does NOT mandate indefinite anticoagulation in standard guidelines, but the unprovoked event in a young patient with strong family history makes indefinite anticoagulation a reasonable shared-decision option. DOACs (apixaban, rivaroxaban) are non-inferior to warfarin for VTE in non-APLAS settings and are the standard of care now. Family screening of first-degree female relatives matters because heterozygous FVL plus oestrogen-containing oral contraception multiplies VTE risk substantially; affected women should be counselled toward progestin-only methods or non-hormonal contraception, especially if also planning pregnancy.

Distractor analysis. (B) Standard treatment is 3 months minimum for any VTE. (C) DOACs are NOT inferior to warfarin in inherited thrombophilia (other than APLAS triple positivity). (D) Heterozygous FVL alone does not mandate lifelong anticoagulation; this is over-treatment. (E) LMWH-only therapy is not standard for chronic VTE management; reserved for cancer and pregnancy.

Vignette 2. A 34-year-old woman with recurrent first-trimester miscarriages

A 34-year-old woman is referred for evaluation of three consecutive first-trimester miscarriages, all between 6 and 9 weeks gestation. She is otherwise well, on no medications. Examination is unremarkable. CBC, thyroid function, prolactin, hysterosalpingography, and karyotyping of both partners are normal. Coagulation screen: PT 12 s, APTT 48 s (mildly prolonged). Mixing study: APTT does not correct on immediate mix. dRVVT: prolonged and confirmed phospholipid-dependent. Anti-cardiolipin IgG 84 GPL units (high titre); anti-β2GPI IgG 65 units (high titre). Repeat testing 12 weeks later confirms persistence of all three antibodies. Which of the following is the most appropriate management for a future pregnancy?

(A) Antiphospholipid syndrome, obstetric form (triple-positive); start low-dose aspirin (75–100 mg daily) preconceptionally, add prophylactic-dose LMWH (enoxaparin 40 mg daily) once pregnancy is confirmed, continue LMWH + aspirin throughout pregnancy and 6 weeks postpartum.

(B) Warfarin throughout pregnancy.

(C) Rivaroxaban from preconception through 6 weeks postpartum.

(D) High-dose corticosteroids alone.

(E) IVF with surrogate carrier; treatment of the antibodies is not effective.

Best answer: (A) Antiphospholipid syndrome, obstetric form (triple-positive); start low-dose aspirin (75–100 mg daily) preconceptionally, add prophylactic-dose LMWH (enoxaparin 40 mg daily) once pregnancy is confirmed, continue LMWH + aspirin throughout pregnancy and 6 weeks postpartum.

Rationale. The patient meets the Sydney revised classification criteria for antiphospholipid syndrome (obstetric form): clinical criterion (≥3 unexplained consecutive spontaneous abortions <10 weeks with exclusion of anatomical, hormonal, and chromosomal causes) AND laboratory criteria (triple-positive antibody profile — lupus anticoagulant, anti-cardiolipin IgG at high titre, and anti-β2GPI IgG, all confirmed on a second occasion 12 weeks apart). The standard for managing future pregnancy in obstetric APS is the combination of low-dose aspirin (started preconceptionally) plus prophylactic-dose LMWH (started once pregnancy is confirmed) and continued through pregnancy and into the puerperium. This combination has been shown in multiple randomised trials to substantially reduce miscarriage rates in obstetric APS. Warfarin is teratogenic in the first trimester (warfarin embryopathy: nasal hypoplasia, stippled epiphyses) and fetotoxic later, so is avoided. DOACs cross the placenta and are not used in pregnancy. Postpartum LMWH continues for 6 weeks at minimum because postpartum is the highest-risk period.

Distractor analysis. (B) Warfarin teratogenic and fetotoxic. (C) DOACs not used in pregnancy. (D) Steroids alone are not the standard for obstetric APS and are not first-line. (E) Treatment with LMWH + aspirin is highly effective and surrogacy is not indicated.

Vignette 3. A 64-year-old postoperative patient with new thrombocytopenia and

a swollen leg

A 64-year-old man is on day 8 following coronary artery bypass grafting. He has been on prophylactic-dose unfractionated heparin since admission. The nurse notes a swollen, painful right calf this morning. CBC: platelets 56,000/µL (had been 320,000/µL on admission and 280,000/µL on day 4; nadir not yet established). Doppler confirms acute right popliteal-to-femoral DVT. CRP not significantly elevated. No fever or signs of sepsis. No DIC (fibrinogen 2.8 g/L, D-dimer modestly raised, PT/APTT normal). 4Ts score: Thrombocytopenia (>50% drop, count 20–100K = 2 points); Timing (5–10 days from heparin start = 2 points); Thrombosis (proven new DVT = 2 points); other Causes excluded (no clear alternative = 2 points) = 8 (high probability). Which of the following is the most appropriate management?

(A) STOP all heparin immediately (UFH, LMWH, heparin flushes, heparin-coated catheters); start non-heparin anticoagulant (argatroban or fondaparinux); send PF4 antibody ELISA and serotonin release assay; document HIT in the medical record permanently; do NOT use warfarin alone in acute HIT.

(B) Continue heparin and add platelet transfusion to raise count.

(C) Switch from UFH to LMWH.

(D) Start warfarin alone for the new DVT.

(E) Hold heparin and observe for spontaneous platelet recovery.

Best answer: (A) STOP all heparin immediately (UFH, LMWH, heparin flushes, heparin-coated catheters); start non-heparin anticoagulant (argatroban or fondaparinux); send PF4 antibody ELISA and serotonin release assay; document HIT in the medical record permanently; do NOT use warfarin alone in acute HIT.

Rationale. The case is classical heparin-induced thrombocytopenia (HIT). All four 4Ts criteria are met at maximum points (8/8 = high probability of HIT). The thrombocytopenia is moderate (50% drop), the timing is 5–10 days from heparin exposure, new thrombosis has occurred, and other causes (sepsis, DIC, drug-induced thrombocytopenia from a different agent) are excluded. The mechanism is IgG antibodies against PF4–heparin complexes activating platelets via FcγRIIa, driving simultaneous thrombocytopenia (consumed in clots) and thrombosis. Management requires immediate cessation of ALL heparin including LMWH (which cross-reacts) and even heparin flushes and heparin-bonded catheters — patients have been killed by ongoing line flushes after UFH discontinuation. Non-heparin anticoagulation must be started immediately because untreated HIT carries 30–50% thrombotic complication risk. Argatroban (direct thrombin inhibitor; hepatic clearance — preferred in renal failure) and fondaparinux (factor Xa inhibitor pentasaccharide; does not cross-react with PF4 antibodies in most cases — though formally off-label for HIT) are the standard first-line options. Bivalirudin is used in cardiac surgery / interventional cardiology contexts. Warfarin alone is dangerous in acute HIT — protein C falls faster than the procoagulants, worsening the prothrombotic state and risking warfarin-induced limb gangrene; warfarin is added only after platelet recovery >150,000/µL with ongoing non-heparin anticoagulant overlap. Confirmatory testing combines PF4 ELISA (sensitive screen) with serotonin release assay or HIPA (functional confirmation, gold standard).

Distractor analysis. (B) Heparin must be STOPPED in HIT, not continued. (C) LMWH cross-reacts with PF4 antibodies. (D) Warfarin alone in acute HIT is dangerous. (E) Observation alone in HIT carries 30–50% thrombotic risk.

Vignette 4. A 22-year-old man with severe DVT and apparent heparin resistance

A 22-year-old man is admitted with massive bilateral lower limb DVT and saddle pulmonary embolism after a long flight. He has no significant medical history but his father had recurrent DVTs from his teens and his elder sister had a postpartum PE. Therapeutic intravenous unfractionated heparin is started at 18 units/kg/h. Despite escalation to 32 units/kg/h, the APTT remains at 1.2× control. Which of the following is the most likely diagnosis and most appropriate next management step?

(A) Antithrombin deficiency; check antithrombin functional level urgently; consider antithrombin concentrate replacement OR switch to argatroban (direct thrombin inhibitor, AT-independent); confirm Factor V Leiden and prothrombin G20210A status as well.

(B) Lupus anticoagulant; switch to LMWH because LMWH is not affected by lupus anticoagulant.

(C) Inadequate dosing only; continue escalating heparin.

(D) Tachyphylaxis; pause heparin for 24 h and re-load.

(E) Drug interaction; check medications.

Best answer: (A) Antithrombin deficiency; check antithrombin functional level urgently; consider antithrombin concentrate replacement OR switch to argatroban (direct thrombin inhibitor, AT-independent); confirm Factor V Leiden and prothrombin G20210A status as well.

Rationale. The clinical presentation — severe early-onset VTE in a young patient, strong autosomal-dominant family history of VTE (father, sister), and apparent heparin resistance (failure to achieve therapeutic APTT despite escalating doses) — is classical antithrombin deficiency. AT deficiency is the rarest but clinically strongest inherited thrombophilia (10- to 50-fold relative risk). Heparin is an indirect thrombin/FXa inhibitor — it accelerates AT-mediated inactivation by ~1000-fold but cannot work without sufficient AT. With AT levels reduced by 50–60% (typical heterozygous deficiency), heparin's effect is markedly attenuated. The diagnostic move is an urgent functional AT assay (chromogenic). Management options include (i) antithrombin concentrate (Atryn — recombinant; or Thrombate — plasma-derived) to replenish AT and restore heparin responsiveness, often used as a bolus to bring AT level above 80% before therapeutic anticoagulation can be achieved; (ii) switch to a direct, AT-independent anticoagulant — argatroban (direct thrombin inhibitor; metabolised hepatically) or bivalirudin. LMWH is also less AT-dependent than UFH but not fully independent. Long-term anticoagulation is indefinite given the severity of presentation, and family screening is indicated. Note: AT cannot be measured during acute thrombosis or on UFH (consumption); for confirmatory testing, repeat the assay 2–4 weeks after stopping anticoagulation.

Distractor analysis. (B) Lupus anticoagulant produces APTT prolongation, not failure to prolong; the case shows the opposite. (C) Pure inadequate dosing is unlikely after dose escalation to 32 units/kg/h with persistent subtherapeutic APTT. (D) Heparin tachyphylaxis is not a recognised mechanism. (E) Drug interaction unlikely in this clinical context.

Vignette 5. A 67-year-old man with pancreatic adenocarcinoma and migratory thrombophlebitis

A 67-year-old man is admitted with three weeks of progressive abdominal pain, weight loss, and migratory tender erythematous cords on different limbs at different times. CT abdomen shows a 4 cm mass in the head of the pancreas with biopsy confirming ductal adenocarcinoma. He has now developed a swollen left calf with Doppler-confirmed acute popliteal-to-femoral DVT. CBC: haemoglobin 11.8 g/dL, platelets 380,000/µL, white blood cells 9,200/µL. Coagulation: D-dimer markedly raised; PT, APTT, fibrinogen normal. CrCl 64 mL/min. Body weight 72 kg. Which of the following is the most appropriate first-line anticoagulation for cancer-associated thrombosis in this patient?

(A) LMWH (enoxaparin 1 mg/kg twice daily or 1.5 mg/kg once daily; or dalteparin 200 IU/kg once daily for the first month, then 150 IU/kg once daily) — preferred over apixaban / edoxaban in this patient because of upper GI bleeding risk from the proximal pancreatic primary. Continue throughout active disease.

(B) Warfarin with target INR 2.0–3.0 indefinitely.

(C) Apixaban 10 mg twice daily for 7 days, then 5 mg twice daily indefinitely.

(D) Aspirin alone.

(E) IVC filter without anticoagulation.

Best answer: (A) LMWH (enoxaparin 1 mg/kg twice daily or 1.5 mg/kg once daily; or dalteparin 200 IU/kg once daily for the first month, then 150 IU/kg once daily) — preferred over apixaban / edoxaban in this patient because of upper GI bleeding risk from the proximal pancreatic primary. Continue throughout active disease.

Rationale. The case is Trousseau's syndrome — migratory superficial thrombophlebitis as a paraneoplastic manifestation of mucin-producing adenocarcinoma (most often pancreatic, also gastric, ovarian, colorectal, lung). Mucinous tumour-derived tissue factor and procoagulant mucins drive the hypercoagulability. Treatment is full anticoagulation. The CLOT trial (2003) established LMWH (dalteparin) as superior to warfarin for cancer-associated VTE for the first 6 months — fewer recurrent thrombi, similar bleeding. The Caravaggio (apixaban) and Hokusai-Cancer (edoxaban) trials subsequently demonstrated DOAC non-inferiority to LMWH in most cancers — but with INCREASED GI bleeding in luminal GI cancers, especially upper GI. In this patient with a pancreatic head primary (peri-ampullary location, with high risk of duodenal erosion), LMWH remains the preferred first-line agent because of the bleeding risk profile. For non-luminal cancers (lung, prostate, breast, gynaecological), apixaban and edoxaban are reasonable alternatives to LMWH. Anticoagulation is continued throughout active cancer (often indefinitely while the cancer is active or in surveillance). Warfarin is INFERIOR to LMWH for cancer-associated VTE per the CLOT trial. IVC filter alone without anticoagulation is reserved for absolute contraindication to anticoagulation; routine use is not supported.

Distractor analysis. (B) Warfarin inferior to LMWH per CLOT. (C) Apixaban acceptable for some cancers but not pancreatic with high upper-GI bleeding risk. (D) Aspirin is not adequate for treatment of established VTE. (E) IVC filter alone leaves the patient unprotected from clot extension and propagation.

Vignette 6. A 42-year-old woman with skin necrosis on day 5 of warfarin

A 42-year-old woman was started on warfarin 5 mg daily four days ago for newly diagnosed unprovoked DVT, without parenteral bridging. On day 5, she develops painful purplish discolouration progressing to necrotic skin lesions on both breasts and the right thigh. Examination: well-demarcated violaceous patches with central black eschar; no other thrombotic features. INR 2.4. CBC: platelets 240,000/µL. CRP not significantly raised. No sepsis. Family history: a brother had unprovoked DVT at age 38. Which of the following is the most likely underlying defect and most appropriate management?

(A) Warfarin-induced skin necrosis from underlying protein C (or protein S) deficiency. STOP warfarin; reverse with vitamin K + activated prothrombin complex concentrate (or fresh frozen plasma); start parenteral anticoagulation (LMWH or UFH) for ongoing VTE management; protein C concentrate (Ceprotin — plasma-derived zymogen, activated in vivo by thrombin–thrombomodulin) for severe necrosis; investigate for protein C and S deficiency 4–6 weeks after stopping warfarin.

(B) Coumarin allergy; corticosteroids and antihistamines.

(C) Calciphylaxis from chronic kidney disease; sodium thiosulfate.

(D) Disseminated intravascular coagulation; cryoprecipitate and platelets.

(E) Increase warfarin dose to push past the hypercoagulable phase.

Best answer: (A) Warfarin-induced skin necrosis from underlying protein C (or protein S) deficiency. STOP warfarin; reverse with vitamin K + activated prothrombin complex concentrate (or fresh frozen plasma); start parenteral anticoagulation (LMWH or UFH) for ongoing VTE management; protein C concentrate (Ceprotin — plasma-derived zymogen, activated in vivo by thrombin–thrombomodulin) for severe necrosis; investigate for protein C and S deficiency 4–6 weeks after stopping warfarin.

Rationale. Warfarin-induced skin necrosis is classical for underlying protein C or protein S deficiency. The mechanism is the differential half-lives of vitamin-K-dependent factors: protein C (~6–8 h) and protein S (~30 h) are depleted faster than the procoagulant factors II (~60 h) and X (~40 h), producing a TRANSIENT hypercoagulable state in the first 3–7 days of warfarin therapy. Patients with already-low baseline protein C or S are pushed into severe transient deficiency with microvascular thrombosis in fatty subcutaneous tissue (breast, thigh, abdomen, buttocks). The presentation is typically days 3–7 of warfarin without bridging. Management requires (i) immediate cessation of warfarin; (ii) reversal with vitamin K plus 4-factor PCC or FFP; (iii) parenteral anticoagulation (LMWH or UFH) to continue VTE protection; (iv) for severe necrosis, exogenous protein C concentrate (Ceprotin) restores anticoagulant function; (v) wound care and surgical debridement as needed; (vi) thrombophilia workup once the patient is stable and 4–6 weeks off warfarin. PREVENTION: always start warfarin with concurrent parenteral anticoagulation and continue parenteral therapy for at least 5 days AND until the INR has been therapeutic for at least 24 hours.

Distractor analysis. (B) Coumarin allergy is rare and presents with rash, not necrosis. (C) Calciphylaxis occurs in advanced CKD and dialysis; this patient has no renal context. (D) DIC has consumptive coagulopathy with low fibrinogen and raised D-dimer. (E) Increasing warfarin worsens the hypercoagulable phase.

Vignette 7. A 36-year-old woman with simultaneous multi-organ thrombosis

A 36-year-old woman with known triple-positive antiphospholipid syndrome (on warfarin, INR 2.5 last week) is admitted after stopping warfarin three days ago for a planned dental extraction. She presents now with progressive headache, confusion, and a swollen right leg. Over the next 72 hours she develops anuria, dyspnoea, chest pain, and abdominal pain. CT: bilateral renal infarcts, splenic infarct, multiple cerebral infarcts in different vascular territories. Echocardiography: new mitral valve thickening with fresh thrombus; right ventricular strain consistent with PE confirmed on CT-PA. Doppler: right popliteal-femoral DVT. CBC: haemoglobin 9.2 g/dL, platelets 78,000/µL, schistocytes on smear, raised LDH. PT and APTT prolonged; D-dimer markedly raised; fibrinogen 1.6 g/L. Antiphospholipid antibodies persistently positive. Which of the following is the most likely diagnosis and most appropriate immediate management?

(A) Catastrophic antiphospholipid syndrome (CAPS); start full-dose anticoagulation (heparin), high-dose corticosteroids, plasma exchange, and IVIg as standard "triple therapy"; consider rituximab and eculizumab for refractory disease.

(B) TTP; urgent plasma exchange.

(C) DIC from sepsis; antibiotics and supportive care.

(D) Warfarin failure due to inadequate INR; restart warfarin alone.

(E) Thrombotic stroke; tPA.

Best answer: (A) Catastrophic antiphospholipid syndrome (CAPS); start full-dose anticoagulation (heparin), high-dose corticosteroids, plasma exchange, and IVIg as standard "triple therapy"; consider rituximab and eculizumab for refractory disease.

Rationale. The case meets the diagnostic criteria for catastrophic antiphospholipid syndrome (CAPS): simultaneous multi-organ thrombosis (≥3 organ systems involved — kidney, spleen, brain, heart, lung, leg) developing rapidly (over <1 week), clinical and imaging evidence of small-vessel thrombosis with end-organ infarction, and confirmed antiphospholipid antibody positivity. The trigger here is anticoagulation cessation for a procedure — a recognised CAPS trigger alongside infection, surgery, malignancy, and pregnancy. The schistocytes and thrombocytopenia reflect microvascular thrombosis and are NOT TTP (ADAMTS13 in CAPS is typically normal; CAPS is the alternative diagnosis when MAHA + thrombocytopenia + multi-organ injury is encountered in a patient with confirmed APS). Mortality in CAPS is approximately 30–50% even with treatment. The standard "triple therapy" combines (i) full-dose anticoagulation (typically therapeutic heparin / LMWH); (ii) high-dose corticosteroids (methylprednisolone 1 g/day for 3 days, then taper); (iii) plasma exchange to remove antibodies; and (iv) IVIg. Rituximab and eculizumab (anti-C5) are added in refractory disease, with eculizumab particularly used given the role of complement activation in CAPS pathogenesis. Long-term anticoagulation must be re-established with warfarin (NOT DOACs in confirmed APS).

Distractor analysis. (B) TTP requires severe ADAMTS13 deficiency; CAPS is the alternative when patients have known APS. (C) DIC requires a clear non-CAPS trigger; this case is anti-coagulation cessation triggering CAPS. (D) Warfarin alone is inadequate in active CAPS. (E) tPA addresses arterial stroke but does not address the multi-organ disease.

Vignette 8. An 82-year-old woman with atrial fibrillation and CrCl 28 mL/min

An 82-year-old woman with newly diagnosed non-valvular atrial fibrillation is referred for anticoagulation. She has hypertension, well-controlled diabetes, prior TIA two years ago, and chronic kidney disease (CrCl 28 mL/min). CHA2DS2-VASc 5 (high stroke risk); HAS-BLED 3 (moderate bleeding risk). Body weight 56 kg. Which of the following is the most appropriate anticoagulant?

(A) Apixaban 2.5 mg twice daily (dose-reduced criterion: ≥2 of age ≥80, weight ≤60 kg, creatinine ≥1.5 mg/dL); preferred DOAC in renal impairment given the lowest renal clearance (~25%) and dose-adjusted regimen for the elderly.

(B) Dabigatran 150 mg twice daily.

(C) Rivaroxaban 20 mg once daily with the evening meal.

(D) Aspirin 81 mg daily.

(E) Warfarin with target INR 2.0–3.0.

Best answer: (A) Apixaban 2.5 mg twice daily (dose-reduced criterion: ≥2 of age ≥80, weight ≤60 kg, creatinine ≥1.5 mg/dL); preferred DOAC in renal impairment given the lowest renal clearance (~25%) and dose-adjusted regimen for the elderly.

Rationale. For atrial fibrillation in an elderly patient with high stroke risk and chronic kidney disease, apixaban is generally the preferred DOAC because of (i) the lowest renal clearance among DOACs (~25% renal vs ~80% for dabigatran); (ii) explicit dose-reduction criteria for the elderly (age ≥80, weight ≤60 kg, creatinine ≥1.5 mg/dL — meet ≥2 of 3 → reduce to 2.5 mg twice daily); and (iii) the lowest major bleeding rate among DOACs in pivotal trials (ARISTOTLE). This patient meets two of the three reduction criteria (age 82, weight 56 kg). Dabigatran is largely renally cleared and is contraindicated at CrCl <30 mL/min. Rivaroxaban at full dose is acceptable down to CrCl 30 mL/min; lower with caution and dose reduction; not recommended at CrCl <15 mL/min. Edoxaban requires CrCl 15–95 mL/min (paradoxically — at CrCl >95 mL/min the drug is excreted too fast and provides inadequate anticoagulation). Aspirin alone is inadequate for stroke prevention in AF with CHA2DS2-VASc ≥2. Warfarin is acceptable but DOACs offer fewer drug-drug interactions, fewer dietary interactions, no INR monitoring, and lower intracranial bleeding rate.

Distractor analysis. (B) Dabigatran contraindicated CrCl <30. (C) Rivaroxaban not preferred in this elderly low-weight patient with CrCl 28. (D) Aspirin alone inadequate. (E) Warfarin acceptable but apixaban preferred per current guidelines.

Vignette 9. A 31-year-old woman planning pregnancy with prior unprovoked DVT

A 31-year-old woman is planning pregnancy and asks for preconception advice. She had an unprovoked left iliofemoral DVT four years ago at age 27, treated with rivaroxaban for 6 months. She has been off anticoagulation for 3.5 years with no recurrence. Thrombophilia workup at the time of the original DVT showed heterozygous Factor V Leiden. Family history: mother had a postpartum PE; maternal aunt had a DVT during pregnancy. Which of the following is the most appropriate VTE prophylaxis plan for pregnancy and postpartum?

(A) Antepartum prophylactic-dose LMWH (enoxaparin 40 mg daily, escalating with weight gain) from confirmation of pregnancy until delivery; intrapartum hold; postpartum LMWH for at least 6 weeks. Switch to warfarin postpartum if breastfeeding-friendly target INR can be maintained, OR continue LMWH; warfarin is compatible with breastfeeding. AVOID DOACs in pregnancy and breastfeeding.

(B) Continue rivaroxaban throughout pregnancy.

(C) No prophylaxis needed because the original DVT was successfully treated.

(D) Warfarin throughout pregnancy.

(E) Aspirin 81 mg daily throughout pregnancy and postpartum.

Best answer: (A) Antepartum prophylactic-dose LMWH (enoxaparin 40 mg daily,

escalating with weight gain) from confirmation of pregnancy until delivery; intrapartum hold; postpartum LMWH for at least 6 weeks. Switch to warfarin postpartum if breastfeeding-friendly target INR can be maintained, OR continue LMWH; warfarin is compatible with breastfeeding. AVOID DOACs in pregnancy and breastfeeding.

Rationale. A woman with prior unprovoked VTE plus heritable thrombophilia plus strong family history is at substantially increased risk during pregnancy and the puerperium. Pregnancy-associated VTE risk is highest in the immediate postpartum (~6 weeks). The standard of care is antepartum prophylactic-dose LMWH starting at confirmation of pregnancy and continuing until delivery, plus 6 weeks of postpartum prophylaxis (LMWH or warfarin). LMWH is the anticoagulant of choice in pregnancy: it does not cross the placenta (unlike warfarin), has predictable kinetics, and is safe for both fetus and mother. DOACs cross the placenta and into breast milk and are not used in pregnancy or breastfeeding. Warfarin is teratogenic in the first trimester (warfarin embryopathy: nasal hypoplasia, stippled epiphyses, CNS malformations) and fetotoxic later (placental and fetal bleeding); avoid antepartum. Warfarin is COMPATIBLE with breastfeeding (the active drug does not enter breast milk in clinically meaningful concentrations) and may be used postpartum if preferred. Aspirin alone is inadequate for established prior VTE. Therapeutic-dose anticoagulation (rather than prophylactic) may be considered in some high-risk profiles but prophylactic-dose LMWH is standard for this clinical pattern.

Distractor analysis. (B) DOACs not used in pregnancy. (C) Past VTE with FVL + family history mandates antepartum prophylaxis. (D) Warfarin teratogenic and fetotoxic. (E) Aspirin alone inadequate.

Vignette 10. A 76-year-old man on dabigatran with major intracranial bleeding

A 76-year-old man on dabigatran 150 mg twice daily for atrial fibrillation is admitted after a fall with confusion and right-sided weakness. CT brain: large left intraparenchymal haemorrhage with mass effect and midline shift. The neurosurgical team is preparing for urgent decompression. Last dabigatran dose was 4 hours ago. CrCl 52 mL/min. Coagulation: APTT 64 s (markedly prolonged); thrombin time markedly prolonged; platelets normal; PT modestly prolonged. Which of the following is the most appropriate immediate reversal strategy?

(A) Idarucizumab (Praxbind) 5 g IV — humanised monoclonal antibody Fab fragment that specifically binds dabigatran with very high affinity, producing complete and rapid reversal of dabigatran effect within minutes. Confirm reversal by repeat APTT or thrombin time. Proceed to surgery once reversal is complete.

(B) Andexanet alfa.

(C) Vitamin K and fresh frozen plasma.

(D) 4-factor prothrombin complex concentrate (PCC) only.

(E) Tranexamic acid only.

Best answer: (A) Idarucizumab (Praxbind) 5 g IV — humanised monoclonal antibody Fab fragment that specifically binds dabigatran with very high affinity, producing complete and rapid reversal of dabigatran effect within minutes. Confirm reversal by repeat APTT or thrombin time. Proceed to surgery once reversal is complete.

Rationale. Idarucizumab is the specific antidote for dabigatran. It is a humanised monoclonal antibody Fab fragment that binds dabigatran with affinity approximately 350-fold greater than dabigatran's affinity for thrombin. The standard dose is 5 g IV (given as two consecutive 2.5 g infusions). Reversal is essentially complete within minutes and the effect lasts for the duration of dabigatran clearance. The REVERSE-AD trial established efficacy in life-threatening bleeding and emergent surgery. Andexanet alfa (Andexxa) is the specific reversal agent for the FXa inhibitors rivaroxaban and apixaban (and partially edoxaban) but does NOT reverse dabigatran. 4-factor PCC has limited efficacy against dabigatran (it provides procoagulant factors but does not neutralise dabigatran in the circulation). Vitamin K and FFP do not reverse dabigatran. Tranexamic acid is an adjunct for fibrinolytic-driven bleeding but does not reverse the anticoagulant. After idarucizumab and bleeding control, dabigatran should not be restarted until clinically appropriate; in some cases switching to a different anticoagulation strategy is preferred.

Distractor analysis. (B) Andexanet reverses FXa inhibitors, not dabigatran. (C) Vitamin K and FFP do not reverse dabigatran. (D) PCC has limited efficacy against dabigatran. (E) Tranexamic acid does not reverse anticoagulant effect.

17.12 Closing Discriminators

HIGH-YIELD PEARL — When does thrombophilia testing change management?

Testing changes management in only a few well-defined scenarios. Reflexive panel testing in every VTE patient is wasteful, generates false-positive results from preanalytical interference, and rarely alters the standard treatment course of 3-month minimum anticoagulation.

- Test antithrombin if there is severe early VTE, strong autosomal-dominant family history, or apparent heparin resistance — result drives consideration of antithrombin replacement or non-heparin anticoagulation.
- Test protein C and S in suspected warfarin-induced skin necrosis (positive history with classical lesions days 3–7 of warfarin) and in neonatal purpura fulminans — result drives use of protein C concentrate.
- Test full APLAS panel (LA + aCL + anti-β2GPI) on two occasions ≥12 weeks apart in unexplained recurrent miscarriage, late fetal loss, severe preeclampsia, unexplained venous OR arterial thrombosis, and any patient with autoimmune disease and thrombosis — result drives drug choice (warfarin, NOT DOAC, in triple-positive).
- Test Factor V Leiden / prothrombin G20210A in young unprovoked VTE with family history — result rarely changes the index treatment but informs family screening (oestrogen contraception in heterozygous female relatives) and pregnancy management.
- Do NOT test routinely in older patients with provoked VTE or in asymptomatic family screening of children. Do NOT test during acute thrombosis or on anticoagulation (other than the genetic markers).

HIGH-YIELD PEARL — Drug-by-drug reversal — exam-ready table

- Warfarin → Vitamin K (oral or IV depending on urgency) + 4-factor prothrombin complex concentrate (PCC) for major bleeding. FFP if PCC unavailable. Vitamin K alone for minor bleeding or asymptomatic high INR.
- Unfractionated heparin → Protamine sulfate 1 mg per 100 IU heparin given within the previous hour. Full reversal.
- Low-molecular-weight heparin → Protamine partially reverses (60–70% of the anti-Xa effect). Andexanet alfa is not approved for LMWH but has been used off-label.
- Fondaparinux → No specific reversal. Activated PCC may be tried for life-threatening bleeding; supportive care otherwise.
- Dabigatran → Idarucizumab (Praxbind) 5 g IV — specific Fab antibody fragment, complete reversal within minutes. PCC has limited efficacy.
- Rivaroxaban / apixaban (and partially edoxaban) → Andexanet alfa (Andexxa) — recombinant inactive FXa decoy. 4-factor PCC at high dose (50 IU/kg) is the off-label alternative when andexanet is unavailable.
- Argatroban / bivalirudin → No specific reversal. Short half-lives (argatroban ~50 min; bivalirudin ~25 min); supportive care, dialysis (bivalirudin partly dialysable), and time.
- Antiplatelet agents (aspirin, P2Y12 inhibitors, GPIIb/IIIa inhibitors) → No specific reversal. Platelet transfusion in major bleeding may help (less effective for ticagrelor — reversibly bound). Tranexamic acid as adjunct.

HIGH-YIELD PEARL — APLAS treatment — DOAC vs warfarin

The TRAPS trial (2018) randomised triple-positive APS patients to rivaroxaban vs warfarin and was stopped early because of significantly more arterial thromboembolic events on rivaroxaban (12% vs 0% in warfarin arm at 1.5 years). Subsequent meta-analyses have confirmed warfarin superiority in triple-positive APS.

Practical implications:

- Triple-positive APS (LA + aCL + anti-β2GPI) → WARFARIN, target INR 2.0–3.0 (some guidelines higher, INR 2.5–3.5, after arterial thrombosis).
- Single-positive APS without arterial events → DOAC may be considered in shared decision-making.
- Any APS with arterial thrombosis → WARFARIN preferred.
- Pregnancy in APS → LMWH + low-dose aspirin (NOT DOACs, NOT warfarin).
- Mechanical heart valves (any cause) → WARFARIN; DOACs CONTRAINDICATED (RE-ALIGN trial).
- Moderate-to-severe mitral stenosis → WARFARIN.

IMG-TRAP — Rifampicin and warfarin: the CYP2C9 induction trap on USMLE pharmacology vignettes

The trap. The classic USMLE pharmacology vignette places a stable warfarin patient on a new drug and asks what happens to the INR. IMGs trained heavily on tuberculosis pharmacology often miss the rifampicin–warfarin interaction because they think of rifampicin as a TB drug rather than as a CYP enzyme inducer. On the exam, rifampicin is one of the canonical inducers (rifampicin, phenytoin, carbamazepine, phenobarbital, St John's wort, chronic alcohol, smoking) and the right answer is: induces CYP2C9 → accelerates warfarin metabolism → INR FALLS → patient becomes subtherapeutic and re-thromboses unless the warfarin dose is increased.

The rule. When a USMLE stem starts an anti-TB regimen, anti-epileptic, or any of the classic inducers in a patient on warfarin, look for falling INR and a thrombotic event. The mirror image — inhibitors (amiodarone, fluconazole, metronidazole, sulfonamides, macrolides, ciprofloxacin, fluoxetine, isoniazid, grapefruit juice) — raises INR and causes bleeding. CYP2C9 and VKORC1 polymorphisms drive much of the inter-individual dose variability, with average therapeutic doses lower in patients of South Asian and East Asian ancestry than in European populations; this is testable Step 1 pharmacogenetics, not a regional aside.

17.13 Quick Recall

QUICK RECALL — Thrombosis, Thrombophilia, and Anticoagulation

Virchow's triad: endothelial injury, stasis, hypercoagulability. Arterial thrombi are platelet-rich (white thrombi, treat with antiplatelet); venous thrombi are fibrin-rich (red thrombi, treat with anticoagulation).

Inherited thrombophilias by frequency in Europeans: Factor V Leiden (3–8%, R506Q makes FVa APC-resistant; APC resistance assay or PCR) > prothrombin G20210A (1–3%, raised prothrombin) > protein C/S deficiency (0.1–0.5%) > antithrombin deficiency (0.02–0.2%, RAREST but STRONGEST risk: 10–50× VTE).

Warfarin-induced skin necrosis: days 3–6 of warfarin in protein C/S deficient patients; transient hypercoagulability from rapid PC/S depletion. Always bridge warfarin with parenteral anticoagulant for 5 days AND until INR therapeutic ≥24 h.

Thrombophilia testing timing: do NOT test AT during acute thrombosis or on UFH (consumed); do NOT test PC/PS on warfarin or in pregnancy/OCP; do NOT test LA on heparin or DOACs. Genetic markers (FVL, PT G20210A) unaffected. APLAS antibodies confirmed on 2 occasions ≥12 weeks apart.

APLAS = Sydney criteria: ≥1 clinical (vascular thrombosis OR obstetric morbidity) + ≥1 lab (LA OR aCL medium/high titre OR anti-β2GPI) confirmed ≥12 weeks apart. Triple positivity = highest risk. CAPS = simultaneous multi-organ thrombosis ≥3 organ systems within 1 week. Treat: anticoagulation + corticosteroids + plasma exchange + IVIg ± rituximab/eculizumab.

APLAS treatment: WARFARIN INR 2.0–3.0 (NOT DOACs in triple-positive — TRAPS trial). Pregnancy: LMWH + low-dose aspirin throughout pregnancy + 6 weeks postpartum.

Acquired hypercoagulable states: cancer (Trousseau's — pancreatic / mucinous adenocarcinoma; LMWH preferred over DOAC in luminal GI/GU cancers), pregnancy (5× risk; LMWH), oestrogen contraception (3–5× risk; FVL combination multiplicative), MPNs (JAK2 V617F; splanchnic thrombosis with normal counts), PNH (FLAER on granulocytes; eculizumab), HIT, IBD, nephrotic syndrome, COVID-19.

Heparins. UFH: AT-mediated thrombin and FXa inhibition (1:1); APTT or anti-Xa monitoring; protamine reversal. LMWH: anti-Xa preference (~3:1); subcut once/twice daily; renal clearance (avoid CrCl <30); protamine partial reversal. Fondaparinux: pure anti-Xa pentasaccharide; subcut once daily; renal (avoid <30); no protamine reversal.

Heparin-induced thrombocytopenia (HIT): 4Ts ≥4 (Thrombocytopenia, Timing 5–10 days, Thrombosis, oTher causes excluded); PF4 ELISA + serotonin release assay; STOP all heparin; start argatroban or fondaparinux; do NOT use warfarin alone in acute HIT.

Warfarin: VKORC1 inhibitor; depletes vitamin-K-dependent factors II, VII, IX, X + PC, PS. INR 2.0–3.0 most indications; 2.5–3.5 mechanical mitral valve and triple-positive APS. Reversal: vitamin K + 4-factor PCC for major bleeding (PCC > FFP).

DOACs. Dabigatran: direct thrombin (FIIa) inhibitor; ~80% renal; idarucizumab reversal. Rivaroxaban / apixaban / edoxaban: direct FXa inhibitors; renal clearance varies (apixaban ~25% — preferred in renal impairment); andexanet alfa or 4-factor PCC reversal. CONTRAINDICATED: mechanical valves, moderate-severe mitral stenosis, triple-positive APS, pregnancy, breastfeeding.

Treatment of VTE. Provoked: 3 months. First unprovoked: 3 months minimum, reassess for indefinite. Recurrent unprovoked: indefinite. Cancer-associated: LMWH OR apixaban/edoxaban (avoid in luminal GI/GU); throughout active cancer. Pregnancy: LMWH + 6 weeks postpartum (no warfarin antepartum, no DOAC). APLAS: warfarin indefinitely. Mechanical valve: warfarin indefinitely.

Drug interactions on warfarin: rifampicin (TB therapy) induces CYP2C9 and reduces warfarin effect (INR falls); amiodarone, sulfonamides, fluconazole, metronidazole, and macrolides inhibit and raise INR. CYP2C9 and VKORC1 polymorphisms drive ethnic variation in dosing — average maintenance doses lower in patients of South and East Asian ancestry than European.

Chapter 18 — Transfusion Medicine

18.1 The ABO Blood Group System

ABO is the single most important system in transfusion medicine because the antibodies are pre-formed, IgM, complement-fixing, and present in every immunocompetent person from the first months of life. An ABO-incompatible transfusion is not merely "reactive" — it is intravascular haemolysis, DIC, and shock within minutes.

Antigens, Genetics, and the H Substance

ABO antigens are carbohydrate epitopes built on a common precursor — the H antigen, made when the FUT1-encoded fucosyltransferase adds fucose to the chain. The A gene then adds N-acetylgalactosamine to H (forming A antigen); the B gene adds galactose (forming B antigen). Group O cells carry the unmodified H antigen — they have neither A nor B transferase activity. Inheritance is codominant: A and B are both expressed when present, O is recessive.

Anti-A and anti-B are naturally occurring (gut bacterial polysaccharides cross-react with A and B), develop by 3–6 months of age, and are predominantly IgM. This is why neonates do not yet have reliable reverse grouping and why ABO-incompatible plasma in a neonate behaves differently from in an adult.

Group	RBC Antigens	Serum Antibodies	US Frequency (approx.)
A	A (and H)	Anti-B	~40%
B	B (and H)	Anti-A	~11%
AB	A, B (and H)	Neither	~4%
O	H only	Anti-A and Anti-B	~45%

Table 18.1 ABO antigen–antibody profile and US population frequencies. Distributions vary by ethnicity (e.g., higher B in East and South Asian populations).

Subgroups, Bombay Phenotype, and Discrepancies

About 80 percent of group A individuals are A1 (high antigen density, agglutinated by Dolichos biflorus lectin); the remaining ~20 percent are A2 (lower density). A2 individuals can produce anti-A1, which is clinically significant only when reactive at 37 °C. Rare subgroups (A3, Ax, Ael, B3, Bx) express antigen so weakly that routine forward grouping may type the patient as O — an important cause of ABO discrepancy.

Bombay phenotype (Oh) is homozygous loss of FUT1 — no H is made, therefore no A or B can be built on it regardless of ABO genotype. Serum contains anti-A, anti-B, and crucially anti-H. Forward grouping reads as group O; reverse grouping reads as not-O because the patient's serum agglutinates ordinary group O (H-rich) cells. The patient can only receive blood from another Bombay donor. Estimated frequency is roughly 1 in 250,000 worldwide, with a regional cluster in western India (~1 in 7,500–10,000) where the phenotype was first described in 1952.

Pearl — Resolving an ABO Discrepancy

Forward and reverse must agree before blood is issued. When they do not, work through this checklist: (1) repeat with a fresh sample; (2) check for cold autoantibodies (warm cells to 37 °C, repeat); (3) check for ABO subgroups using anti-A1 lectin and saliva secretor studies; (4) ask about recent transfusion (mixed-field reaction); (5) consider age extremes (neonate or elderly with weak antibody) and immunocompromise; (6) consider Bombay phenotype if anti-H is present. Until resolved: issue group O red cells (least likely to cause haemolysis) and AB plasma if needed, but do not finalise the patient's blood group.

IMG-Trap — Do not Reach for Bombay on Every ABO Discrepancy

IMGs trained in Mumbai often over-prioritise Bombay phenotype on USMLE because of its local prevalence (1 in 7,500–10,000 in Mumbai versus ~1 in 250,000 globally). USMLE tests it rarely; when it does, the discriminator is anti-H in serum reacting with group O screening cells. Do not reach for Oh on every ABO discrepancy vignette — the USMLE answer key is usually an A subgroup (A2 with anti-A1, or A3/Ax typing weakly), recent transfusion with mixed-field agglutination, or a cold autoantibody. Reserve Bombay for the vignette that explicitly tests anti-H reactivity with group O cells, not every "types as O but crossmatch incompatible" scenario.

18.2 The Rh Blood Group System

Rh is the second-most-important system. It is encoded by two closely linked genes on chromosome 1: RHD (encodes D antigen) and RHCE (encodes C/c and E/e). Unlike ABO, Rh antibodies are IgG and immune (require prior exposure through transfusion or pregnancy). The D antigen is the most immunogenic non-ABO antigen — a single unit of D-positive red cells transfused into a D-negative recipient leads to anti-D in 50–80 percent.

RhD-negative frequency varies by ethnicity: ~15% in non-Hispanic Whites, ~8% in African Americans, ~5–8% in South Asians, and <1% in East Asians. The variation matters most in obstetrics — anti-D immunoglobulin prophylaxis (RhIG, 300 µg at 28 weeks and within 72 hours of delivery for RhD-negative mothers carrying RhD-positive fetuses) is a standing USMLE topic.

Antigen	Significance	Notes
D	Most immunogenic non-ABO antigen; principal cause of HDFN	D-positive ~85% Whites, ~92% African Americans, ~99% East Asians
C / c	HDFN and acute/delayed haemolytic reactions	Anti-c is the most clinically significant Rh antibody after anti-D
E / e	HDFN; delayed haemolytic transfusion reactions	Anti-E common in multiply-transfused patients (e.g., sickle cell, thalassaemia)

Table 18.2 Clinically relevant Rh antigens.

Weak D versus Partial D

Weak D (formerly Du) means a quantitative reduction in normal D antigen — fewer copies per cell, but each copy is structurally complete. Cells react weakly or negatively at immediate spin and become positive only at the IAT phase. Weak D individuals do not make anti-D and can usually receive D-positive blood.

Partial D means a qualitative defect — some D epitopes are missing. Partial D individuals can produce anti-D against the missing epitopes when exposed to fully-D-positive blood, and should therefore receive D-negative units. The two cannot be reliably separated by serology alone; molecular RHD genotyping is the discriminator.

Pearl — Weak D vs Partial D — Clinical Rule
Donor weak D = call positive (transfuse only to D+ recipients). Recipient weak D = call positive (can receive D+). Recipient partial D = treat as D− (can make anti-D). Pregnant woman with weak D type 1, 2, or 3 (the common European variants identified by RHD genotyping): treat as D-positive, no Rh-immunoglobulin needed. All other weak/partial D pregnancies, or where genotyping is unavailable: treat as D-negative and give RhIG.

18.3 Other Clinically Important Blood Group Systems

Beyond ABO and Rh, the ISBT recognises over 40 systems and 360+ antigens. Five systems generate most of the clinically significant problems.

System	Principal Antigens	Antibody Class	Clinical Significance
Kell	K (KEL1), k (KEL2)	IgG	Anti-K is highly immunogenic; severe HDFN and HTRs. K-negative blood for transfusion-dependent thalassaemia and SCD.
Duffy	Fy(a), Fy(b)	IgG	Fy(a−b−) common in West Africans → resistance to Plasmodium vivax (Duffy is the merozoite receptor).
Kidd	Jk(a), Jk(b)	IgG (complement-fixing)	"Notorious" for delayed haemolytic reactions; antibody titers fall rapidly between exposures.
MNS	M, N, S, s	Mixed	Anti-M/N usually clinically insignificant (cold IgM). Anti-S/s are IgG and can cause HDFN.
Lewis	Le(a), Le(b)	IgM (mostly)	Naturally occurring; usually clinically insignificant. Lewis antigens are adsorbed onto RBCs from plasma.
P1PK / Globoside	P1, P, P(k)	IgM/IgG	Anti-PP1Pk in p phenotype — intravascular haemolysis and recurrent first-trimester miscarriage.

Table 18.3 Other clinically important blood group systems.

Pearl — Three Buzzwords That Win Vignettes
(1) "Notorious for delayed haemolytic reactions with falling antibody titers" → Kidd (anti-Jka). (2) "Highly immunogenic, second only to D, severe HDFN, K-negative blood policy in chronic transfusion programs" → Kell. (3) "Confers resistance to Plasmodium vivax" → Duffy Fy(a−b−).

18.4 Pre-transfusion Testing

Pre-transfusion testing exists to ensure that the donor unit is compatible with the recipient at the antigen–antibody level. The standard sequence is sample collection with positive patient identification, recipient ABO and Rh(D) typing, antibody screen, and crossmatch.

The Sample — Why Identification Beats Chemistry

Patient misidentification at the bedside is the leading cause of fatal haemolytic transfusion reactions worldwide. The blood bank cannot detect the error — the sample is correctly typed and the unit is correctly issued; the patient on whose chart the sample was drawn is simply not the patient on the bed. The defences are procedural: two-person identification, wristband checks, sample labelling at the bedside (never away from the patient), and a second-sample policy in critical transfusions. Group-and-screen samples must be drawn and labelled in front of the patient, never batched at the nurses' station.

Forward and Reverse Grouping

Forward grouping (cell typing) tests recipient red cells against known anti-A and anti-B reagents. Reverse grouping (serum typing) tests recipient serum against known A1 and B reagent cells. Both must agree. Reverse grouping is unreliable in neonates (antibodies not yet developed), in elderly or immunocompromised patients (weak antibodies), and in patients with hypogammaglobulinaemia or recent IVIG. Forward grouping can fail in ABO subgroups, mixed-field reactions after recent transfusion, and Bombay phenotype.

Antibody Screen (Indirect Antiglobulin Test)

The antibody screen detects clinically significant unexpected alloantibodies in recipient serum. A panel of two or three group O screening cells with known antigen profiles (covering D, C, c, E, e, K, k, Fya, Fyb, Jka, Jkb, M, N, S, s, P1, Lea, Leb) is incubated with patient serum at 37 °C with an enhancement medium (LISS — low-ionic-strength saline; or PEG — polyethylene glycol), washed, and tested with anti-human globulin (AHG, Coombs reagent). Agglutination at the AHG phase indicates an IgG alloantibody. A positive screen prompts antibody identification with an extended 10–16 cell panel and consideration of antigen-negative units.

Crossmatch — Three Flavours

Crossmatch Type	What It Detects	When Used
Full (AHG) crossmatch	ABO incompatibility AND IgG alloantibodies against donor cells	Antibody screen positive; history of clinically significant antibody
Immediate spin (IS)	ABO incompatibility only (IgM-mediated agglutination at room temp)	Antibody screen negative AND no antibody history
Electronic (computer)	Computerised verification of ABO/Rh compatibility — no serological testing of the unit	Two concordant typings on file, negative screen, validated computer system

Table 18.4 Crossmatch types — what each one tests for.

An incompatible crossmatch in warm autoimmune haemolytic anaemia is a special case. The autoantibody reacts with all donor units. The decision to transfuse is clinical — using the "least incompatible" units and accepting accelerated red cell destruction — never serological. Steroid therapy, IVIG, and minimum effective transfusion volume are the framework; do not delay transfusion in a symptomatic AIHA patient because the crossmatch is positive.

Step 2 Bridge — Type and Screen vs Type and Crossmatch
On the wards, "type and screen" (ABO/Rh + antibody screen, no crossmatch) is ordered when transfusion is possible but not certain. "Type and crossmatch" reserves a specific unit for a specific patient. The maximum surgical blood ordering schedule (MSBOS) sets institutional norms — e.g., elective cholecystectomy = T&S only, total knee replacement = T&S, AAA repair = crossmatch 4 units. This reduces unnecessary unit reservation and the crossmatch-to-transfusion ratio.

Recent Advances

Molecular blood group typing (PCR, NGS) resolves complex serological problems — multiply transfused patients with mixed populations, warm autoantibodies masking alloantibodies, prenatal fetal RhD genotyping from cell-free fetal DNA in maternal plasma. Extended antigen matching (Rh, Kell, Duffy, Kidd, MNS) for chronically transfused patients reduces alloimmunisation rates significantly in sickle cell disease and thalassaemia. Column agglutination technology (gel cards) has replaced tube testing in most modern blood banks — it offers standardised endpoints, photographic documentation, and reduced subjective error.

18.5 Blood Components — Preparation, Storage, and Clinical Use

Modern transfusion practice rests on component therapy. Whole blood is rarely transfused as such; it is fractionated by differential centrifugation into red cells, platelets, plasma, and cryoprecipitate, each stored at conditions that preserve the relevant function. The patient receives only the deficient component. This is the single most heavily examined section of the chapter — USMLE expects you to know preparation, storage temperature and shelf life, indication, and the expected post-transfusion increment for each component.

From Whole Blood to Components — The Centrifugation Pathway

A whole-blood unit (450–500 mL drawn into CPDA-1 or CPD with SAGM additive) is processed within 6–8 hours of collection. The first soft spin (~1,500 g for 5–7 minutes) sediments red cells; the supernatant is platelet-rich plasma (PRP). The PRP undergoes a hard spin (~5,000 g for 10–15 minutes), producing a platelet button (resuspended in 50–60 mL plasma) and a cell-free plasma supernatant. Plasma frozen rapidly within 6–8 hours of collection is fresh frozen plasma (FFP). Slow thawing of FFP at 1–6 °C precipitates a cold-insoluble fraction rich in factor VIII, von Willebrand factor, fibrinogen, factor XIII, and fibronectin — this is cryoprecipitate. Each whole-blood donation therefore yields one unit each of PRBC, RDP, FFP, and cryoprecipitate.

An alternative buffy-coat method (more common in Europe) layers four whole-blood units, pools the buffy coats, and produces a pooled platelet concentrate. Apheresis (single-donor) platelets and plasma are collected directly from the donor by an automated cell separator and bypass the whole-blood pathway entirely.

Component	Preparation	Storage	Shelf Life	Indication / Expected Effect
Packed RBCs (PRBC)	Centrifuge whole blood; remove most plasma. Hct 55–75%.	2–6 °C	35 d (CPDA-1) / 42 d (SAGM)	Symptomatic anaemia. Adult: 1 unit raises Hb ≈ 1 g/dL or Hct ≈ 3%. Paediatric dose 10–15 mL/kg.
Random donor platelets (RDP)	PRP or buffy-coat method from whole blood.	20–24 °C with continuous gentle agitation	5 d (7 d if pathogen-reduced)	Bleeding with thrombocytopenia; prophylactic if platelets <10 × 10^9/L. 1 RDP raises count by ~5–10 × 10^9/L.
Single donor platelets (SDP / apheresis)	Apheresis from one donor — yields 3 × 10^{11} platelets in 200–300 mL plasma.	20–24 °C with agitation	5 d (7 d if PR)	Equivalent to 4–6 RDP units; fewer donor exposures, lower HLA alloimmunisation risk. Choice for chronic transfusion.
Fresh frozen plasma (FFP)	Plasma frozen within 6–8 h of collection. Volume 200–250 mL.	≤ -18 °C	1 year	Multiple coagulation factor deficiency (DIC, liver disease, massive transfusion, warfarin reversal when 4F-PCC unavailable). TTP — replacement fluid in TPE. Dose 10–15 mL/kg.
Cryoprecipitate	Slow-thaw FFP at 1–6 °C; collect the cold-insoluble	≤ -18 °C	1 year	Hypofibrinogenaemia (<100 mg/dL with bleeding), DIC, congenital

Component	Preparation	Storage	Shelf Life	Indication / Expected Effect
	precipitate. ≥80 IU FVIII and ≥150 mg fibrinogen per unit.			fibrinogen disorders, factor XIII deficiency, vWD type 3 if no concentrate. Dose 1 unit/10 kg raises fibrinogen by ~50–100 mg/dL.
Granulocyte concentrate	Apheresis from G-CSF and dexamethasone-stimulated donor. Must be irradiated.	20–24 °C, transfuse within 24 h	24 h	Severe neutropenia (ANC <500) with documented infection refractory to antimicrobials. Rare and falling out of use as antifungals improve.
Whole blood	Unprocessed donation in anticoagulant. Increasingly used as low-titer group O whole blood (LTOWB) in trauma resuscitation.	2–6 °C	21–35 d	Massive haemorrhage; exchange transfusion in neonatal HDFN. LTOWB protocols at major US trauma centres.

Table 18.5 Blood components — preparation, storage, shelf life, and clinical use. Highest-yield table in the chapter.

Special Processing

Three modifications upgrade standard components to meet specific clinical needs.

Modification	Method	Indication
Leukoreduction	Pre-storage filtration (preferred) or bedside filter — reduces leukocyte count to $<5 \times 10^6$ per unit (3-log reduction).	FNHTR prevention, HLA alloimmunisation prevention, CMV risk reduction. Universal pre-storage leukoreduction is now standard in most US blood centres.
Irradiation	Gamma (Cs-137 / Co-60) or X-ray, ≥25 Gy mid-plane (max 50 Gy). Inactivates donor T lymphocytes.	Prevents TA-GVHD. Mandatory in HSCT recipients, congenital T-cell immunodeficiency, intrauterine and neonatal exchange transfusion, Hodgkin lymphoma, fludarabine/cladribine therapy, and any directed donation from a relative. Irradiated PRBCs expire 14 d after irradiation due to potassium leak.
Washing	Saline wash removes plasma proteins (3 wash cycles, ~80% protein removal).	Severe / recurrent allergic reactions, IgA deficiency with anti-IgA, neonatal alloimmune thrombocytopenia. 24-hour outdate after washing.

Table 18.6 Special component processing — when standard is not enough.

Pearl — Cryoprecipitate Dose Calculation

One unit of cryoprecipitate contains ≥80 IU factor VIII and ≥150 mg fibrinogen in roughly 15–20 mL. Adult dose = 1 unit per 10 kg body weight (typically 8–10 units pooled), expected to raise plasma fibrinogen by 50–100 mg/dL. For factor VIII replacement in haemophilia A when concentrate is unavailable: 1 unit/10 kg raises FVIII activity by ~30–50 percent. Fibrinogen target in obstetric haemorrhage and DIC: ≥150–200 mg/dL.

Pearl — Massive Transfusion Protocol — 1:1:1

Defined as transfusion of ≥10 units PRBC in 24 hours, or replacement of one circulating blood volume. Modern practice (PROPPR trial, 2015) replaces blood loss in a 1:1:1 ratio of PRBC : FFP : platelets to avoid the dilutional coagulopathy seen with crystalloid-and-RBC-only resuscitation. Tranexamic acid 1 g IV within 3 hours of trauma (CRASH-2). Replace calcium (citrate from massive plasma load chelates Ca^{2+} → tetany, hypotension, prolonged QT). Watch the lethal triad: hypothermia, acidosis, coagulopathy — each amplifies the others.

18.6 Transfusion Reactions

Reactions are classified by timing (acute, within 24 hours; delayed, beyond 24 hours) and mechanism (immune vs non-immune). Acute haemolytic reactions are emergencies; TA-GVHD is nearly uniformly fatal and entirely preventable; TRALI–TACO discrimination changes management.

Classification Table

Timing / Type	Reaction	Mechanism	Key Clinical Features
Acute immune	Acute haemolytic (AHTR)	ABO-incompatible transfusion → preformed anti-A/anti-B + complement → intravascular haemolysis	Within minutes. Fever, rigors, flank/back pain, haemoglobinuria (pink urine), DIC, hypotension, oliguria. Mortality 10–50% if a full unit is transfused. Emergency.
Acute immune	Febrile non-haemolytic (FNHTR)	Cytokines accumulated in stored unit (IL-1, IL-6, TNF) and/or recipient antibodies vs donor leukocytes	Temperature rise ≥1 °C with chills during/after transfusion, no haemolysis. Diagnosis of exclusion. Largely prevented by pre-storage leukoreduction.
Acute immune	Allergic / urticarial	Recipient IgE against donor plasma proteins	Urticaria, pruritus, mild flushing. Stop briefly, give antihistamine, restart slowly. The only reaction where transfusion may be resumed.

Timing / Type	Reaction	Mechanism	Key Clinical Features
Acute immune	Anaphylaxis	Anti-IgA antibodies in IgA-deficient recipient OR severe atopic donor allergens	Bronchospasm, hypotension, angioedema within minutes. Stop, IM epinephrine, washed cellular products + IgA-deficient plasma for future transfusions.
Acute immune	TRALI	Donor anti-HLA / anti-neutrophil antibodies (typically multiparous female donor) activate recipient lung neutrophils	Acute hypoxaemia + bilateral pulmonary infiltrates within 6 h of transfusion. Normal cardiac filling pressures, normal/mildly elevated BNP. Supportive (often needs ventilation). Donor deferred.
Acute non-immune	TACO	Volume overload — too much, too fast	Dyspnea, raised JVP, S3 gallop, pulmonary oedema. Elevated BNP. Responds to diuretics. Risk: elderly, cardiac, renal, paediatric.
Acute non-immune	Bacterial / septic	Yersinia enterocolitica in PRBC (cold-tolerant); skin staph/strep in platelets (room temp)	High fever (>2 °C rise), rigors, hypotension, shock during/just after transfusion. Cultures of patient and unit. Broad-spectrum antibiotics.
Delayed immune	Delayed haemolytic (DHTR)	Anamnestic alloantibody response (Kidd > Rh > Duffy > Kell)	Falling Hb 3–14 d post-transfusion, jaundice, positive DAT, new alloantibody on screen. Usually self-limiting; antigen-negative units for future transfusions.
Delayed immune	Post-transfusion purpura (PTP)	Anti-HPA-1a in HPA-1a-negative recipient (typically multiparous female) — destroys both donor and own platelets by bystander mechanism	Severe thrombocytopenia 5–12 d after transfusion. IVIG is first-line. Self-limited.
Delayed immune	TA-GVHD	Viable donor T cells engraft in immunocompromised recipient and attack host tissues	Rash, diarrhoea, hepatitis, pancytopenia 1–6 weeks post-transfusion. >90% mortality. Prevented by ≥25 Gy gamma irradiation.
Delayed non-immune	Iron overload	Cumulative iron from chronic transfusion (~250 mg per unit)	After ~20 units lifetime — endocrine, cardiac, hepatic dysfunction. Manage with chelation (deferasirox, deferiprone, deferoxamine).

Table 18.7 Classification of transfusion reactions — timing, mechanism, and clinical features.

TRALI versus TACO — The Distinction That Changes Management

Both present with acute respiratory distress during or shortly after transfusion. Mistaking TRALI for TACO leads to diuresis of an already volume-depleted patient; mistaking TACO for TRALI delays the diuretic that would resolve it. The discriminators are cardiac filling pressures and BNP.

Feature	TRALI	TACO
Onset	Within 6 h of transfusion	During or within 6–12 h of transfusion
Mechanism	Donor anti-HLA/neutrophil Ab → pulmonary capillary leak	Volume overload
JVP	Normal	Elevated
S3 gallop	Absent	Often present
BNP	Normal or mildly elevated (<200 pg/mL)	Markedly elevated (>1,200 pg/mL typical)
Cardiac filling pressures (PCWP)	Normal (<18 mmHg)	Elevated (>18 mmHg)
CXR	Bilateral fluffy infiltrates, normal heart size	Bilateral infiltrates + cardiomegaly + Kerley B lines
Response to diuretics	No improvement (may worsen)	Rapid improvement
Treatment	Supportive; ventilation if needed; protective lung strategy	Slow/stop transfusion; loop diuretic; upright posture; oxygen

Table 18.8 TRALI vs TACO — the discriminators.

Trap — TA-GVHD — Preventable, Almost Always Fatal

Do not miss this on a vignette. Donor T cells engraft in immunocompromised recipient → attack skin (rash), gut (diarrhoea), liver (hepatitis), and crucially marrow (pancytopenia — distinguishes from solid-organ-transplant GVHD where marrow is spared). Onset 1–6 weeks post-transfusion. Mortality >90 percent. Prevention is simple and absolute: ≥25 Gy gamma irradiation of cellular components for at-risk recipients (HSCT, congenital T-cell immunodeficiency, Hodgkin lymphoma, fludarabine therapy, intrauterine and neonatal exchange transfusion, directed donation from any blood relative — even a fully ABO-matched sibling).

Workup of a Suspected Acute Reaction

Six steps in order, started the moment a reaction is suspected:

- Stop the transfusion immediately. Keep the line open with normal saline (never dextrose, which haemolyses any residual red cells).
- Bedside clerical check — verify patient identity, unit label, compatibility tag. The single most informative step in catching wrong-blood errors.

- Notify the blood bank. Send post-transfusion EDTA and clotted samples + the implicated unit with its giving set + post-transfusion urine sample (haemoglobinuria suggests intravascular haemolysis).
- Visual inspection of post-transfusion plasma for pink discolouration (free haemoglobin = intravascular haemolysis). Repeat ABO/Rh on pre- and post-samples and the unit. Direct antiglobulin test on post-sample (positive in AHTR and DHTR).
- Targeted investigation — LDH, indirect bilirubin, haptoglobin (low in haemolysis), plasma free haemoglobin, urine haemoglobin, creatinine; coagulation screen and fibrinogen if DIC suspected; blood cultures of patient and unit if sepsis suspected; chest X-ray + BNP for respiratory presentations.
- Haemovigilance reporting — in the US, fatal reactions are reported to the FDA within 24 hours; non-fatal serious adverse reactions are reported through the AABB Haemovigilance Module of CDC's NHSN.

18.7 Transfusion-Transmitted Infections

Despite layered screening, residual risk remains because of the window period — the interval between donor infection and detectability. The standard US screening panel includes HIV-1/2, HBV (HBsAg + anti-HBc + HBV NAT), HCV (anti-HCV + HCV NAT), HTLV-I/II, syphilis, West Nile virus (NAT, seasonal), Trypanosoma cruzi (Chagas, one-time per lifetime donor screen), and Zika (selectively). Bacterial detection of platelets is mandated by FDA. CMV testing is selective for at-risk recipients (or replaced functionally by leukoreduction).

Pathogen	Window (NAT)	Window (Serology)	US Screening
HIV-1/2	5–10 d	15–22 d (4th-gen Ag/Ab combo detects p24 + Ab)	4th-gen Ag/Ab + HIV-1 NAT
HBV	15–35 d (HBV DNA)	30–38 d (HBsAg)	HBsAg + anti-HBc + HBV NAT
HCV	3–5 d (HCV RNA)	26–38 d (anti-HCV)	Anti-HCV + HCV NAT
HTLV-I/II	Not used routinely	30–60 d	Anti-HTLV-I/II (one-time on first donation)
Syphilis	Not applicable	Treponemal serology	Treponemal CIA / RPR
West Nile	~3 d (NAT)	Late seroconversion	Seasonal NAT (peaks summer)
T. cruzi (Chagas)	Not applicable	Anti-T. cruzi serology	One-time serology on first donation
CMV	—	Serology	Not universal; leukoreduction is functionally equivalent for at-risk recipients

Table 18.9 TTIs — window periods and US screening framework.

NAT — ID-NAT and MP-NAT

NAT detects viral nucleic acid directly (by RT-PCR or transcription-mediated amplification), narrowing the window period markedly compared with serology. It runs in two formats: ID-NAT (individual donation) tests every donation singly — highest sensitivity, highest cost; MP-NAT (mini-pool, typically 6 or 16 donations) pools samples to reduce cost at some loss of sensitivity for low-titer viraemia. Multiplex platforms (Roche cobas TaqScreen MPX, Grifols Procleix Ultrio Elite) detect HIV, HCV, and HBV simultaneously from a single sample. In the US, NAT for HIV and HCV is FDA-required; HBV NAT is now also standard.

Pathogen Reduction Technology

PRT inactivates residual viruses, bacteria, parasites, and donor leukocytes in platelet and plasma components by photochemical (amotosalen + UVA — INTERCEPT; riboflavin + UVB — Mirasol) or UVC-only treatment. Treated platelets carry an extended 7-day shelf life. PRT functionally replaces leukoreduction, irradiation, and bacterial culture for treated components. INTERCEPT-treated platelets and plasma are FDA-approved and increasingly used in the US.

18.8 Paediatric and Neonatal Transfusion

Neonates and infants are not small adults. Smaller blood volume (~80 mL/kg in term neonate, ~100 mL/kg in preterm), immature immunity, immature liver and kidney, and an incompletely developed antibody repertoire all change transfusion practice. USMLE expects you to recognise the distinct rules: irradiated, fresh, leukoreduced, CMV-risk-reduced — and to know why each matters.

Neonatal Particulars

Reverse grouping is unreliable for the first 4–6 months because anti-A and anti-B antibodies are not yet developed; ABO grouping in a neonate is forward only, with the maternal sample used for serum antibody screen. ABO and Rh typing performed on the mother's sample stays valid for the neonate's transfusion needs through the first 4 months unless the neonate has received non-O cellular products.

Component selection follows specific neonatal rules. PRBCs for neonatal transfusion should be group O (or ABO-identical), Rh-matched, leukoreduced, irradiated (mandatory for IUT and exchange transfusion; recommended for low-birth-weight transfusions), CMV-risk-reduced (leukoreduced or seronegative), Hb S–negative, and ideally <7 days old (lower potassium load — fresh PRBCs avoid hyperkalaemic cardiac arrest in rapid large-volume transfusion). Aliquoting one parent unit into multiple paediatric satellite bags reduces donor exposure across multiple top-up transfusions.

Indication	Component / Dose	Special Requirements
Top-up transfusion (anaemia of prematurity)	PRBC 10–15 mL/kg over 3–4 h	Leukoreduced, CMV-risk-reduced, irradiated if <1,200 g birth weight or prior IUT. Restrictive Hb thresholds (PINT, ETTNO trials).
Exchange transfusion	Whole blood	Group O Rh-negative (or ABO-compatible

Indication	Component / Dose	Special Requirements
(HDFN)	(reconstituted PRBC + AB FFP to Hct 50–60%); volume = 2 × blood volume	with both mother and neonate), <5 days old, irradiated, CMV-risk-reduced, Hb S-negative, warmed to 37 °C.
Intrauterine transfusion (IUT)	PRBC, group O Rh-negative, fresh (<5 d), Hct 75–85%, irradiated	Compatible with maternal serum (not fetal). Irradiation mandatory. Volume calculated from estimated fetal blood volume and target Hct.
Neonatal thrombocytopenia	Platelets 10–20 mL/kg	ABO-identical or compatible. NAIT (neonatal alloimmune thrombocytopenia): HPA-1a-negative platelets if anti-HPA-1a maternal Ab present; washed maternal platelets as backup.
Disseminated intravascular coagulation	FFP 10–15 mL/kg + cryoprecipitate 5–10 mL/kg	ABO-compatible plasma. Treat underlying cause (sepsis, asphyxia, NEC).

Table 18.10 Paediatric and neonatal transfusion — component, dose, and special requirements.

Pearl — Why Neonatal PRBCs Must Be Fresh and Irradiated
Fresh (<7 days, ideally <5 days for exchange) — to avoid the supernatant potassium load that accumulates during storage. A unit at end-of-shelf-life can have plasma K^+ >25 mmol/L; rapid large-volume transfusion in a 1.5 kg neonate can cause hyperkalaemic cardiac arrest. Irradiated — because neonates (especially preterm) have immature T-cell function and are at risk of TA-GVHD even from unrelated donors. Both rules are absolute for IUT and exchange transfusion.

18.9 Therapeutic and Donor Apheresis

Apheresis (Greek aphairesis, "to take away") selectively removes one blood component using an automated cell separator and returns the rest to the donor or patient. Therapeutic apheresis treats disease; donor apheresis collects components for transfusion.

ASFA Categories

The American Society for Apheresis classifies indications by evidence strength and is the framework USMLE expects.

Category	Definition	Examples
I	First-line therapy, alone or with other modalities	TTP (TPE with FFP replacement), Guillain–Barré syndrome (TPE), myasthenia gravis crisis, hyperviscosity syndrome, sickle cell acute chest syndrome (RBC exchange), severe babesiosis

Category	Definition	Examples
		(RBC exchange)
II	Accepted as second-line therapy	ANCA-associated RPGN with severe renal failure, ABO-incompatible solid organ transplant desensitisation, antibody-mediated rejection
III	Optimum role not established; individualised decision	Sepsis with multi-organ failure, HLA-antibody desensitisation in renal transplant
IV	Ineffective or harmful — IRB approval needed if performed	Active SLE without renal involvement, plasmapheresis alone for lupus nephritis

Table 18.11 ASFA categories — therapeutic apheresis evidence framework.

Types of Therapeutic Apheresis

Procedure	Removed	Replacement	Key Indications
Therapeutic plasma exchange (TPE)	Patient plasma — antibodies, immune complexes, paraproteins, toxins	FFP (mandatory in TTP, replaces ADAMTS13), 5% albumin, or combination	TTP (Cat I), GBS, myasthenia crisis, anti-GBM disease (Goodpasture), catastrophic APS, hyperviscosity
Leukapheresis	White blood cells (mostly blasts in leukaemia)	None or saline	Hyperleukocytosis (WBC >100 × 10^9/L) with leukostasis (CNS or pulmonary symptoms) — bridge to chemotherapy
Plateletpheresis (therapeutic)	Platelets	None	Symptomatic thrombocytosis in MPN (platelets >1,000 × 10^9/L with thrombosis or bleeding) — bridge to cytoreduction
Red cell exchange (erythrocytapheresis)	Patient red cells	Donor PRBCs	Sickle cell — acute chest syndrome, stroke, prevention. Severe falciparum malaria with parasitaemia >10%. Severe babesiosis.
LDL apheresis	LDL-cholesterol (selective adsorption)	None	Familial hypercholesterolaemia refractory to statins — homozygous and severe heterozygous
Photopheresis (ECP)	Mononuclear cells, treated with 8-MOP + UVA, then reinfused	—	Cutaneous T-cell lymphoma (Sézary syndrome), steroid-refractory chronic GVHD

Table 18.12 Types of therapeutic apheresis.

Pearl — Plasma Volume and the 63% Rule

Estimated plasma volume (mL) = body weight (kg) × 70 mL/kg × (1 − haematocrit). For a 70 kg patient with Hct 0.40: PV = 70 × 70 × 0.60 = 2,940 mL. One plasma volume exchange removes ≈63% of an intravascular substance (one half-life), two volumes ≈86%. Diminishing returns mean 1.0–1.5 PV per session is the standard. TPE schedule for TTP: daily until platelet count >150 × 10^9/L for two consecutive days and clinical resolution.

Donor Apheresis and Citrate Toxicity

Donor apheresis (single-donor platelets, plasma, or stem cells) uses citrate as the anticoagulant in the extracorporeal circuit. Citrate chelates ionised calcium → perioral tingling, finger paresthesias, muscle cramps, and in severe cases tetany or cardiac arrhythmia. Treatment: slow the return rate, oral calcium during the procedure, IV calcium gluconate if symptomatic. The most common donor reaction is vasovagal (pallor, sweating, hypotension, occasionally syncope) — managed by Trendelenburg position and supportive care.

18.10 Haematopoietic Stem Cell Transplantation

HSCT replaces a diseased or destroyed marrow with haematopoietic stem cells from the patient (autologous) or a donor (allogeneic). From the transfusion medicine perspective the practical questions are: where do the stem cells come from, what blood support is needed during the aplastic phase, and what blood-group rules apply when donor and recipient are ABO-mismatched.

Auto versus Allo

Feature	Autologous HSCT	Allogeneic HSCT
Stem cell source	Patient's own (harvested before myeloablation)	HLA-matched sibling, matched unrelated donor (MUD), haploidentical relative, cord blood
Conditioning	High-dose chemotherapy (e.g., melphalan, BEAM)	Myeloablative (busulfan/cyclophosphamide, TBI) or reduced-intensity (fludarabine-based)
Graft-vs-host disease	None (own cells)	Acute (≤100 d) and chronic (>100 d) — major complication
Graft-vs-tumour effect	None	Present — contributes substantially to cure (mediated by donor T cells and NK cells)
TRM (transplant-related mortality)	1–5% (mostly infection, organ toxicity)	10–30% depending on donor type and conditioning
Indications	Multiple myeloma, relapsed	AML/ALL high-risk, MDS, severe

Feature	Autologous HSCT	Allogeneic HSCT
	lymphoma (HL, NHL), neuroblastoma, severe autoimmune disease (refractory)	aplastic anaemia, thalassaemia major, sickle cell, primary immunodeficiency, Hurler, ALD

Table 18.13 Autologous versus allogeneic HSCT.

Stem Cell Sources and Mobilisation

Three sources: bone marrow (multiple posterior iliac aspirations under GA, ~10–15 mL/kg target), peripheral blood stem cells (most common — G-CSF mobilisation followed by leukapheresis), and umbilical cord blood (collected at delivery, cryopreserved). PBSC engraft fastest (neutrophils ~10–14 days), cord blood slowest (~21–28 days) but with permissive HLA mismatch.

PBSC mobilisation: G-CSF (filgrastim 10 µg/kg/day for 4–5 days). Plerixafor (CXCR4 antagonist) is added for poor mobilisers — it disrupts the CXCR4/CXCL12 anchor that holds $CD34^+$ cells in the marrow niche. Peripheral $CD34^+$ count is checked on day 4 or 5; apheresis is initiated when $CD34^+$ exceeds ~10–20/µL. Target dose $\geq 2 \times 10^6$ $CD34^+$ cells/kg (autologous), ideally $\geq 5 \times 10^6$/kg; allogeneic targets are similar or higher.

ABO-Incompatible HSCT

Up to 30 percent of allogeneic transplants are ABO-mismatched (HLA matching takes priority). Three categories:

- Major incompatibility — recipient has antibody against donor RBC antigens (e.g., recipient O, donor A). Risk: immediate haemolysis of donor red cells in the graft; delayed donor red cell engraftment.
- Minor incompatibility — donor has antibody against recipient RBC antigens (e.g., donor O, recipient A). Risk: passenger lymphocyte syndrome — donor B cells in the graft produce antibody against recipient red cells 7–14 days post-transplant, causing haemolysis.
- Bidirectional — both directions (e.g., recipient A, donor B). Combines risks of both.

Phase / Incompatibility	Red Cells	Platelets / Plasma
Pre-engraftment, major incompatibility	Recipient ABO type	Donor type (or AB plasma if uncertain)
Pre-engraftment, minor incompatibility	Donor type (or group O)	Recipient type
Pre-engraftment, bidirectional	Group O	AB plasma
Post-engraftment (full chimerism)	Donor type	Donor type

Table 18.14 Blood product selection in ABO-incompatible HSCT.

Acute GVHD — Glucksberg Grading

Acute GVHD occurs within 100 days post-allogeneic transplant (the NIH 2014 consensus also recognises late-onset acute GVHD). Three target organs: skin, gut, and liver. Grade by individual organ stage (1–4) then assemble overall grade (I–IV).

Organ	Stage 1	Stage 2	Stage 3	Stage 4
Skin (rash)	<25% BSA	25–50%	Generalised erythroderma	Erythroderma + bullae / desquamation
Gut (diarrhoea)	500–1,000 mL/d (or persistent nausea)	1,000–1,500 mL/d	1,500–2,500 mL/d	>2,500 mL/d, severe pain ± ileus
Liver (bilirubin)	34–51 µmol/L (2–3 mg/dL)	51–102 (3–6)	102–255 (6–15)	>255 (>15)

Table 18.15 Acute GVHD — Glucksberg organ staging.

Overall grade. I (mild): skin stage 1–2 only. II (moderate): skin 1–3 plus gut 1 and/or liver 1. III (severe): gut 2–3 and/or liver 2–3 (skin variable). IV (life-threatening): any organ stage 4. First-line treatment is high-dose methylprednisolone (1–2 mg/kg/day). Steroid-refractory acute GVHD has high mortality; ruxolitinib (REACH-1, REACH-2 trials) is now standard second-line.

Quick Recall — Non-Malignant HSCT Indications ("SHIP")
• S — Severe aplastic anaemia (matched sibling first-line if age <40). • H — Haemoglobinopathies: thalassaemia major (Pesaro Class I best outcomes), sickle cell with recurrent VOC/stroke despite hydroxyurea. • I — Immunodeficiencies: SCID (transplant emergency, do before 3 months of age), WAS, CGD, HLH. • P — Plus metabolic / storage disorders: Hurler (MPS I), adrenoleukodystrophy, osteopetrosis, Krabbe.

18.11 Special Transfusion Topics

Irradiated Blood Products — Who, Why, How

Gamma (Cs-137 or Co-60) or X-irradiation at ≥25 Gy mid-plane (max 50 Gy, beyond which red cell damage exceeds therapeutic benefit) inactivates donor T-lymphocyte proliferation, preventing TA-GVHD. Indications include: HSCT recipients (from start of conditioning indefinitely after allogeneic; until 6 months after autologous), congenital T-cell immunodeficiency (DiGeorge, SCID), Hodgkin lymphoma (treatment-induced T-cell suppression), patients on purine analogues (fludarabine, cladribine, pentostatin, bendamustine), patients on alemtuzumab or ATG, intrauterine transfusion and neonatal exchange transfusion, low-birth-weight neonates (<1,200 g, institutional variation), HLA-matched or HLA-selected platelet products, and any directed donation from a first- or second-degree relative.

Irradiation increases potassium leakage from red cells; irradiated PRBCs expire 14 days after irradiation or by original expiry, whichever is sooner. Platelet function is essentially unaffected.

CMV-Risk-Reduced Components

CMV is harboured intracellularly in leukocytes. Two strategies achieve CMV-risk reduction: (1) CMV-seronegative donor selection — most reliable in seronegative populations but in the US CMV seroprevalence is roughly 50–70 percent in adults, so seronegative units have limited supply; (2) leukoreduction — pre-storage filtration to $<5 \times 10^6$ leukocytes per unit reduces CMV transmission to levels equivalent to seronegative units. Current US consensus: leukoreduction is functionally equivalent. Indications: CMV-seronegative HSCT and solid organ transplant recipients, neonates (especially preterm and low birth weight), CMV-seronegative pregnant women, and patients with severe T-cell deficiency.

Donor Haemovigilance

Surveillance of adverse donor reactions. Most common is vasovagal (~1–3 percent of donations) — pallor, sweating, hypotension, occasionally syncope; managed by Trendelenburg, oral fluids, and reassurance. Less common: haematoma at venipuncture (1 percent), nerve injury, arterial puncture, and during apheresis citrate toxicity (perioral tingling → tetany if severe). In the US, transfusion-related fatalities are reported to FDA within 24 hours; non-fatal serious adverse reactions are reported through the AABB Haemovigilance Module of the CDC NHSN.

Artificial Blood / Oxygen Carriers

Two approaches investigated for decades. Haemoglobin-based oxygen carriers (HBOCs — modified human, bovine, or recombinant Hb): free Hb scavenges nitric oxide → vasoconstriction and hypertension, which has limited clinical development; only Hemopure has had limited approval (South Africa, veterinary). Perfluorocarbon emulsions dissolve oxygen physically but require very high inspired oxygen concentrations. Next-generation encapsulated haemoglobin (Hb in liposomes or polymerised) addresses NO scavenging but remains investigational.

Quality Control in the Blood Bank

Vein-to-vein quality control. Mandatory monitored parameters include: visual inspection of every issued unit (clots, discolouration, leaks); sterility cultures of platelet units (highest contamination risk because of room-temperature storage; FDA mandates bacterial detection on all platelet products); haemoglobin content of PRBC (≥45 g per unit); platelet count of RDP ($\geq 5.5 \times 10^{10}$), SDP ($\geq 3 \times 10^{11}$); leukocyte count in leukoreduced products ($<5 \times 10^6$); factor VIII content of FFP (≥0.7 IU/mL in 75% of units tested); fibrinogen content of cryoprecipitate (≥150 mg per unit). Equipment calibration (centrifuge, refrigerator, freezer, platelet incubator) must be documented continuously; alarms and backup systems are essential. AABB accreditation and FDA CFR Title 21 compliance are the regulatory backbone in the US.

18.12 Buzzwords — Vignette Triggers

Phrases that should trigger a specific diagnosis on first read. Memorise the right column.

Buzzword / Clue	Diagnosis
Patient types as O on forward grouping but reverse grouping shows agglutination with O cells	Bombay phenotype (Oh) — anti-H
Anti-A1 lectin / Dolichos biflorus	A1 vs A2 subgroup discrimination
Falling Hb 3–14 days post-transfusion, jaundice, positive DAT, antibody titer dropping	Delayed haemolytic transfusion reaction (anti-Jka — Kidd)
"Notorious for delayed haemolytic reactions"	Kidd (Jka)
Highly immunogenic, second only to D, severe HDFN, K-negative blood policy	Kell (anti-K)
Fy(a−b−) phenotype, resistance to Plasmodium vivax	Duffy (West African origin)
Recurrent first-trimester miscarriage + intravascular haemolysis on transfusion	p phenotype with anti-PP1Pk
Pink urine + flank pain + fever within minutes of transfusion	Acute haemolytic transfusion reaction (ABO mismatch)
Multiparous female donor; bilateral pulmonary infiltrates within 6 h; normal BNP; non-cardiogenic oedema	TRALI
Elderly cardiac patient; raised JVP; S3; elevated BNP; responds to furosemide	TACO
Severe thrombocytopenia 5–12 days post-transfusion in multiparous woman	Post-transfusion purpura (anti-HPA-1a)
Rash + diarrhoea + hepatitis + pancytopenia 1–6 weeks post-transfusion in immunocompromised host	Transfusion-associated GVHD
Anaphylaxis on first transfusion in young patient with recurrent sinopulmonary infections	IgA deficiency with anti-IgA
Yersinia enterocolitica septic shock from cold-stored unit	PRBC bacterial contamination
Garlic-like body odour after stem cell infusion	DMSO (cryopreservative) — physiological, not a reaction
Perioral tingling + finger paresthesias during apheresis	Citrate toxicity (hypocalcaemia)
Plasma exchange with FFP replacement for falling platelets, MAHA, neurological signs, fever, renal involvement	TTP — TPE Cat I indication; FFP replaces ADAMTS13
Sickle cell with acute chest syndrome — best transfusion strategy	Red cell exchange (erythrocytapheresis), Cat I indication

Buzzword / Clue	Diagnosis
Donor-derived B cells produce antibody → recipient red cell haemolysis 7–14 d post-allo HSCT	Passenger lymphocyte syndrome (minor ABO incompatibility)
Hyperkalaemic cardiac arrest in a neonate after large-volume PRBC transfusion	Old/end-of-shelf-life unit; use fresh PRBC (<7 d) for neonatal large-volume transfusion

Table 18.16 Vignette buzzwords — quick-trigger map.

18.13 Vignettes — USMLE Style

Ten case-based questions spanning the chapter. Each carries five options with correct answer rationale and short distractor analysis.

Vignette 1
A 24-year-old woman of South Asian ancestry is admitted for elective caesarean delivery. Pre-operative type and screen shows no agglutination with anti-A or anti-B (forward grouping types as O). Reverse grouping shows agglutination with both A1 and B reagent cells AND with the laboratory's group O screening cells. Anti-D testing is negative. Which of the following is the most likely blood group? A. Group O Rh-negative B. Bombay phenotype (Oh) C. Group A2 with anti-A1 D. Group AB with cold autoantibody E. Group O with cold agglutinin disease

Answer: B (Bombay phenotype)
The diagnostic finding is agglutination of patient serum with group O screening cells. Group O cells carry H antigen; only a person with anti-H (i.e., Bombay phenotype, lacking the H gene FUT1) will agglutinate them. (A) Plain group O Rh− would have anti-A and anti-B but no anti-H, so reverse grouping with O cells would be negative. (C) A2 with anti-A1: forward grouping would be positive with anti-A. (D, E) Cold autoantibodies usually react across all reagent cells including the patient's own — but here the H-specific reactivity at 37 °C in a serologic workup points to Oh.

Vignette 2
A 45-year-old man with no significant past history develops fever to 39.5 °C, lumbar pain, hypotension, and pink-tinged urine 10 minutes into a packed red cell transfusion for a Hb of 6 g/dL. The transfusion is stopped immediately. Which is the single most informative next step in the bedside investigation? A. Direct antiglobulin test on a post-transfusion sample B. Verify patient identity, unit label, and compatibility tag C. Send blood cultures of patient and unit D. Chest X-ray and BNP E. Send post-transfusion plasma for visual inspection of free haemoglobin

Answer: B (Bedside identity check)

Acute haemolytic transfusion reactions are almost always due to ABO incompatibility, and ABO incompatibility is almost always a clerical error (wrong patient, wrong unit). The single bedside step most likely to identify the cause is the identity check. (A) DAT and (E) plasma inspection are useful and standard but they confirm haemolysis rather than identify why it happened. (C) Cultures address bacterial contamination — possible but less likely in this presentation. (D) is for respiratory presentations. The clerical check both diagnoses the error and prevents a second wrong unit being issued to another patient.

Vignette 3

A 68-year-old woman with chronic kidney disease receives 2 units of PRBC for symptomatic anaemia. Two hours into the second unit she develops dyspnea, raised JVP, bilateral basal crackles, and a third heart sound. SpO_2 is 88% on room air. BNP is 2,400 pg/mL. Chest X-ray shows bilateral infiltrates and cardiomegaly with Kerley B lines. Which is the most likely diagnosis and the most appropriate immediate management? A. TRALI — supportive care, no diuretics B. TACO — slow/stop transfusion, IV furosemide, upright posture, oxygen C. Acute haemolytic transfusion reaction — stop, fluids, send post-samples D. Anaphylaxis — IM epinephrine, antihistamine, stop E. FNHTR — antipyretic, slow restart

Answer: B (TACO)

Elevated JVP, S3, and BNP >1,200 with cardiomegaly + Kerley B lines on CXR are classic TACO. The patient is elderly with CKD — a high-risk substrate. (A) TRALI has normal BNP, no JVP elevation, and does not respond to diuretics. (C) AHTR would present with fever, flank pain, haemoglobinuria. (D) and (E) do not fit the volume-overload picture.

Vignette 4

A 32-year-old woman, gravida 3 para 2, undergoes platelet transfusion for chemotherapy-induced thrombocytopenia. One hour into the transfusion she develops sudden severe dyspnea, hypoxia (SpO_2 82%), and bilateral pulmonary infiltrates. JVP is normal. BNP is 95 pg/mL. Echocardiogram shows normal left ventricular function. The platelet unit was an apheresis unit collected from a 38-year-old multiparous female donor. What is the most likely mechanism? A. Volume overload B. Recipient anti-IgA antibodies reacting with donor IgA C. Donor anti-HLA antibodies activating recipient pulmonary neutrophils D. Bacterial contamination of the platelet unit E. Cytokine accumulation in stored platelets

Answer: C (TRALI from donor anti-HLA)

Classic TRALI: bilateral infiltrates within 6 hours, hypoxia, normal cardiac filling pressures, normal BNP, normal LV function. The multiparous female donor is the textbook source — pregnancy-induced anti-HLA antibodies in donor plasma activate recipient neutrophils in the pulmonary capillary bed. Most US blood services now defer multiparous female donors from plasma-rich component donation (male-predominant plasma policy). (A) is TACO — BNP would be elevated. (B) anaphylaxis presents with bronchospasm and hypotension, not isolated lung injury. (D) bacterial sepsis presents with fever and shock. (E) FNHTR is fever without lung injury.

Vignette 5

A 28-year-old man with sickle cell disease and chronic transfusion dependence receives a PRBC transfusion. He is asymptomatic. Eight days later he presents with jaundice and falling Hb (from 9.2 to 6.8 g/dL). Direct antiglobulin test is now positive (was negative before transfusion). Antibody screen identifies a new anti-Jka. What is the most likely diagnosis? A. Acute haemolytic transfusion reaction B. Delayed haemolytic transfusion reaction C. Hyperhemolysis syndrome D. Autoimmune haemolytic anaemia E. Sickle cell crisis with intramedullary haemolysis

Answer: B (Delayed haemolytic transfusion reaction)

Falling Hb 3–14 days post-transfusion, new alloantibody (anti-Jka — the Kidd antibody is "notorious" for delayed reactions because its titer falls between exposures and is missed on screen), positive DAT — textbook DHTR. (A) is within minutes to hours, intravascular, ABO-driven. (C) hyperhemolysis is severe and includes bystander destruction of recipient red cells; possible in chronic SCD transfusion but the classic anti-Jka picture here is DHTR. (D, E) do not explain a new alloantibody.

Vignette 6

A 35-year-old woman presents with fever, fluctuating neurological signs, microangiopathic haemolytic anaemia (LDH 1,800; schistocytes on smear), thrombocytopenia (platelets 18 × 10^9/L), and AKI. ADAMTS13 activity is <10%. What is the most appropriate first-line therapy? A. Platelet transfusion to keep platelets >20 × 10^9/L B. Therapeutic plasma exchange with FFP replacement C. Therapeutic plasma exchange with 5% albumin replacement D. Rituximab monotherapy E. Splenectomy

Answer: B (TPE with FFP replacement)

TTP is an ASFA Category I indication for plasma exchange. The replacement fluid must be FFP (or cryosupernatant) because it replaces the missing ADAMTS13. (C) Albumin replacement does not provide ADAMTS13 and would worsen the deficiency. (A) Platelet transfusion is contraindicated in TTP without life-threatening bleeding — it adds substrate to ongoing microvascular thrombosis. (D) Rituximab and caplacizumab are adjuncts for refractory or relapsing disease. (E) Splenectomy is salvage in chronic refractory cases.

Vignette 7

A 40-year-old man with multiple myeloma undergoes autologous haematopoietic stem cell transplantation. The blood bank requests irradiated and CMV-risk-reduced blood products for the transplant period. Which is the principal reason irradiation is required? A. To inactivate residual myeloma cells in the unit B. To reduce CMV transmission C. To prevent transfusion-associated graft-versus-host disease D. To prolong red cell shelf life E. To reduce HLA alloimmunisation

Answer: C (Prevent TA-GVHD)
Gamma irradiation at ≥25 Gy inactivates donor T-lymphocyte proliferation, preventing TA-GVHD. The HSCT recipient is profoundly immunocompromised by conditioning therapy and cannot reject engrafting donor T cells. TA-GVHD has >90% mortality and is entirely preventable by irradiation. (A) Irradiation does not reliably kill tumour cells in components. (B) CMV reduction is achieved by leukoreduction or seronegative selection, not irradiation. (D) Irradiation shortens shelf life (potassium leak — 14 days max for PRBC). (E) HLA alloimmunisation is reduced by leukoreduction.

Vignette 8
A 55-year-old man undergoes HLA-matched sibling allogeneic HSCT. The recipient is blood group O Rh-positive; the donor is blood group A Rh-positive. On day 10 post-transplant the recipient's Hb is falling and a new positive DAT is noted with anti-A specificity. Which type of ABO incompatibility is this and what is the explanation? A. Major incompatibility — recipient anti-A destroying donor red cells in graft B. Minor incompatibility — passenger lymphocyte syndrome C. Bidirectional incompatibility — both directions D. Rh incompatibility — anti-D E. Autoimmune haemolytic anaemia from conditioning

Answer: A (Major incompatibility)
Recipient O has anti-A antibodies; donor is A. This is major incompatibility. In the early post-transplant period the recipient's pre-existing anti-A may persist and can haemolyse residual donor red cells in the graft and any donor-type red cells transfused. Pre-engraftment red cell selection: recipient ABO type (group O) until engraftment is established. (B) Passenger lymphocyte syndrome is the minor scenario — donor B cells in the graft producing antibody against recipient red cells. (C, D, E) do not fit the donor-recipient mismatch pattern given.

Vignette 9
A 1,100 g preterm neonate at day 14 of life requires top-up red cell transfusion for anaemia of prematurity. The neonate is in the NICU on minimal respiratory support. Mother is group A Rh-positive; baby is group A Rh-positive. Mother is CMV seronegative. Which combination of component selection is most appropriate? A. Group A Rh-positive PRBC, leukoreduced, irradiated, CMV-risk-reduced, fresh (<7 d) B. Group O Rh-negative PRBC, fresh, no irradiation needed C. Group A Rh-positive whole blood, no special processing D.

Group A Rh-positive PRBC, washed, no irradiation E. Group AB Rh-positive PRBC, leukoreduced, no CMV reduction

Answer: A

Low-birth-weight preterm neonates need: ABO/Rh-matched (or group O if maternal anti-A/B titer is high) PRBCs; leukoreduced; irradiated (immature T-cell function → risk of TA-GVHD); CMV-risk-reduced (especially if mother is seronegative); fresh (<7 days, ideally <5 days for large-volume transfusion) to avoid hyperkalaemic cardiac events from accumulated supernatant K^+. (B) Group O Rh-negative is reserved for emergency or unknown group; if A-positive type is confirmed, ABO-identical is preferred. (C, D) Whole blood and washed PRBC do not address the irradiation requirement. (E) Group AB is plasma type, not appropriate for red cell selection.

Vignette 10

A 60-year-old man with Waldenström macroglobulinaemia presents with confusion, blurred vision, mucosal bleeding, and serum viscosity 6.5 cP (normal <1.8). IgM is 7.5 g/dL. Plasma exchange with 5% albumin replacement is initiated as a bridge to chemotherapy. The patient weighs 80 kg and his haematocrit is 0.30. Approximately what fraction of the IgM will be removed after a single 1.0 plasma volume exchange? A. ~25% B. ~50% C. ~63% D. ~86% E. ~95%

Answer: C (~63%)

A single plasma volume exchange follows first-order kinetics — it removes one half-life worth of an intravascular substance, which is approximately 63% (1 − 1/e). Two plasma volumes remove ~86%. Plasma volume = 80 × 70 × (1 − 0.30) = 3,920 mL. The 63% rule is the most commonly tested apheresis calculation on USMLE. Hyperviscosity from IgM (Waldenström) is an ASFA Category I indication for TPE; albumin (not FFP) is the replacement fluid because there is no missing factor to replace, unlike TTP. Diminishing returns mean 1.0–1.5 PV per session is the standard.

18.14 Closing Discriminators

Five high-yield distinctions to lock in before exam day.

Discriminator 1 — Forward vs Reverse Grouping Discrepancy

Forward typing tests cells with anti-sera; reverse typing tests serum with reagent cells. Both must agree. Discrepancy → never issue blood until resolved. Common causes of forward weak/missing reaction: ABO subgroup, recent transfusion mixed-field, leukaemia with antigen loss. Common causes of reverse weak/missing reaction: neonate, elderly, immunocompromised, IVIG, hypogammaglobulinaemia. Reverse showing extra reactivity with O cells = anti-H = Bombay.

Discriminator 2 — TRALI vs TACO

Both: respiratory distress, bilateral infiltrates, hypoxia within 6 h of transfusion. TRALI has normal BNP, normal JVP, normal LV function on echo, no response to diuretics, classic donor history (multiparous female anti-HLA). TACO has elevated BNP, raised JVP, often S3, cardiomegaly + Kerley B lines, brisk response to furosemide. Get this wrong and you diurese a TRALI patient or fail to diurese a TACO patient.

Discriminator 3 — Weak D vs Partial D

Weak D = quantitative reduction (fewer copies, structurally intact). Reacts at IAT phase. Does NOT make anti-D. Can receive D-positive blood. Partial D = qualitative defect (missing epitopes). CAN make anti-D against missing epitopes when exposed to fully-D blood. Should receive D-negative blood. Serology cannot reliably separate them — molecular RHD genotyping does. In practice, treat any unclear weak/partial D pregnant woman as D-negative and give RhIG.

Discriminator 4 — Major vs Minor ABO-Incompatible HSCT

Major: recipient has antibody against donor antigens (recipient O, donor A) → recipient anti-A destroys donor red cells in graft + delayed donor red cell engraftment. Pre-engraftment red cells = recipient type. Minor: donor has antibody against recipient antigens (donor O, recipient A) → passenger lymphocyte syndrome at day 7–14 (donor B cells in graft make antibody against recipient red cells). Pre-engraftment red cells = donor type or group O.

IMG-Trap — Discriminator 5 — Three Pitfalls IMGs Carry into USMLE

(1) Bombay over-anchoring. Mumbai-trained candidates over-pick Oh on every ABO discrepancy because of local prevalence (1 in 7,500–10,000 vs 1 in 250,000 globally). USMLE answer for "types as O but crossmatch incompatible" is more often subgroup, mixed-field from recent transfusion, or cold autoantibody. Reserve Oh for serum reactivity with group O cells. (2) D-negative frequencies. Do not default to "5–8%" — USMLE obstetrics questions assume ~15% in non-Hispanic Whites and <1% in East Asians; ethnicity in the stem is the cue. (3) Adrenaline ≠ epinephrine. The USMLE drug name for the anaphylaxis answer is epinephrine, IM, given immediately when transfusion-related anaphylaxis is suspected (anti-IgA in IgA-deficient recipient). Stem language and answer language must match.

18.15 Quick Recall

Quick Recall — Transfusion Medicine in 16 Lines

- ABO antibodies = naturally occurring IgM, complement-fixing → ABO mismatch causes intravascular haemolysis (AHTR). US ABO frequencies: O ~45%, A ~40%, B ~11%, AB ~4%. • Bombay phenotype (Oh): h/h homozygous, no H antigen, makes anti-H. Worldwide ~1 in 250,000; only Bombay-donor blood compatible. • Rh: D most immunogenic non-ABO antigen. D-negative ~15% Whites, ~8% African Americans, <1% East Asians. Weak D = quantitative (give D+); partial D = qualitative (give D−). • Other systems: Kell anti-K severe HDFN; Kidd anti-Jka delayed haemolytic; Duffy Fy(a−b−) Plasmodium vivax resistance. • Pre-transfusion testing: forward + reverse grouping (must agree), antibody screen (IAT), crossmatch (full AHG / immediate spin / electronic). • Components: PRBC 2–6 °C, 35 d (CPDA-1) / 42 d (SAGM); platelets 20–24 °C with agitation, 5 d; FFP and cryo ≤−18 °C, 1 yr. • 1 unit PRBC raises Hb ~1 g/dL. 1 RDP raises platelets ~5–10 × 10^9/L. 1 unit cryo per 10 kg raises fibrinogen 50–100 mg/dL. • MTP 1:1:1 ratio (PRBC:FFP:platelets). Calcium replacement (citrate). Tranexamic acid in trauma (CRASH-2). Watch lethal triad. • AHTR = ABO mismatch, intravascular haemolysis, DIC. FNHTR = cytokines, prevented by leukoreduction. Anaphylaxis = anti-IgA in IgA-deficient → IM epinephrine. • TRALI: normal BNP, no response to diuretics. TACO: elevated BNP, responds to diuretics. • TA-GVHD >90% mortality, prevented by ≥25 Gy gamma irradiation. Mandatory in HSCT, IUT, neonatal exchange, Hodgkin, fludarabine, related-donor units. • TTI window with NAT: HIV 5–10 d, HBV 15–35 d, HCV 3–5 d. US screening: HIV-1/2, HBV, HCV (all NAT + serology), HTLV-I/II, syphilis, WNV (seasonal), T. cruzi (one-time). • Paediatric/neonatal: PRBC fresh (<7 d), leukoreduced, irradiated, CMV-risk-reduced. Reverse grouping unreliable <4 months. • TPE: 1 PV exchange removes ~63%; FFP replacement mandatory in TTP. ASFA Cat I: TTP, GBS, MG crisis, hyperviscosity, sickle ACS, severe babesiosis. • HSCT: PBSC mobilisation G-CSF ± plerixafor; target CD34 ≥2 × 10^6/kg auto, similar allo. Major ABO incomp = recipient-type RBC pre-engraft; minor = donor-type or O. • Haemovigilance: fatal reactions reported to FDA within 24 h; non-fatal SARs through AABB Haemovigilance Module / CDC NHSN.

— End of Chapter 18 —

Index

Pathway to USMLE — Volume 2: Haematology and Transfusion Medicine. Page numbers refer to printed body pages. Principal discussions are marked in boldface where applicable.

A

B

C

D

E

F

G

H

I

J

K

L

M

N

P

R

S

T

V

W

www.ingramcontent.com/pod-product-compliance
Lightning Source LLC
Chambersburg PA
CBHW061353240926
51846CB00007B/1391
* 9 7 8 8 1 6 8 6 7 3 0 4 5 *